Prostate Cancer

Contemporary Issues in Cancer Imaging

A Multidisciplinary Approach

Series editor

Rodney H. Reznek,

Cancer Imaging, St Bartholomew's Hospital, London

Editorial adviser

Janet E. Husband,

Diagnostic Radiology, Royal Marsden Hospital, Surrey

Current titles in the series

Cancer of the Ovary
Lung Cancer
Colorectal Cancer
Carcinoma of the Kidney
Carcinoma of the Esophagus
Carcinoma of the Bladder

Forthcoming titles in the series

Squamous Cell Cancer of the Neck
Pancreatic Cancer
Interventional Radiological Treatment of Liver Tumors
Gastric Cancer
Primary Carcinomas of the Liver
Breast Cancer

Prostate Cancer

Edited by

Hedvig Hricak

and

Peter T. Scardino

Series editor

Rodney H. Reznek

Editorial adviser

Janet E. Husband

CAMBRIDGE
UNIVERSITY PRESS

CAMBRIDGE UNIVERSITY PRESS
Cambridge, New York, Melbourne, Madrid, Cape Town, Singapore, São Paulo, Delhi

Cambridge University Press
The Edinburgh Building, Cambridge CB2 8RU, UK

Published in the United States of America by Cambridge University Press, New York

www.cambridge.org
Information on this title: www.cambridge.org/9780521887045

First published 2009

Printed in the United Kingdom at the University Press, Cambridge

A catalog record for this publication is available from the British Library

Library of Congress Cataloging in Publication data
Prostate cancer / edited by Hedwig Hricak and Peter T. Scardino.
   p.   ;   cm. – (Contemporary issues in cancer imaging)
Includes bibliographical references and index.
ISBN 978-0-521-88704-5
1. Prostate – Cancer.   2. Prostate – Cancer – Imaging.   I. Hricak, Hedvig.   II. Scardino, Peter T.   III. Series.
[DNLM: 1.   Prostatic Neoplasms – therapy.   2.   Diagnostic Imaging – methods.   3.   Prostatic Neoplasms –
diagnosis.   WJ 762 P965425 2008]
RC280.P7P7415   2008
616.99'463–dc22

                                                                                                    2008025533

ISBN 978-0-521-88704-5 hardback

Contents

The color plates can be found between pages 148 and 149.

Contributors

Oguz Akin, M.D.
Assistant Professor of Radiology
Department of Radiology
Radiology Service
Memorial Sloan-Kettering Cancer Center
New York, USA

Gustavo E. Ayala, M.D.
Baylor College of Medicine
Houston
TX, USA

James A. Eastham, M.D.
Sidney Kimmel Center for Prostate and
   Urologic Cancers
Urology Service
Memorial Sloan-Kettering Cancer Center
New York, USA

Mark Garzotto, M.D.
Department of Surgery
Division of Urology
Oregon Health and Science University
Oregon, USA

Ethan J. Halpern, M.D.
Department of Radiology
Jefferson Prostate Diagnostic Center
Kimmel Cancer Center
Thomas Jefferson University
Philadelphia, USA

Kai H. Hammerich, M.D., Ph.D.
Baylor College of Medicine
Department of Pathology
Houston
TX, USA

Hedvig Hricak, M.D., Ph.D., Dr. h.c.
Department of Radiology
Radiology Service
Memorial Sloan-Kettering Cancer Center
New York, USA

Marisa A. Kollmeier, M.D.
Department of Radiation Oncology
Memorial Sloan-Kettering Cancer Center
New York, USA

Steven M. Larson, M.D.
Nuclear Medicine Service
Department of Radiology
Memorial Sloan-Kettering Cancer Center
New York, USA

Timothy A. Masterson, M.D.
Sidney Kimmel Center for Prostate and
Urologic Cancers
Urology Service
Memorial Sloan-Kettering Cancer Center
New York, USA

Michael J. Morris, M.D.
Memorial Sloan-Kettering Cancer Center
New York, USA

Neeta Pandit-Taskar, M.D.
Asst Attending Physician and Asst Member
Nuclear Medicine Service
Department of Radiology
Memorial Sloan-Kettering Cancer Center
New York, USA

Mark L. Pe, M.D.
Department of Urology
Jefferson Prostate Diagnostic Center
Kimmel Cancer Center
Thomas Jefferson University
Philadelphia, USA

Darko Pucar, M.D.
Department of Radiology
Memorial Sloan-Kettering Cancer Center
New York, USA

Peter T. Scardino, M.D., F.A.C.S.
Department of Surgery
Memorial Sloan-Kettering Cancer Center
New York, USA

Lawrence H. Schwartz, M.D.
Department of Radiology
Memorial Sloan-Kettering Cancer Center
New York, USA

Tamar Sella, M.D.
Department of Radiology
Hadassah-Hebrew University Medical Center
Jerusalem, Israel

Amita Shukla-Dave, Ph.D
Assistant Attending Physicist
Departments of Medical Physics and Radiology
Memorial Sloan-Kettering Cancer Center
New York, USA

Edouard J. Trabulsi, M.D
Department of Urology
Jefferson Prostate Diagnostic Center
Kimmel Cancer Center
Thomas Jefferson University
Philadelphia, USA

Thomas M. Wheeler, M.D.
Professor and Chair
Baylor College of Medicine
Houston
TX, USA

Kristen L. Zakian
Associate Attending Physicist
Departments of Medical Physics and Radiology
Memorial Sloan-Kettering Cancer Center
New York, USA

Michael J. Zelefsky, M.D.
Department of Radiation Oncology
Memorial Sloan-Kettering Cancer Center
New York, USA

Jingbo Zhang, M.D.
Department of Radiology
Memorial Sloan-Kettering Cancer Center
Weill Cornell Medical College
New York, USA

Series Foreword

Imaging has become pivotal in all aspects of the management of patients with cancer. At the same time it is acknowledged that optimal patient care is best achieved by a multidisciplinary team approach. The explosion of technological developments in imaging over the past years has meant that all members of the multidisciplinary team should understand the potential applications, limitations and advantages of all the evolving and exciting imaging techniques. Equally, to understand the significance of the imaging findings and to contribute actively to management decisions and to the development of new clinical applications for imaging, it is critical that the radiologist should have sufficient background knowledge of different tumors. Thus the radiologist should understand the pathology, the clinical background, the therapeutic options, and prognostic indicators of malignancy.

Contemporary Issues in Cancer Imaging – A Multidisciplinary Approach aims to meet the growing requirement for radiologists to have detailed knowledge of the individual tumors in which they are involved in making management decisions. A series of single subject issues, each of which will be dedicated to a single tumor site and edited by recognized expert guest editors, will include contributions from basic scientists, pathologists, surgeons, oncologists, radiologists, and others.

While the series is written predominantly for the radiologist, it is hoped that individual issues will contain sufficient varied information so as to be of interest to all medical disciplines and to other health professionals managing patients with cancer. As with imaging, advances have occurred in all these disciplines related to cancer management and it is our fervent hope that this series, bringing together expertise from such a range of related specialties, will not only promote the understanding and rational application of modern imaging but will also help to achieve the ultimate goal of improving outcomes of patient with cancer.

Rodney H. Reznek

Preface

Prostate cancer remains the most common internal malignancy in adult men in the western world. While there are many available treatment regimens for prostate cancer, there are few evidence-based guidelines for treatment selection, and the rationale behind common decision practices prior to localized primary or systemic therapy is continuously evolving. Providing optimal treatment selection and the most accurate outcome prediction requires the consideration and synthesis of multiple patient characteristics, which may include demographics (e.g., age, ethnicity), clinical variables (e.g., laboratory values, imaging features), pathologic findings (e.g., stage and grade), and the molecular characteristics of the tumor (e.g., receptor status, gene expression profiling). The multitude of parameters and diversity of expertise required mean that there has been a paradigm shift in the management of patients with prostate cancer, with a multidisciplinary disease management approach becoming more attractive to patients. For the radiologist, understanding the pathophysiology of prostate cancer, the critical clinical issues, and the advantages and limitations of different treatment approaches is essential for meaningful interpretation of imaging studies, be they ultrasound, computed tomography, magnetic resonance imaging or nuclear medicine studies. Similarly, for the practicing clinician, understanding the advantages and limitations of each imaging modality and appreciating the importance of optimal technique are crucial to rational incorporation of imaging studies into the care of the patient with prostate cancer. Promoting the spirit of a multidisciplinary approach, this volume includes detailed descriptions of anatomy, the natural history of prostate cancer, treatment options and imaging modalities. The series *Contemporary Issues in Cancer Imaging* has been designed not only to help radiologists understand the goals and requirements of oncologic imaging, but also to serve as a valuable reference for all those involved in the management of cancer.

Hedvig Hricak
Peter T. Scardino

1

Anatomy of the prostate gland and surgical pathology of prostate cancer

Kai H. Hammerich, Gustavo E. Ayala, and Thomas M. Wheeler

Introduction

Urologists and pathologists have focused more and more on the anatomic structures of the human prostate gland and their relationship to prostate carcinoma development and prognosis since the resurgence of radical prostatectomy in the late 1980s. The accessibility of whole-mount slide preparation in the study of the prostate has greatly simplified this analysis.

This chapter concentrates on the anatomy of the prostate gland and analyzes how anatomic structures relate to the origin, development, and evolution of prostate carcinoma. The concept of zonal anatomy and its role in prostate carcinoma will also be described.

Anatomy and histology of the normal prostate gland

Embryology and development of the prostate gland

During the third month of gestation, the prostate gland develops from epithelial invaginations from the posterior urogenital sinus under the influence of the underlying mesenchyme [1]. The normal formation of the prostate gland requires the presence of 5α-dihydrotestosterone, which is synthesized from fetal testosterone by the action of 5α-reductase [2]. This enzyme is localized in the urogenital sinus and external genitalia of humans [3]. Consequently, deficiencies of 5α-reductase will cause a rudimentary or undetectable prostate in addition to severe abnormalities of the external genitalia, although the epididymides, vasa deferentia, and seminal vesicles remain normal [4].

During the prepubertal period, the constitution of the human prostate remains more or less identical but begins to undergo morphologic changes into the adult phenotype with the beginning of puberty. The gland enlarges continuously in size to reach the adult weight of approximately 20 g by 25–30 years of age [1].

Prostate Cancer, eds. Hedvig Hricak and Peter T. Scardino. Published by Cambridge University Press.
© Cambridge University Press 2009.

Normal anatomy and histology of the prostate

The base of the prostate is at the bladder neck and the apex at the urogenital diaphragm [5]. The Denonvilliers' fascia, a thin, filmy layer of connective tissue, separates the prostate and seminal vesicles from the rectum posteriorly. Skeletal muscle fibers from the urogenital diaphragm extend into the prostate at the apex and up to the midprostate anteriorly [6].

In the twentieth century, several investigators maintained that the prostate gland was composed of diverse lobes by analogy with laboratory animals [1, 7]. This concept became popular even though no distinct lobes can be seen in the human. Thereupon, McNeal established the current and most widely accepted concept of various zones rather than lobes of the prostate [8, 9, 10].

The peripheral zone comprises all the prostatic glandular tissue at the apex as well as all of the tissue located posteriorly near the capsule (Figure 1.1). In this zone, carcinoma, chronic prostatitis, and postinflammatory atrophy are relatively more

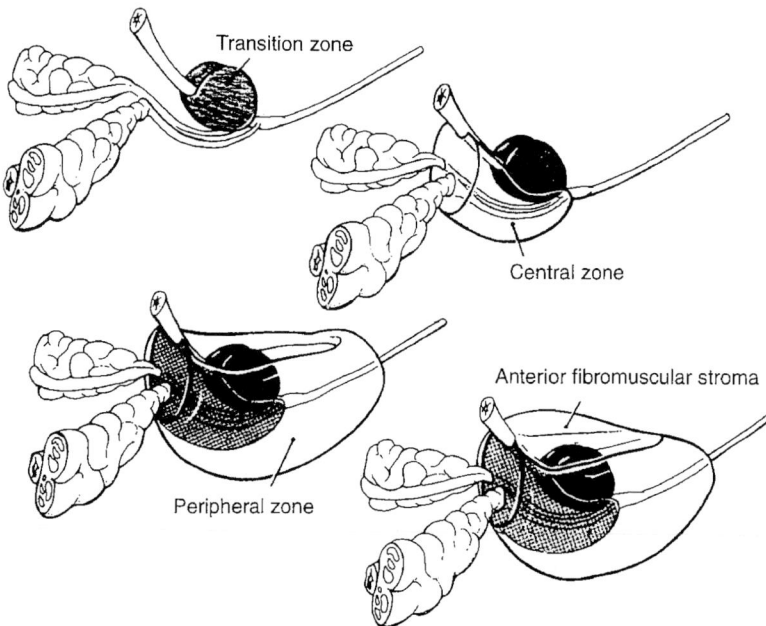

Figure 1.1. Zonal anatomy of the normal prostate as described by McNeal [8, 9, 10]. The transition zone comprises only 5%–10% of the glandular tissue in the young male. The central zone forms part of the base of the prostate and it is traversed by the ejaculatory ducts. The prostate is constituted by the peripheral zone, particularly distal to the verumontanum. (From Greene D R, Shabsigh R, Scardino P T. Urologic ultrasonography. In: Walsh P C, Retik A B, Stamey T A et al. eds. *Campbell's Urology*, 6th edn. Philadephia: WB Saunders, 1992; 342–393, with permission.)

common than in the other zones. The central zone is a cone-shaped area of the adult gland, with the apex of the cone at the confluence of the ejaculatory ducts and the prostatic urethra at the verumontanum (Figure 1.1). The transition zone consists of two equal portions of glandular tissue lateral to the urethra in the midgland (Figure 1.1). This portion of the prostate is involved in the development of age-related benign prostatic hyperplasia (BPH) and, less commonly, adenocarcinoma. The anterior fibromuscular stroma (AFMS) forms the convexity of the anterior external surface. The apical half of this area is rich in striated muscle, which blends into the gland and the muscle of the pelvic diaphragm (Figure 1.1). Toward the base, smooth muscle cells become predominant, blending into the fibers of the bladder neck [11]. The distal portion of the AFMS is important in voluntary sphincter functions, whereas the proximal portion plays a central role in involuntary sphincter functions.

The histologic architecture of the prostate is that of a branched duct gland. Two cell layers, a luminal secretory columnar cell layer and an underlying basal cell layer, line each gland or duct. The lumens of otherwise normal prostatic glands and ducts frequently contain multilaminated eosinophilic concretions, termed corpora amylacea, that become more common in older men. Calculi are larger than those corpora with a predilection for the ducts that traverse the length of the surgical capsule, separating the transition and peripheral zones.

The prostatic capsule is composed of fibrous tissue surrounding the gland. Although the term "capsule" is embedded in the current literature and common parlance, there is no consensus about the presence of a true capsule [12]. This capsule is best appreciated posteriorly and posterolaterally as a layer more fibrous than muscular, between the prostatic stroma and extraprostatic fat.

The seminal vesicles are located superior to the base of the prostate. They undergo confluence with the vas deferens on each side to form the ejaculatory ducts. The ejaculatory duct complex consists of the two ejaculatory ducts along with a second loose stroma rich in vascular spaces. The utricle (when present) is located between the ejaculatory ducts. The remnants of the utricle occasionally form cystic structures in the midline posteriorly. The seminal vesicles are resistant to nearly all of the disease processes that affect the prostate. Seminal vesicle involvement (SVI) by prostate cancer (PCa) is one of the most important predictors for PCa progression (Figure 1.2) [13, 14].

Metastatic PCa oftentimes involves pelvic lymph nodes. The prognostic significance of this feature has been documented by several investigators [15]. In some individuals, periprostatic (PP) and periseminal vesicle (PSV) lymph nodes are

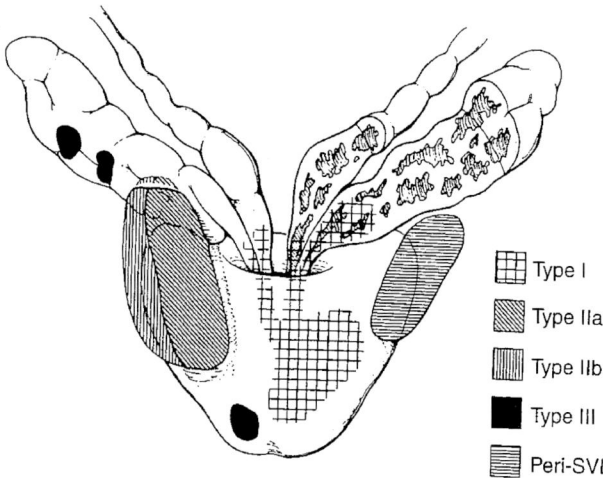

Figure 1.2. Diagrammatic representation of the three patterns of seminal vesicle involvement (SVI) and peri-SVI. The combination of types I and II is categorized as type I + II. (From Ohori M, Scardino P T, Lapin S L *et al.* The mechanisms and prognostic significance of seminal vesicle involvement by prostate cancer. *Am J Surg Pathol* 1993; 17: 1253 [14], with permission.)

Type I
Type IIa
Type IIb
Type III
Peri-SVI

present and, although uncommon, they may be involved by metastatic PCa as well, sometimes in the absence of pelvic lymph node metastases [16].

Neural anatomy

The prostate is an extraordinarily well-innervated organ. Two neurovascular bundles are located posterolaterally adjacent to the gland and form the superior and inferior pedicles on each side. These nerves are important in regulating the physiology, morphology, and growth maturation of the gland [17, 18, 19, 20]. The prostate receives both parasympathetic and sympathetic innervation, the former from the hypogastric and pelvic nerves, and the latter from a peripheral hypogastric ganglion [21]. Walsh and Donker previously demonstrated the importance of these nerves in penile erection, so urologists as well as patients have put an increasing interest on nerve-sparing surgical treatment of PCa [22].

Surgical pathology of the prostate gland

Epidemiology, clinical aspects

Prostate cancer remains the most common malignancy affecting men and the second leading cause of cancer-related death of men in the United States [23]. In 2007, there were 218 890 new cases of PCa, resulting in 27 050 deaths in the United States [23]. Adenocarcinoma accounts for about 95% of prostatic neoplasms, and frequently has no specific presenting symptoms. More often than not, PCa is clinically silent, although it sometimes mimics obstructive symptoms of BPH. Therefore, patients may be diagnosed with advanced PCa with metastases without symptoms related to the region of prostate. Consequently, in the past two decades the diagnostic value of patient screening by using early detection programs has come to the forefront of focus. With the introduction of widespread screening with serum prostate-specific antigen (PSA), the incidence of stage IV PCa at presentation has dramatically lessened, although the number of PCa detected has increased as well [24].

Morphologic diagnosis of prostate adenocarcinoma

The identification on gross inspection of PCa diagnosed today is often difficult or impossible. Although the color of most grossly visible tumors is tan-white, a minority of PCa cases are yellow, a more specific gross feature of PCa. In prosta-tectomies, PCa tends to be multifocal, mainly found in the peripheral zone [25, 26], followed by the transition zone and then central zone. In the authors' experience, PCa foci must be at least 5 mm in diameter for reliable gross identification, although much larger tumor areas may be difficult or impossible to accurately identify grossly. Most grossly recognizable tumors are firm to palpation and the minority are fleshy and soft. Most tumors palpable by digital rectal examination (DRE) are visualized by ultrasound and gross inspection.

Histology of prostate cancer and Gleason grading

In both radical prostatectomy specimens and needle biopsy samples, histologic grading of PCa by the Gleason system is the strongest prognostic factor of a patient's time to progression [27, 28, 29]. The Gleason system describes the histologic appearance of PCa under low magnification (architectural as opposed to cytologic grading) (Figure 1.3). The Gleason scoring system is defined by a scale of 1 to 5. Well-differentiated PCa (Gleason grade 1 or 2) is characterized by a proliferation of microacinar structures lined by prostatic luminal cells without an accompanying basal cell layer. At least some of the neoplastic cells contain prominent nucleoli, defined as at least 1 μm in diameter by Gleason but defined as larger by other investigators [28, 30]. Gleason pattern 5 is the highest grade and includes a solid pattern with central necrosis or infiltrating individual cells.

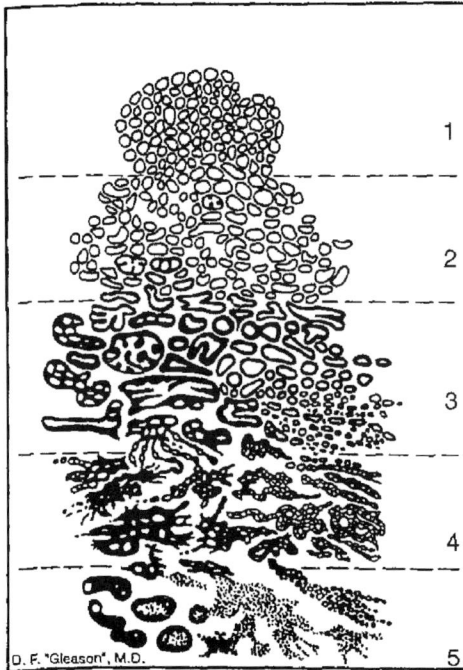

Figure 1.3. Simplified drawing of histologic patterns of prostatic adenocarcinoma, emphasizing the degree of glandular differentiation and relation to stroma. All black in the drawing represents tumor tissue, with all cytologic detail obscured except in the right side of pattern 4, where tiny structures are intended to suggest the hypernephroid pattern. (From Gleason D F. Histologic grading of prostatic adenocarcinoma. In: Tannenbaum M, ed. *Urologic Pathology: The Prostate*. Philadelphia: Lea & Febiger. 1977; 181, with permission).

As PCa is usually heterogeneous with two or more grades in a given cancer, Gleason chose to incorporate both a primary (most prevalent) and a secondary (next most prevalent) grade into the system [31]. The primary pattern is added to the secondary grade to arrive at a Gleason score. Consequently, the Gleason score possibilities range from 2 (1 + 1) up to 10 (5 + 5).

Although the Gleason system is now internationally accepted, there are several issues concerning it as a grading system. Most notably Gleason grading is observer dependent and may vary depending on the level of experience. Also, it is controversial whether to grade PCa after treatment (androgen ablation or radiation). Another limitation is that the majority of patients diagnosed today fall into the Gleason 6–7 category, an intermediate prognostic range limiting the potential usefulness of a 10-point scale. That said, several studies have confirmed that the time to progression in patients with a Gleason 4 + 3 is significantly less compared to that for Gleason 3 + 4 patients [32, 33].

Other histologic parameters such as the presence of extracapsular extension, perineural invasion, surgical margin status, lymph node status and SVI hold prognostic information and have been added to postoperative nomograms in order to optimize the prediction of time to progression (Figure 1.4).

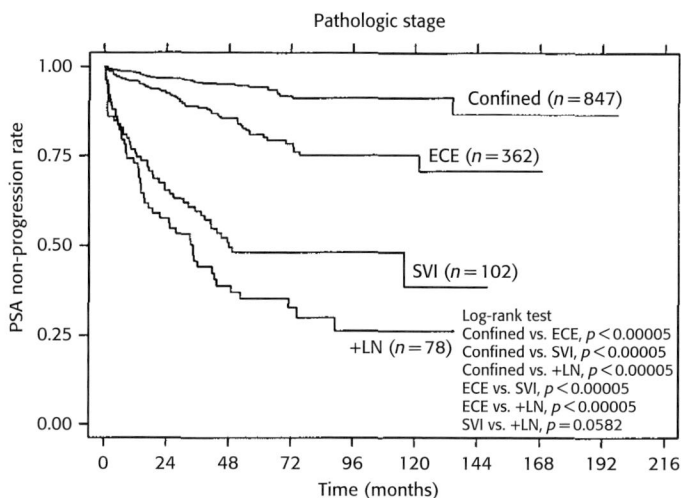

Figure 1.4. Kaplan Meier disease-free probability plot by pathologic stage. ECE, extracapsular extension; LN, lymph node; SVI, seminal vesicle involvement.

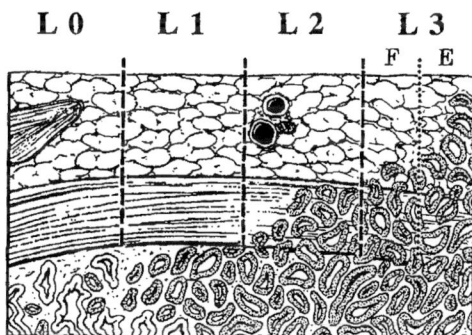

Figure 1.5. Levels of prostatic capsular invasion (see text for definitions.) Extraprostatic extension designated as L3 signifies extension of tumor into periprostatic soft tissue, which may be subclassified as focal (L3F) or established (L3E). The sharpness of the boundaries between prostatic stroma, capsule, and adipose tissue is exaggerated for clarity. (From Stamey T A, McNeal J E, Freiha F S et al. Morphometric and clinical studies on 68 consecutive radical prostatectomies. *J Urol* 1988; 129: 1245–1241; [34] and from Wheeler TM. Anatomic consideration in carcinoma of the prostate. *Urol Clin North Am* 1989; 16: 623–634, with permission.)

Several investigations have been done analyzing the prognostic significance of the level of PCa invasion with respect to the prostatic capsule [34, 35, 36]. According to the staging of the International Union Against Cancer (UICC) and also the American Joint Commission on Cancer (AJCC), tumors at levels 0–2 would be considered pathologically confined, whereas tumors that are at level 3 (L3), focal (L3F) or established (L3E) are considered pathologically not confined to the prostate (Figure 1.5) [37].

Various studies have demonstrated the importance of the prostatic neuroanatomy due to its relationship with PCa in the process of perineural invasion

(PNI). Indeed, PNI is highly prevalent in PCa, being reported in about 85% of radical prostatectomy cases [38, 39, 40]. It has been shown to be the primary mechanism by which PCa penetrates the capsule and/or metastasizes [41]. One study has shown that the volume of PCa in the perineural space is closely correlated with prognosis [42].

Recently, a new system based on the quantification of intratumoral reactive stroma, also named "stromogenic cancer," has been introduced as another way to grade PCa. Stromogenic cancer is the phenomenon of dedifferentiation of smooth muscle cells into myofibroblasts that have the capability to promote PCa growth [43, 44]. Reactive stroma (RS) was classified into four groups (Grade 0, up to 5% RS; Grade 1, 6%–15% RS; Grade 2, 16%–50% RS; and Grade 3, >50% RS). Quantification of RS Grades 0 and 3 in PCa was determined to be an independent predictor of recurrence-free survival, and correlated significantly with other clinicopathologic parameters of PCa [45, 46].

Zonal anatomy and prostate adenocarcinoma

Based upon the pioneering work of McNeal beginning in the 1960s, much has been written about the different neoplastic potential of the zones of the prostate, and of the effect of zonal origin on prognosis [47, 48]. At one time the predominant thought was that PCa arose nearly exclusively in the posterior part of the prostate (now known as the peripheral zone) close to the prostatic capsule [16, 49]. However, later studies confirmed that in prostates removed for PCa a significant minority of PCa foci arise in the transition zone and central zone [36, 50]. The periurethral portion of the prostate had been considered to be resistant to the development of PCa, although it was known to be quite susceptible to the development of nodular hyperplasia. McNeal is also credited with describing the unique well-differentiated nature of tumors arising in the transition zone (Gleason pattern 1 and 2) [26]. These tumors were characterized as having a low risk of progression and of being rarely associated with capsular invasion or SVI [26].

Treatment effects on primary prostate adenocarcinoma

Radiation and hormone therapy may cause artifactual elevation of the Gleason score due to collapse of the glandular architecture [51, 52]. At the time of writing, there is no consensus about grading results after treatment [53, 54].

Radiation therapy induces profound changes in the non-neoplastic ducts and acini as well as the prostatic stroma, and the former changes may be confused with adenocarcinoma histologically by the uninitiated [55]. Often, the individual tumor cells appear so damaged by the radiation therapy as to appear non-viable. This latter change may also be seen after endocrine therapy, which can be performed in different ways: orchiectomy, estrogen administration, or androgen deprivation [51, 56].

Other novel therapies have been utilized, such as gene therapy, for PCa. The resulting morphologic changes described associated with HSV-tk ganciclovir gene therapy have been loss of glandular architecture, increased inflammation and apoptosis/necrosis, as well as areas of degenerating tumor cells [57].

Staging systems for prostatic adenocarcinoma

In the twentieth century, several different staging systems for PCa were established. The first internationally accepted staging system for PCa was introduced by Whitmore in 1956. Stages were classified in letters (A–D) [58]. This staging system was modified by Jewett, subdividing level B. Jewett demonstrated that patients with a palpable nodule had increased cancer-free survival [59]. In the early 1950s, staging systems for solid tumors began to consider the TNM (Tumor – Lymph node – Metastasis) classification to analyze patients' prognosis and to determine the tumor's definite level of development. Within each category of TNM, there are several sublevels based on tumor volume or extent (T1–T4), amount and/or size of lymph node metastases (N0–N3), and distant metastases (M0–M1) (Table 1.1) [60]. Since its inception, several enhancements have been made to the TNM staging system to allow more precise analysis of the clinico-pathologic stage of the tumor [61]. In 1992, the AJCC staging system mirrored the TNM staging system [37, 62, 63]. The AJCC staging system is based primarily on a particular clinico-pathologic classification of each tumor, allowing for more precise stratification of patients into prognostically distinct groups [60].

Although many different areas of metastases of a PCa have been described (kidney, breast, brain, liver), metastatic spread most commonly occurs into the pelvic lymph nodes, bones, and lungs [64, 65]. Bony metastases are mainly an osteoblastic process. However, the development and improvement of staging systems is a complex procedure and, today, clinical subspecialties are focusing on the improvement of staging systems for different neoplastic disease to precisely demonstrate each patient's prognosis.

Table 1.1. The 2002 American Joint Committee on Cancer/International Union Against Cancer TNM Staging Classification

Stage	Definition
Primary tumor, clinical (T)	
TX	Primary tumor cannot be assessed
T0	No evidence of primary tumor
T1	Clinically inapparent tumor not palpable or visible by imaging
	T1a: Tumor incidental histologic finding in 5% or less of tissue resected
	T1b: Tumor incidental histology finding in more than 5% of tissue resected
	T1c: Tumor identified by needle biopsy [e.g., because of elevated prostate-specific antigen (PSA) levels]
T2	Tumor confined within the prostate[a]
	T2a: Tumor involves half of one lobe or less
	T2b: Tumor involves more than half of one lobe but not both
	T2c: Tumor involves both lobes
T3	Tumor extends through the prostate capsule[b]
	T3a: Extracapsular extension (unilateral or bilateral)
	T3b: Tumor invades seminal vesicle(s)
T4	Tumor is fixed or invades adjacent structures other than the seminal vesicle(s): bladder neck, external sphincter, rectum, levator muscles, pelvic wall, or all the above
Primary tumor, pathologic (pT)	
pT2[c]	Organ confined
	pT2a: Unilateral, involving half of one lobe or less
	pT2b: Unilateral, involving more than half of one lobe but not both lobes
	pT2c: Bilateral
pT3	Extraprostatic extension
	pT3a: Extraprostatic extension
	pT3b: Seminal vesicle invasion
pT4	Invasion of bladder, rectum
Regional lymph nodes (N)	
NX	Regional lymph nodes cannot be assessed
N0	No regional lymph node metastasis
N1	Metastasis in regional lymph node or nodes

Table 1.1. (cont.)

Stage	Definition
Distant metastases^d (M)	
MX	Distant metastasis cannot be assessed
M0	No distant metastasis
M1	Distant metastasis
	M1a: Non-regional lymph node(s)
	M1b: Bone(s)
	M1c: Other site(s)

^{a} Tumor that is found in one or both lobes by needle biopsy, but not palpable or reliably visible by imaging, is classified as T1c.

^{b} Invasion into the prostatic apex or into (but not beyond) the prostatic capsule is classified as T2, not T3.

^{c} There is no pathologic T1 classification.

^{d} When more than one site of metastasis is present, the most advanced category is used; pM1c is most advanced.

Source: Adapted with permission from Greene F L, Page D L, Fleming I D, *et al. Cancer Staging Manual*, 6th edn. New York: Springer, 2002 [37].

Summary

Since the resurgence of radical prostatectomy in the early 1980s, urologists and pathologists have focused more and more attention on the relationship of prostate cancer foci to anatomic landmarks in the prostate gland and have correlated these with the origin of prostate carcinoma and patient prognosis.

Histologic grading of prostate cancer by the Gleason system is the strongest prognostic factor for a patient's time to progression. Stage is also critically important in prognosis and involves pathologic staging of the cancer with respect to capsular invasion, extracapsular extension, seminal vesicle involvement, lymphovascular involvement, and perineural invasion diameter.

In the twentieth century, several different staging systems for PCa were established. The current worldwide-accepted AJCC staging system presently allows for a reasonable degree of stratification of patients into prognostically distinct groups. However, despite these advances, the prediction of prognosis for the individual patient remains somewhat imprecise. New biomarker development will be important in the future for precisely predicting prognosis as well as predicting response to specific therapies.

REFERENCES

1. O. Lowsley, The development of the human prostate gland with reference to the development of other structures at the neck of the urinary bladder. *Am J Anat*, **13** (1912), 299–350.

2. D. Coffey, The molecular biology, endocrinology, and physiology of the prostate and seminal vesicles. In: *Campbell's Urology*, 6th edn., ed. P. C. Walsh, A. B. Retik, T. A. Stamley, *et al.*, Philadelphia: W B Saunders, 1992; 49–52.

3. J. D. Wilson, J. E. Griffin, M. Leshin, *et al.*, Role of gonadal hormones in development of the sexual phenotypes. *Hum Genet*, **58**:1 (1981), 78–84.

4. J. Imperato-McGinley, L. Guerrero, T Gautier, *et al.*, Steroid 5alpha-reductase deficiency in man. An inherited form of male pseudohermaphroditism. *Birth Defects Orig Artic Ser*, **11**:4 (1975), 91–103.

5. S. J. Berry, D. S. Coffey, P. C. Walsh, *et al.*, The development of human benign prostatic hyperplasia with age. *J Urol*, **132**:3 (1984), 474–9.

6. L. V. Kost, G. W. Evans, Occurrence and significance of striated muscle within the prostate. *J Urol*, **92** (1964), 703–4.

7. L. M. Franks, Atrophy and hyperplasia in the prostate proper. *J Pathol Bacteriol*, **68**:2 (1954), 617–21.

8. J. E. McNeal, Anatomy of the prostate: an historical survey of divergent views. *The Prostate*, **1**:1 (1980), 3–13.

9. J. E. McNeal, Normal histology of the prostate. *Am J Surg Pathol*, **12**:8 (1988), 619–33.

10. J. E. McNeal, Normal and pathologic anatomy of prostate. *Urology*, **17**:Suppl 3 (1981), 11–16.

11. J. E. McNeal, The prostate and prostatic urethra: a morphologic synthesis. *J Urol*, **107**:6 (1972), 1008–16.

12. A. G. Ayala, J. Y. Ro, R. Babaian, *et al.*, The prostatic capsule: does it exist? Its importance in the staging and treatment of prostatic carcinoma. *Am J Surg Pathol*, **13**:1 (1989), 21–7.

13. A. A. Villers, J. E. McNeal, E. A. Redwine, *et al.*, Pathogenesis and biological significance of seminal vesicle invasion in prostatic adenocarcinoma. *J Urol*, **143**:6 (1990), 1183–7.

14. M. Ohori, P. T. Scardino, S. L. Lapin, *et al.*, The mechanisms and prognostic significance of seminal vesicle involvement by prostate cancer. *Am J Surg Pathol*, **17**:12 (1993), 1252–61.

15. L. Cheng, E. J. Bergstralh, J. C. Cheville, *et al.*, Cancer volume of lymph node metastasis predicts progression in prostate cancer. *Am J Surg Pathol*, **22**:12 (1998), 1491–500.

16. P. S. Kothari, P. T. Scardino, M. Ohori, *et al.*, Incidence, location, and significance of periprostatic and periseminal vesicle lymph nodes in prostate cancer. *Am J Surg Pathol*, **25**:11 (2001), 1429–32.

17. M. Lujan, A. Paez, L. Llanes, *et al.*, Role of autonomic innervation in rat prostatic structure maintenance: a morphometric analysis. *J Urol*, **160**:5 (1998), 1919–23.

18. H. Watanabe, M. Shima, M. Kojima, *et al.*, Dynamic study of nervous control on prostatic contraction and fluid excretion in the dog. *J Urol*, **140**:6 (1988), 1567–70.

19. J. M. Wang, K. E. McKenna, K. T. McVary, *et al.*, Requirement of innervation for maintenance of structural and functional integrity in the rat prostate. *Biol Reprod*, **44**:6 (1991), 1171–6.

20. P. C. Walsh, H. Lepor, J. C. Eggleston, Radical prostatectomy with preservation of sexual function: anatomical and pathological considerations. *The Prostate*, **4**:5 (1983), 473–85.

21. H. Lepor, M. Gregerman, R. Crosby, *et al.*, Precise localization of the autonomic nerves from the pelvic plexus to the corpora cavernosa: a detailed anatomical study of the adult male pelvis. *J Urol*, **133**:2 (1985), 207–12.

22. P. C. Walsh, P. J. Donker, Impotence following radical prostatectomy: insight into etiology and prevention. *J Urol*, **128**:3 (1982), 492–7.

23. A. Jemal, R. Siegel, E. Ward, *et al.*, Cancer statistics, 2007. *CA Cancer J Clin*, **57**:1 (2007), 43–66.

24. S. H. Landis, T. Murray, S. Bolden, *et al.*, Cancer statistics, 1999. *CA Cancer J Clin*, **49**:1 (1999), 8–31.

25. A. Villers, J. E. McNeal, F. S. Freiha, *et al.*, Multiple cancers in the prostate. Morphologic features of clinically recognized versus incidental tumors. *Cancer*, **70**:9 (1992), 2313–18.

26. J. E. McNeal, E. A. Redwine, F. S. Freiha, *et al.*, Zonal distribution of prostatic adenocarcinoma. Correlation with histologic pattern and direction of spread. *Am J Surg Pathol*, **12**:12 (1988), 897–906.

27. J. E. Oesterling, C. B. Brendler, J. I. Epstein, *et al.*, Correlation of clinical stage, serum prostatic acid phosphatase and preoperative Gleason grade with final pathological stage in 275 patients with clinically localized adenocarcinoma of the prostate. *J Urol*, **138**:1 (1987), 92–8.

28. D. F. Gleason, Atypical hyperplasia, benign hyperplasia, and well-differentiated adenocarcinoma of the prostate. *Am J Surg Pathol*, **9**:Suppl 5–6 (1985), 53–67.

29. D. F. Gleason, The Veterans Administration Cooperative Research Group. Histologic grading and clinical staging of prostatic carcinoma. In *Urologic Pathology: The Prostate*, ed. M. Tannenbaum, Philadelphia: Lea & Febinger, 1977; 171–4.

30. A. Bocking, W. Auffermann, H. Schwarz, *et al.*, Cytology of prostatic carcinoma. Quantification and validation of diagnostic criteria. *Anal Quant Cytol*, **6**:2 (1984), 74–88.

31. R. Arora, M. O. Koch, J. N. Eble, *et al.*, Heterogeneity of Gleason grade in multifocal adenocarcinoma of the prostate. *Cancer*, **100**:11 (2004), 2362–6.

32. T. Y. Chan, A. W. Partin, P. C. Walsh, *et al.*, Prognostic significance of Gleason score 3 + 4 versus Gleason score 4 + 3 tumor at radical prostatectomy. *Urology*, **56**:5 (2000), 823–7.

33. C. M. Herman, M. W. Kattan, M. Ohori, *et al.*, Primary Gleason pattern as a predictor of disease progression in Gleason score 7 prostate cancer: a multivariate analysis of 823 men treated with radical prostatectomy. *Am J Surg Pathol*, **25**:5 (2001), 657–60.

34. T. A. Stamey, J. E. McNeal, F. S. Freiha, *et al.*, Morphometric and clinical studies on 68 consecutive radical prostatectomies. *J Urol*, **139**:6 (1988), 1235–41.

35. J. I. Epstein, M. J. Carmichael, G. Pizov, *et al.*, Influence of capsular penetration on progression following radical prostatectomy: a study of 196 cases with long-term followup. *J Urol*, **150**:1 (1993), 135–41.

36. T. M. Wheeler, O. Dillioglugil, M. W. Kattan, *et al.*, Clinical and pathological significance of the level and extent of capsular invasion in clinical stage T1–2 prostate cancer. *Hum Pathol*, **29**:8 (1988), 856–62.

37. F. L. Greene, D. L. Page, I. D. Fleming, *et al.*, eds. *AJCC Cancer Staging Manual*, 6th edn. New York: Springer-Verlag, 2002.

38. P. Ernst, Uber das Wachstum und die Verbreitung Bosartiger Geschwulste insbesondere des Krebses in die Lymphbahnen der Nerven. *Beitr Pathol Anat*, **7**:Suppl (1905), 29.

39. G. E. Ayala, H. Dai, M. Ittmann, *et al.*, Growth and survival mechanisms associated with perineural invasion in prostate cancer. *Cancer Res*, **64**:17 (2004), 6082–90.

40. G. E. Ayala, H. Dai, S. A. Tahir, *et al.*, Stromal antiapoptotic paracrine loop in perineural invasion of prostatic carcinoma. *Cancer Res*, **66**:10 (2006), 5159–64.

41. A. Villers, J. E. McNeal, E. A. Redwine, *et al.*, The role of perineural space invasion in the local spread of prostatic adenocarcinoma. *J Urol*, **142**:3 (1989), 763–8.

42. N. Maru, M. Ohori, M. W. Kattan, *et al.*, Prognostic significance of the diameter of perineural invasion in radical prostatectomy specimens. *Hum Pathol*, **32**:8 (2001), 828–33.

43. J. A. Tuxhorn, G. E. Ayala, D. R. Rowley, Reactive stroma in prostate cancer progression. *J Urol*, **166**:6 (2001), 2472–83.

44. J. A. Tuxhorn, S. J. McAlhany, T. D. Dang, *et al.*, Stromal cells promote angiogenesis and growth of human prostate tumors in a differential reactive stroma (DRS) xenograft model. *Cancer Res*, **62**:11 (2002), 3298–307.

45. G. Ayala, J. A. Tuxhorn, T. M. Wheeler, *et al.*, Reactive stroma as a predictor of biochemical-free

recurrence in prostate cancer. *Clin Cancer Res*, **15**:9 (2003), 4792–801.

46. N. Yanagisawa, R. Li, D. Rowley, *et al.*, Stromogenic prostatic carcinoma pattern (carcinomas with reactive stromal grade 3) in needle biopsies predicts biochemical recurrence-free survival in patients after radical prostatectomy. *Hum Pathol*, **38**:11 (2007), 1611–20.

47. D. R. Greene, T. M. Wheeler, S. Egawa, *et al.*, Relationship between clinical stage and histological zone of origin in early prostate cancer: morphometric analysis. *Br J Urol*, **68**:5 (1991), 499–509.

48. J. E. McNeal. Origin and development of carcinoma in the prostate. *Cancer*, **23**:1 (1969), 24–34.

49. R. A. Moore. The morphology of small prostatic carcinoma. *J Urol*, **33** (1935), 224–34.

50. D. R. Greene, T. M. Wheeler, S. Egawa, *et al.*, A comparison of the morphological features of cancer arising in the transition zone and in the peripheral zone of the prostate. *J Urol*, **146**:4 (1991), 1069–76.

51. W. M. Murphy, M. S. Soloway, G. H. Barrows, Pathologic changes associated with androgen deprivation therapy for prostate cancer. *Cancer*, **68**:4 (1991), 821–8.

52. M. Hellstrom, M. Haggman, S. Brandstedt, *et al.*, Histopathological changes in androgen-deprived localized prostatic cancer. A study in total prostatectomy specimens. *Eur Urol*, **24**:4 (1993), 461–5.

53. B. Helpap, V. Koch, Histological and immunohistochemical findings of prostatic carcinoma after external or interstitial radiotherapy. *J Cancer Res Clin Oncol*, **117**:6 (1991), 608–14.

54. J. A. Wheeler, G. K. Zagars, A. G. Ayala, Dedifferentiation of locally recurrent prostate cancer after radiation therapy. Evidence for tumor progression. *Cancer*, **71**:11 (1993), 3783–7.

55. D. G. Bostwick, B. M. Egbert, L. F. Fajardo, Radiation injury of the normal and neoplastic prostate. *Am J Surg Pathol*, **6**:6 (1982), 541–51.

56. L. M. Franks, Estrogen-treated prostatic cancer: the variation in responsiveness of tumor cells. *Cancer*, **13** (1960), 490–501.

57. G. Ayala, T. Satoh, R. Li, *et al.*, Biological response determinants in HSV-tk + ganciclovir gene therapy for prostate cancer. *Mol Ther*, **13**:4 (2006), 716–28.

58. W. F. Whitmore, Jr., Natural history and staging of prostate cancer. *Urol Clin North Am*, **11**:2 (1984), 205–20.

59. H. J. Jewett, Significance of the palpable prostatic nodule. *JAMA*, **160**:10 (1956), 838–9.

60. H. B. Burke, D. E. Henson, The American Joint Committee on Cancer. Criteria for prognostic factors and for an enhanced prognostic system. *Cancer*, **72**:10 (1993), 3131–5.

61. D. G. Bostwick, Staging prostate cancer – 1997: current methods and limitations. *Eur Urol*, **32**: Suppl 3 (1997), 2–14.

62. F. H. Schroder, P. Hermanek, L. Denis, *et al.*, The TNM classification of prostate cancer. *Prostate Suppl*, **4** (1992), 129–38.

63. M. Ohori, T. M. Wheeler, P. T. Scardino, The New American Joint Committee on Cancer and International Union Against Cancer TNM classification of prostate cancer. Clinicopathologic correlations. *Cancer*, **74**:1 (1994), 104–14.

64. L. Bubendorf, A. Schopfer, U. Wagner, *et al.*, Metastatic patterns of prostate cancer: an autopsy study of 1,589 patients. *Hum Pathol*, **31**:5 (2000), 578–83.

65. S. M. de la Monte, G. W. Moore, G. M. Hutchins, Metastatic behavior of prostate cancer. Cluster analysis of patterns with respect to estrogen treatment. *Cancer*, **58**:4 (1986), 985–93.

2

The natural and treated history of prostate cancer

Mark Garzotto

Introduction

Adenocarcinoma of the prostate is the most common visceral cancer of industri-
alized nations and the second most lethal cancer among men. In the United States
alone, 186 000 new cases are expected and over 28 000 men will die from this disease
in 2008 [1]. Therefore, while prostate cancer is a leading cause of cancer death,
the vast majority of men survive the disease and ultimately die of other causes.
Currently it is estimated that a man's lifetime risk of being diagnosed with prostate
cancer is 1 in 6. These odds are expected to increase as the combination of improved
medical therapy and lifestyle modifications lead to prolonged population longevity.
It is well known that not all prostate cancer patients will benefit from interventions
with curative intent as many tumors will remain indolent throughout the patient's
life. In fact it is estimated that only 3% of all men, or about 1 in 6 of all prostate
cancer patients, will die of this disease. Nevertheless, a significant proportion of
prostate cancer patients who die of other causes may well suffer from disease
progression or treatment complications during their lifetime. Thus, the clinical
sequelae of prostate cancer can be quite variable, ranging from the tumor being
discovered incidentally without any symptoms, to patients presenting with widely
metastatic, treatment-resistant disease that is rapidly fatal. Thus prostate cancer
often presents perplexing management questions to clinicians who treat this disease.

Given the divergence in potential outcomes, it is imperative to be able to harness
clinical information to accurately risk-stratify patients into distinct groups. One of
the challenges is to identify patients at a curable stage who are most likely to benefit
from therapy, while sparing those from treatment who harbor indolent cancers.
Successful characterization of prostate cancer cases will undoubtedly lead to improvements in the application of appropriate therapies and in counseling patients about

Prostate Cancer, eds. Hedvig Hricak and Peter T. Scardino. Published by Cambridge University Press.
© Cambridge University Press 2009.

the progression of disease. A better understanding of the prostate cancer outcomes will also lead to improvements in health-related quality of life and a systematic reduction in medical expenditure. Furthermore, in-depth knowledge of the natural history of prostate cancer will serve as a basis for future trial design with specific disease states in mind.

In this chapter, the natural history of treated and untreated prostate cancer in the eras both before and since the introduction of widespread screening for prostate-specific antigen (PSA) will be reviewed. This information is intended to provide the reader with a framework for understanding the rationale for the various clinical approaches to prostate cancer that are outlined in subsequent chapters of this text.

Historical series

The concept of large-scale watchful waiting for prostate cancer grew out of several early reports showing the feasibility of observation alone for early staged prostate cancer [2, 3, 4, 5]. These findings were bolstered by improvements in the histologic categorization of prostate tumors by using the Gleason scoring system [6], which improved the prediction of prostate cancer outcomes over all other available patho-logic variables and remains the benchmark by which patients are classified in routine medical practice [7, 8, 9].

Studies with extended follow-up of localized prostate cancer patients have pre-viously been published and these serve as a foundation for our understanding of the natural history of untreated prostate cancer. In a population-based, retrospective study by Albertsen *et al.* [10, 11], the long-term outcomes of men primarily under-going no therapy for clinically localized disease were examined. This study consisted of 767 men diagnosed prior to the introduction of serum prostate-specific antigen (PSA) testing into the field. The effect of Gleason score, age and co-morbidities were closely examined in this study. In each age group, Gleason score was found to reliably predict the rate of death from prostate cancer, with increasing scores predicting increased mortality from prostate cancer. These predictive indices were tabulated in graph form for easy applicability to clinical use (Figure 2.1) [11]. For example, men with low Gleason scores (e.g., 2, 3, or 4), aged 60–64 years, had only a 5% chance of dying of prostate cancer within 15 years. Conversely, the presence of a tumor with a Gleason score of 8 or higher tumor in this age group increased the prostate cancer mortality to 81% within 15 years – a 16-fold difference. This study also examined the role that co-morbidities play in affecting the cause of death in men with prostate cancer. The results showed that men with significant co-morbidities

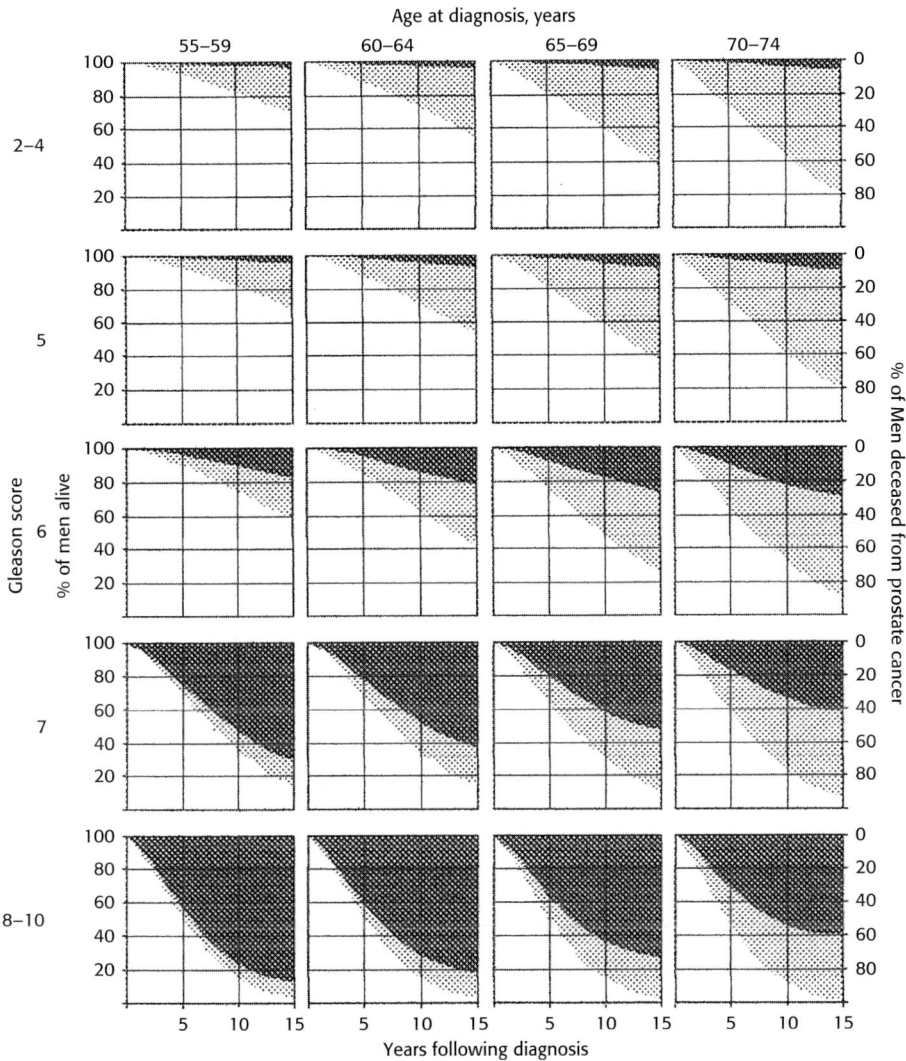

Figure 2.1. Competing risk analysis by age in men with localized prostate cancer. Graph shows the overall survival (in white), death from competing morbidities (in gray) and death from prostate cancer (in black) in men diagnosed with clinical prostate cancer. Reprinted with permission from [11] (*JAMA*; September 16, 1998; Vol. 280:11; Copyright © (1998), American Medical Association. All Rights reserved.)

had a 2-fold greater chance of death due to all causes than men without significant illnesses. Also, increasing age was strongly associated with increased death from other causes. This important study clearly demonstrates the need to consider both tumor and patient factors when counseling patients regarding treatment options for prostate cancer.

The results of observation alone for localized prostate cancer were also analyzed in a prospective trial carried out in Sweden [12, 13]. Johansson and colleagues have reported the 20-year results of a well-characterized cohort of 223 men with organ-confined, non-metastatic prostate cancer. Approximately half of these tumors were incidentally diagnosed by transurethral prostate resection and the mean age at diagnosis was 72 years [12]. Tumors were found to be well- or moderately differentiated in 96% of cases, thus only 4% were poorly differentiated at diagnosis. Patients were observed until symptomatic progression, when they were primarily offered androgen deprivation therapy – curative therapy was not routinely administered [13]. With over 20 years of follow-up, clinical tumor progression occurred in 40% of all patients, with 17% of patients developing metastatic disease. Prostate cancer was considered to be the cause of death in 16% of patients; however, this number increased to 22% in men younger than 70 years of age at diagnosis. The effects of grade, tumor stage, age, and follow-up length on clinical outcomes were examined. In this analysis, increased tumor grade was found to be the strongest clinical predictor of both prostate cancer mortality and local tumor progression [12]. The authors also noted a sharp reduction in prostate-cancer-specific survival in men after 15 years of follow-up, suggesting that prostate carcinomas maintain the capacity to rapidly degenerate to a more aggressive phenotype [12]. Based on this finding, the authors concluded that early treatment may be the most appropriate for those with a long life expectancy. With respect to patients on watchful waiting protocols, these findings highlight the stringent need for continuous, extended monitoring for cancer progression.

These series offer insights into the potential clinical outcomes of prostate cancer patients. However, their utility in current practice is limited by the fact that these cases were diagnosed prior to the introduction of PSA testing in the late 1980s. Thus contemporary studies are needed to guide the management of patients in today's practice setting.

Several approaches towards observing prostate cancer have been described. These are similar in the fact that therapeutic intervention is initially withheld; however, they differ in rigor of surveillance, as well as threshold for and type of intervention. Traditionally watchful waiting or expectant management was observation of the patient until the development of metastatic disease or localized symptomatic progression, at which point the patient was offered palliative hormonal therapy. Alternatively, active surveillance (or expectant management with curative intent) includes active prostate cancer monitoring with scheduled attention to both local and PSA progression. Upon progression, the patient is typically recommended to undergo local treatment with curative intent.

Natural history of prostate in the PSA era

The introduction of PSA testing into clinical practice had an unprecedented effect on prostate cancer detection, staging, and awareness. After its approval in 1986 by the US Food and Drug Administration, the use of PSA testing became widespread for prostate cancer screening. In the period from 1989 to 1992, the number of new cases increased by a rate of 20% per year [14]. After a peak in incident cases in 1992, the number of new cases decreased by 10.8% per year before becoming relatively stable. Associated with this change was a subsequent reduction in the absolute number of patients presenting with distant disease [14] and an overall reduction in prostate cancer mortality [15]. Based on an analysis of the results from the Physician's Health Study, it is estimated that PSA testing improves the lead time for cancer detection over clinical detection by 5.5 years [16]. Others have shown lead times due to PSA testing could be over 10 years [17]. Given these dramatic changes in the presentation and detection of prostate cancer, it is essential to re-evaluate the natural history of prostate cancer in the modern era.

Several observational studies have reviewed the intermediate outcomes of watchful waiting alone for prostate cancer in the PSA era [18, 19, 20, 21, 22, 23, 24] (Table 2.1). From these studies, it is clear that many of the men who initially choose observation tend to be older and have significant other co-morbid conditions [18, 24]. The median PSA in these studies ranged from 4.8 to 7.4 ng/ml. Some studies excluded patients with higher grade tumors [18, 19, 20], whereas others included these cases [22, 23, 24]. These reports show that despite there being careful selection of patients for observation, a higher proportion of patients than expected subsequently chose cancer-directed treatment. Rates of cancer-directed treatment in these series ranged from 39% up to 74%. The stated reasons for the initiation of treatment were biochemical progression in 23%–77% of cases, and clinical progression in 18%–29% of cases [20, 23, 24]. Interestingly, treatment was begun due to patient preference alone (no documented progression) in over 20% of patients [20, 23], which highlights the difficulties in trying to maintain patients on a course of observation. Cancer-specific survival in these case series has been high [21, 23]; however, additional follow-up is needed before any conclusions can be drawn. Thus, despite the fact that these men were the most appropriate candidates for watchful waiting to be selected from a larger base of patients, this approach appears to have been one of mostly deferred therapy for the majority of men.

In order for an expectant management approach to become more accepted in clinical practice, improvements in the prediction of disease progression rates

Table 2.1. Results of observation for clinically localized prostate cancer during the prostate-specific antigen era

Study	Number of patients	Median follow-up (years)	Median PSA (ng/ml)	Tx initiated (%)	Tx initiated due to biochemical progression (%)	Tx initiated due to clinical progression (%)	Predictors of secondary treatment
Koppie et al. [22]	329	2.3	7.4	39	N/A	N/A	Age, PSA, stage
Zietman et al. [24]	198	3.4	6.6	44 (actuarial at 5 years)	77	18	none
Carter et al. [18]	313	3.8	5.1	74	N/A	N/A	PSADT, stage
Panagiotou et al. [23]	192	3.6	6.9	48	42.2	28.9	Gleason score, percent positive biopsy cores, PSADT
Klotz [21]	299	3.0	6.5	40	23	29	N/A
Carter et al. [19]	407	2.8	4.8	41	N/A	N/A	PSA, %fPSA, PSAD, PSAV, year of diagnosis

Abbreviations: PSA, prostate-specific antigen; PSADT, PSA doubling time; % fPSA, percentage free PSA; PSAD, PSA density; PSAV, PSA velocity; Tx, treatment.

are needed. Models for the prediction of tumor indolence have been developed for patients who have been diagnosed with prostate cancer [25, 26, 27]. These have shown that the presence of small non-aggressive tumors in prostatectomy specimens can be predicted using pre-treatment models based on clinical factors alone. In the future, ongoing prospective trials will perhaps be able to confirm the validity of these predictive tools by examining clinical outcomes. Importantly data regarding survival, quality of life, secondary treatment, and other outcomes are needed in men who opt for expectant management in the PSA era. Furthermore, the discovery of additional biomarkers based on both blood and tissue markers and improved imaging of prostate cancer will likely strengthen our ability to predict the clinical course of prostate cancer in individual patients.

Delayed curative therapy after choosing watchful waiting

Before wide-range acceptance of observation as an individual approach to prostate cancer can become well established, secondary treatment results must be considered as patients are unlikely to accept a course of observation if delayed interventions are ineffective. Prior to the use of PSA testing in clinical practice, few patients who initially elected observation went on to curative therapies [3, 5, 11]. The results of delayed secondary treatment with curative intent in the PSA era have been reported by several groups [28, 29, 30] (Table 2.2). Disease control rates in these series ranged from 77% to 97% [29, 30]. In a study by El-Geneidy et al., [28], factors that predicted subsequent curative treatment included: younger age, increased proportion of positive biopsy cores, and a shorter PSA doubling time in the follow-up phase [28]. Notably, although the study sizes were small, the oncologic results of therapy in this scenario were found to be comparable to those for patients undergoing primary treatment without delay after the diagnosis was made. Warlick and colleagues [30] compared results of men undergoing delayed curative radical prostatectomy to a matched cohort of men undergoing immediate radical prostatectomy [30]. They found that rates of finding curable cancer were not different between the two groups. Thus, in highly selected patients, a potential alternative approach to the standard of immediate therapy is to delay treatment until tumor progression. This option potentially holds the promise of a reduction in treatment-related morbidity and cost without an apparent reduction in cancer control. These findings will require prospective validation in a large cohort before definite treatment recommendations can be made.

Table 2.2. Results of delayed therapy with curative intent for prostate cancer in the PSA era

Study	Number of patients	Mean time to secondary treatment (years)	Median PSA at diagnosis (ng/ml)	Treatment initiated	Disease-free rate (%)	Predictors of delayed curative treatment
Patel *et al.* [29]	31	N/A	5.9	RT = 14 RP = 17	97	Per protocol
El-Geneidy *et al.* [28]	38	3.3	6.9	RT = 15 RP = 23	N/A	Age, percent positive biopsy cores, PSADT
Warlick *et al.* [30]	38	2.2	4.9	RP = 38	77[a]	N/A

Abbreviations: PSA, prostate-specific antigen; PSADT, PSA doubling time; %fPSA, percent free PSA; PSAD, PSA density; RP, radical prostatectomy; N/A, not available.
[a] Based on surgical pathology findings.

The natural history of treated prostate cancer

Among men who undergo a radical prostatectomy for localized disease, it is estimated that 20%–40% of men will experience a PSA recurrence with extended follow-up [31, 32, 33]. The treatment of recurrent disease is often driven by early detection with PSA testing. In the post-operative setting, with early salvage, therapies such as radiation and hormones are commonly employed. However, some surgical series have examined the results of expectant management for post-prostatectomy recurrences. In a study by Pound *et al.* [34] of 1997 patients, it was shown that the metastases-free rate was 82% at 15 years post-prostatectomy. The median time to metastases after the first rise in PSA was 8 years and median time to death after the development of metastases was 5 years. Significant predictors of both the development of metastatic disease and overall survival were Gleason score (8 or above), a rapid PSA recurrence and rate of PSA rise (i.e., PSA doubling time) [33, 34]. In a subsequent study by Yossepowitch and colleagues [35], the rate of the development of metastases was examined in 4054 non-castrate patients treated at Memorial Sloan-Kettering Cancer Center. Ninety-five patients (2.3% of cohort) were found to have presented with metastases before the institution of hormone therapy. In this study, median survival was 6.6 years after the development of metastases. It was demonstrated that, in addition to PSA doubling time, the type of metastatic disease seen at presentation (minimal versus extensive) was a strong predictor of death after the development of metastases [35]. These studies high-light the significance of a PSA recurrence in the post-operative period and identify those at greatest risk for prostate cancer metastases and death. Furthermore, these data identify those who are most appropriate candidates for experimental ther-apies designed to prevent the development of metastases or extend patient survival.

The direct impact of curative therapy on the natural history of prostate cancer has been studied in only a limited number of completed trials. The most important of these has been the Scandinavian Prostate Cancer Study – 4. In this trial, 695 men with prostate cancer were randomized to either observation alone or radical prosta-tectomy [36]. At baseline, the mean PSA was about 13 ng/ml with nearly half of all patients having PSA values over 10 ng/ml [36]. With a median follow-up of 8.2 years, significant improvements in cancer outcomes have been reported for men entered onto the surgical intervention arm of the trial [37]. At 10 years, this study showed a 44% improvement in disease-specific mortality and a 26% improvement in overall survival (Figure 2.2). Surgical intervention resulted in a 67% reduction in local progression and a 40% reduction in the spread of metas-tases. This landmark study was the first to unequivocally show the salient benefits of curative intervention for localized prostate cancer and this study sets a standard by which new treatments should be evaluated.

Despite these results showing the clear benefits of surgery, it is important to point out that many of these men had more advanced tumors than are typically detected using screening algorithms. In this trial only 5% of all cases were screen-detected cancers. Thus it is important to continue to study the effect of screening on prostate cancer presentation and response to therapy. Randomized trials are currently underway to study the effect of screening on prostate cancer outcomes.

Ongoing randomized controlled trials

To define the PSA-era outcomes for observation of prostate cancer, several co-operative group trials have been instituted in both North America and Europe. The Prostate Cancer Intervention Versus Observation Trial (PIVOT) is a multi-center trial sponsored by the National Cancer Institute and the Department of Veterans Affairs [38]. Patients with localized prostate cancer have been randomized to either surgical removal of the prostate or observation alone. The study objective is to compare early radical prostatectomy to expectant management with reservation

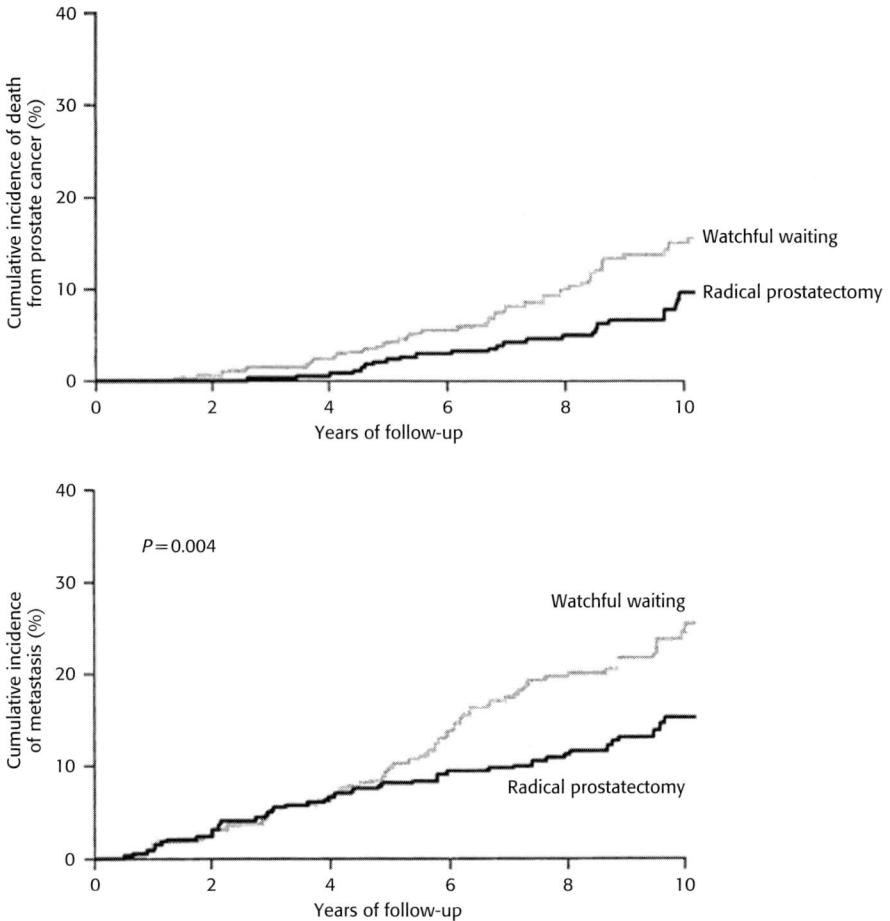

Figure 2.2. Cumulative incidence of death from prostate cancer (upper panel) and metastases (lower panel) in men treated with radical prostatectomy versus observation alone. Reprinted with permission from [37] (*NEJM*; May 12, 2005; Vol. 352:19; Copyright © (2005), Massachusetts Medical Society. All Rights reserved.)

of therapy for palliative treatment of symptomatic or metastatic disease progression. Secondary endpoints include prostate-cancer-specific mortality, quality of life, as well as histologic, laboratory, and demographic predictors of cancer outcomes. Accrual to this trial has been completed with 731 patients enrolled, and follow-up will continue through 2009. This study will determine the effect that surgery has on the natural history of prostate cancer when applied at an early stage in the disease course.

In a multigroup trial conducted in Canada and the USA by the National Cancer Institute of Canada, immediate curative treatment will be compared to delayed curative therapy in patients with localized prostate cancer (A Phase III Study of Active Surveillance *T*herapy *A*gainst *R*adical *T*reatment in Patients Diagnosed with Favorable Risk Prostate Cancer, i.e., *START* Trial). Participants of this study must have organ-confined disease, a PSA of ≤10 ng/ml, and a Gleason score of ≤6 on prostate biopsy at enrolment. Patients will be randomized to radical intervention (either prostatectomy or radiation per patient preference) or to a program of active surveillance (with plans for radical intervention if disease progression occurs). Progression is to be defined per protocol as: (1) biochemical progression = PSA doubling time of less than 3 years; (2) an increase in Gleason score with a predominant pattern of 4 (i.e., $4 + 3 = 7$ or greater); or (3) signs of clinical progression including urinary retention, hematuria, or hydronephrosis. Patients in each treatment arm will undergo routine periodic evaluations; however, patients in the active surveillance arm will submit to repeat scheduled prostate biopsies from which tumor histology will be re-evaluated. The primary endpoint of the trial is disease-specific survival. The accrual goal is 2130 patients to be followed for a minimum of 10 years. Once completed this study will provide information about the effectiveness of delayed therapy compared to immediate treatment. It will also allow for the prospective description of the natural history of prostate cancer in the PSA era. Lastly, correlative studies can be carried out on biopsy and prostatectomy specimens that will allow for the delineation of tumor progression at specific phases in the evolution of prostate cancer pathogenesis.

Finally, in the United Kingdom, the ProtecT Trial (i.e., *Pro*state *Te*sting for *C*ancer and *T*reatment Trial) will evaluate the effectiveness of standard therapies (surgery and radiation) for clinically localized prostate cancer compared to active surveillance. Subjects with localized, early prostate cancer will be randomized to monitoring, surgery or radiation therapy. Study endpoints include patient survival, disease progression, safety, quality of life, and economic impact. Study results from ProtecT are expected in the year 2015.

Summary

Over the last decade predictive models have become available that allow for the clinician to predict the natural history of prostate cancer. It is clear that for select patients surgical intervention is effective at preventing this history from unfolding. Further salvage treatments, in particular radiation therapy, may alter the progression of disease in those with recurrent disease. Studies are ongoing which will help determine the effectiveness of surgery and radiation at earlier stages in the disease progression and whether delayed interventions can be efficacious. These trials will include analyses of quality of life and costs to healthcare systems. These studies will include molecular analyses that will search for novel biomarkers that improve upon existing disease prediction models. Future studies will also include novel imaging techniques that will allow for real-time assessment of disease progression of small-volume localized prostate cancer.

REFERENCES

1. A. Jemal, R. Siegel, E. Ward, *et al.*, Cancer statistics, 2008. *CA Cancer J Clin*, **58**:2 (2008), 71–96.

2. W. F. Whitmore, Jr., J. A. Warner, I. M. Thompson, Jr. Expectant management of localized prostatic cancer. *Cancer*, **67**:4 (1991), 1091–6.

3. J. E. Johansson, H. O. Adami, S. O. Andersson, *et al.*, Natural history of localised prostatic cancer. A population-based study in 223 untreated patients. *Lancet*, **1**:8642 (1989), 799–803.

4. P. O. Madsen, P. H. Graversen, T. C. Gasser, *et al.*, Treatment of localized prostatic cancer. Radical prostatectomy versus placebo. A 15-year follow-up. *Scand J Urol Nephrol Suppl*, **110** (1988), 95–100.

5. G. W. Chodak, R. A. Thisted, G. S. Gerber, *et al.*, Results of conservative management of clinically localized prostate cancer. *New Engl J Med* **33**:4 (1994), 242–8.

6. D. F. Gleason, Histologic grade, clinical stage, and patient age in prostate cancer. *NCI Monogr*, **7** (1988), 15–18.

7. A. V. D'Amico, R. Whittington, S. B. Malkowicz, *et al.*, Biochemical outcome after radical prostatectomy, external beam radiation therapy, or interstitial radiation therapy for clinically localized prostate cancer. *JAMA*, **280**:11 (1998), 969–74.

8. M. W. Kattan, T. M. Wheeler, P. T. Scardino, Postoperative nomogram for disease recurrence after radical prostatectomy for prostate cancer. *J Clin Oncol*, **5** (1999), 1499–507.

9. M. W. Kattan, M. J. Zelefsky, P. A. Kupelian, *et al.*, Pretreatment nomogram for predicting the outcome of three-dimensional conformal radiotherapy in prostate cancer. *J Clin Oncol*, **18**:19 (2000), 3352–9.

10. P. C. Albertsen, J. A. Hanley, J. Fine, 20-year outcomes following conservative management of clinically localized prostate cancer. *JAMA*, **293**:17 (2005), 2095–101.

11. P. C. Albertsen, J. A. Hanley, D. F. Gleason, *et al.*, Competing risk analysis of men aged 55 to 74 years at diagnosis managed conservatively for clinically localized prostate cancer. *JAMA*, **280**:11 (1998), 975–80.

12. J. E. Johansson, O. Andren, S. O. Andersson, *et al.*, Natural history of early, localized prostate cancer. *JAMA*, **291**:22 (2004), 2713–19.

13. J. E. Johansson, L. Holmberg, S. Johansson, *et al.*, Fifteen-year survival in prostate cancer. A prospective, population-based study in Sweden. *JAMA*, **277**:6 (1997), 467–71.

14. B. F. Hankey, E. J. Feuer, L. X. Clegg, *et al.*, Cancer surveillance series: interpreting trends in prostate cancer. Part I: evidence of the effects of screening in recent prostate cancer incidence, mortality, and survival rates. *J Natl Cancer Inst*, **91**:12 (1999), 1017–24.

15. K. McDavid, J. Lee, J. P. Fulton, *et al.*, Prostate cancer incidence and mortality rates and trends in the United States and Canada. *Public Health Rep*, **119**:2 (2004), 174–86.

16. P. H. Gann, C. H. Hennekens, M. J. Stampfer, A prospective evaluation of plasma prostate-specific antigen for detection of prostatic cancer. *JAMA*, **273**:4 (1995), 289–94.

17. G. Draisma, R. Boer, S. J. Otto, *et al.*, Lead times and overdetection due to prostate-specific antigen screening: estimates from the European Randomized Study of Screening for Prostate Cancer. *J Natl Cancer Inst*, **95**:12 (2003), 868–78.

18. C. A. Carter, T. Donahue, L. Sun, *et al.*, Temporarily deferred therapy (watchful waiting) for men younger than 70 years and with low-risk localized prostate cancer in the prostate-specific antigen era. *J Clin Oncol*, **21**:21 (2003), 4001–8.

19. H. B. Carter, A. Kettermann, C. Warlick, *et al.*, Expectant management of prostate cancer with curative intent: an update of The Johns Hopkins Experience. *J Urol*, **178**:6 (2007), 2359–64; discussion 2364–5.

20. R. Choo, L. Klotz, C. Danjoux, *et al.*, Feasibility study: watchful waiting for localized low to intermediate grade prostate carcinoma with selective delayed intervention based on prostate specific antigen, histological and/or clinical progression. *J Urol*, **167**:4 (2002), 1664–9.

21. L. Klotz, Active surveillance with selective delayed intervention: using natural history to guide treatment in good risk prostate cancer. *J Urol*, **172**:5(2) (2004), S48–50; discussion S-1.

22. T. M. Koppie, G. D. Grossfeld, D. Miller, *et al.*, Patterns of treatment of patients with prostate cancer initially managed with surveillance: results from The CaPSURE database. Cancer of the Prostate Strategic Urological Research Endeavor. *J Urol*, **164**:1 (2000), 81–8.

23. I. Panagiotou, T. M. Beer, Y. C. Hsieh, *et al.*, Predictors of delayed therapy after expectant management for localized prostate cancer in the era of prostate-specific antigen. *Oncology*, **67**:3–4 (2004), 194–202.

24. A. L. Zietman, H. Thakral, L. Wilson, *et al.*, Conservative management of prostate cancer in the prostate specific antigen era: the incidence and time course of subsequent therapy. *J Urol*, **166**:5 (2001), 1702–6.

25. J. I. Epstein, P. C. Walsh, M. Carmichael, *et al.*, Pathologic and clinical findings to predict tumor extent of nonpalpable (stage T1c) prostate cancer. *JAMA*, **271**:5 (1994), 368–74.

26. M. W. Kattan, J. A. Eastham, T. M. Wheeler, *et al.*, Counseling men with prostate cancer: a nomogram for predicting the presence of small, moderately differentiated, confined tumors. *J Urol*, **170**:5 (2003), 1792–7.

27. E. W. Steyerberg, M. J. Roobol, M. W. Kattan, *et al.*, Prediction of indolent prostate cancer: validation and updating of a prognostic nomogram. *J Urol*, **177**:1 (2007), 107–12; discussion 12.

28. M. El-Geneidy, M. Garzotto, I. Panagiotou, *et al.*, Delayed therapy with curative intent in a contemporary prostate cancer watchful-waiting cohort. *BJU Int*, **93**:4 (2004), 510–15.

29. M. I. Patel, D. T. DeConcini, E. Lopez-Corona, *et al.*, An analysis of men with clinically localized prostate cancer who deferred definitive therapy. *J Urol*, **171**:4 (2004), 1520–4.

30. C. Warlick, B. J. Trock, P. Landis, *et al.*, Delayed versus immediate surgical intervention and prostate cancer outcome. *J Natl Cancer Inst*, **98**:5 (2006), 355–7.

31. M. Han, A. W. Partin, C. R. Pound, *et al.*, Long-term biochemical disease-free and cancer-specific survival following anatomic radical retropubic prostatectomy. The 15-year Johns Hopkins experience. *Urol Clin North Am*, **28**:3 (2001), 555–65.

32. A. J. Stephenson, K. M. Slawin, F. J. Bianco, Jr., *et al.*, Perspectives on the natural history of recurrent prostate cancer after radical prostatectomy, based on the response to salvage radiotherapy. *BJU Int*, **94**:9 (2004), 1210–12.

33. S. J. Freedland, E. B. Humphreys, L. A. Mangold, *et al.*, Risk of prostate cancer-specific mortality following biochemical recurrence after radical prostatectomy. *JAMA*, **294**:4 (2005), 433–9.

34. C. R. Pound, A. W. Partin, M. A. Eisenberger, *et al.*, Natural history of progression after PSA elevation following radical prostatectomy. *JAMA*, **281**:17 (1999), 1591–7.

35. O. Yossepowitch, F. J. Bianco, Jr., S. E. Eggener, *et al.*, The natural history of noncastrate metastatic prostate cancer after radical prostatectomy. *Eur Urol*, **51**:4 (2007), 940–7; discussion 7–8.

36. L. Holmberg, A. Bill-Axelson, F. Helgesen, *et al.*, A randomized trial comparing radical prostatectomy

with watchful waiting in early prostate cancer. *New Engl J Med*, **347**:11 (2002), 781–9.

37. A. Bill-Axelson, L. Holmberg, M. Ruutu, *et al.*, Radical prostatectomy versus watchful waiting in early prostate cancer. *New Engl J Med*, **352**:19 (2005), 1977–84.

38. T. J. Wilt, M. K. Brawer, The Prostate Cancer Intervention Versus Observation Trial: a randomized trial comparing radical prostatectomy versus expectant management for the treatment of clinically localized prostate cancer. *J Urol*, **152**:5(2) (1994), 1910–14.

3

Current clinical issues in prostate cancer that can be addressed by imaging

Hedvig Hricak and Peter T. Scardino

Introduction

The role of imaging in the management of prostate cancer has long been controversial, and imaging continues to be both overused and underused. Guidelines are available regarding the use of imaging for the assessment of advanced disease. However, in recent years, imaging technology has matured, image acquisition and interpretation have improved, and a host of clinical studies have demonstrated the potential of imaging for improving other aspects of prostate cancer care, including the detection of local primary or recurrent disease and surgical or radiation treatment planning. This review will discuss the many ways in which imaging can contribute to the evidence-based clinical management of prostate cancer, focusing on the most commonly used cross-sectional imaging modalities: transrectal ultrasound (TRUS), computed tomography (CT), magnetic resonance imaging (MRI), radionuclide bone scanning, positron-emission tomography (PET), and combined PET/CT.

Imaging in diagnosis

Prostate-specific antigen (PSA) testing and digital rectal examination (DRE) continue to be the mainstays of prostate cancer detection. When either of these yields abnormal results, TRUS-guided biopsy is performed. The initial biopsy session will detect cancer in about 29% of patients who undergo biopsy for suspected prostate cancer, depending on the PSA level and DRE results. However, the sensitivity for detection is about 80%–90%, depending on the biopsy scheme used [1, 2]. Cancers missed by systematic transrectal biopsy may be small or located in the anterior part of the gland, an area rarely sampled [3]. If repeated biopsies are negative in a patient

Prostate Cancer, eds. Hedvig Hricak and Peter T. Scardino. Published by Cambridge University Press.
© Cambridge University Press 2009.

at high risk for prostate cancer, MRI may be used to identify appropriate targets for an additional repeat biopsy [4]. Magnetic resonance imaging has been found to perform better than DRE in localizing cancer throughout the prostate gland and better than TRUS in localizing cancer in the middle and base of the gland [5]. It is also reasonably sensitive for detecting large cancers (>1 cm) in the anterior prostate gland [5].

Optimal MRI for prostate cancer detection requires the use of an endorectal coil and a pelvic phased-array coil on a mid- to high-field magnet, with thin (3 mm) slices and a small (14 cm) field of view [6]. On T_2-weighted MR images, the zonal anatomy of the prostate can be seen. Cancer most commonly demonstrates decreased signal intensity within the high-signal-intensity peripheral zone, but it may also be detected in the transition zone [7, 8]. New technology that allows co-registration of MRI with real-time TRUS to guide prostate biopsies appears promising [9].

Imaging in treatment selection

The goal in cancer care is evidence-based rather than empirical treatment selection. When the biopsy results are positive for prostate cancer, a wide variety of options for treatment may be considered, ranging from radical prostatectomy, to various forms of radiation therapy, to deferred treatment (i.e., "active surveillance," a plan to defer definitive treatment until evidence of cancer progression). Treatment selection should depend on the health and life expectancy of the patient, the patient's preferences, and the risk posed by the cancer. Imaging can help to assess this risk.

Identifying potentially insignificant cancer

Earlier detection of prostate cancer with PSA screening [10] has raised concerns about overdiagnosis and overtreatment [11, 12]. It is estimated that in the USA more than 30% of prostate cancer patients are overtreated [13]. Thus it is important to distinguish cancers that pose little or no risk to life and health (clinically "indolent" or insignificant cancers) from those that are potentially lethal (clinically significant) if left untreated.

A number of clinical variables (e.g., PSA, clinical stage, biopsy Gleason score) have proven to be valuable for assessing the risk of prostate cancer progression [14].

Nomograms that combine these variables are more accurate than any single variable alone for predicting the pathologic stage of prostate cancer or the outcome of treatment [14, 15, 16], and they are often used for counseling patients during treatment selection. Several nomograms have been designed that use clinical variables to predict the presence of indolent prostate cancer (defined as organ-confined cancer with a total volume of 0.5 cm^3 or less and no poorly differentiated component on histology) [17, 18, 19, 20, 21, 22, 23].

Recently, Shukla-Dave *et al.* [24] developed nomogram models to predict the presence of insignificant prostate cancer in patients with clinically low-risk disease based on a combination of clinical variables and findings from MRI or combined MRI/MR spectroscopic imaging (MRSI) [24]. MRSI, which can be performed in the same examination as MRI using commercially available software, provides information about metabolic activity in the prostate and has been shown to increase the accuracy of MRI in prostate cancer detection, staging, and tumor volume estimation [25, 26, 27]. In the study by Shukla-Dave *et al.*, MRI/MRSI findings were scored on a scale from 0 (definitely insignificant prostate cancer) to 3 (definitely significant prostate cancer) [24]. The nomogram models that incorporated MRI or MRI/MRSI scores performed significantly better than models based on clinical variables alone. Whereas the most comprehensive clinical model tested yielded an area under the receiver-operating characteristic curve (AUC) of 0.726, the models combining clinical variables with MRI and MRI/MRSI yielded AUCs of 0.803 ($p < 0.018$) and 0.854 ($p < 0.001$), respectively [24]. Although the new MR-based models are not sufficiently accurate to identify an indolent cancer unequivocally, if validated prospectively, they may prove useful for counseling patients who are considering active surveillance [24].

For patients who choose active surveillance (e.g., every 2 years), serial MRI or MRI/MRSI can be used to identify new or growing lesions that should be assessed by biopsy. Furthermore, in patients with clinically low-risk, localized cancer, MRI may prove useful for identifying lesions suitable for focal therapy in the future.

Assessing clinically significant prostate cancer

For patients with clinically significant prostate cancer, imaging – in particular MRI or MRI/MRSI – can provide useful information for the selection and planning of treatment.

The reported accuracy of MRI in the local staging of prostate cancer ranges from 54% to 93% [8, 28, 29, 30, 31, 32, 33]. On the whole, the accuracy of MRI in local staging has increased with time, most likely because of the maturation of MRI technology (e.g., faster imaging sequences, more powerful gradient coils, and post-processing image correction), better understanding of the morphologic criteria for diagnosing extracapsular extension and seminal vesicle invasion, and greater reader experience. The inclusion of findings from MRI or combined MRI/MRSI in prostate cancer staging nomograms has been shown to significantly improve the prediction of organ-confined disease and seminal vesicle invasion [34, 35]. Furthermore, two studies found that the addition of MRI to clinical variables improved the prediction of extracapsular extension, although the improvement was only significant when image interpretation was done by specialists in genitourinary MRI [31, 36].

Imaging in treatment planning

In patients who choose radical prostatectomy, MRI can provide invaluable information for surgical planning. By demonstrating the location, size, and extent of the cancer MRI helps the surgeon to avoid leaving positive surgical margins or unnecessarily damaging surrounding structures that are essential for the recovery of normal urinary and sexual function.

For example, with accurate information about the location of the cancer, the surgeon can modify the operation to resect more widely in areas of suspected extracapsular extension, or to dissect closer to the prostate in the areas of the neurovascular bundles when extracapsular extension appears unlikely. A study [37] of 76 patients showed that pre-operative reviews of endorectal MR images significantly improved the surgeon's decisions regarding whether to preserve or resect the neurovascular bundles at radical prostatectomy ($p < 0.01$). Similarly, by predicting the presence and location of seminal vesicle invasion, MRI can assist the surgeon in deciding whether to remove the seminal vesicles completely.

Magnetic resonance imaging can also be of assistance by demonstrating the location of cancer within the gland. For example, visualization of a large, anterior transition zone tumor on the pre-operative MRI will alert the surgeon to the need for more distal transection of the dorsal vein complex over the urethra [38], whereas demonstration of a prominent tumor in the posterior apex will warn the surgeon to dissect more widely in that area.

Magnetic resonance imaging may help predict substantial intraoperative blood loss, as the prominence of the apical periprostatic veins on MRI has been positively associated with blood loss [39]. In addition, the length of the membranous urethra on coronal endorectal MRI can help to predict the time to recovery of urinary continence [40]. It has been found that patients with a longer than average (14 mm) membranous urethra experience a more rapid return to complete continence [40].

There is no question that lymph node metastasis is one of the most important negative prognostic factors in prostate cancer. For many years, CT was the only imaging modality used to identify lymph node metastases. The results were disappointing, as detection depends on size criteria (generally, a short-axis diameter greater than 7–8 mm), even though lymph node metastases may be present in normal-sized nodes or absent from enlarged nodes. The detection of metastatic lymph nodes by MRI depends on the same size criteria as CT and therefore is similarly limited, with high specificity but low sensitivity. However, the use of MRI before treatment has the advantage of allowing the primary tumor and the pelvic lymph nodes to be assessed simultaneously. A recent study has shown that the prediction of lymph node metastasis by MRI improved when MRI findings for seminal vesicle invasion, extracapsular extension and nodal metastasis were combined in a model [41]. By identifying specific enlarged nodes that may harbor cancer and by helping to predict the pathologic tumor stage, and therefore the likelihood of lymph node metastasis, MRI can improve surgical planning and help determine whether systemic therapy should be administered before surgery. If radiation therapy is planned, MRI may help the radiation oncologist to decide whether the pelvic lymph nodes should be included in the radiation field.

Detection of recurrence

Regardless of the type of treatment administered, serial measurements of PSA and DRE are the standard tools used to monitor for tumor recurrence. When recurrence is suspected due to a rising PSA or because a nodule or induration has been felt on DRE, imaging may be useful to confirm the presence of recurrence and to determine whether it is local or systemic.

Detection of local recurrence after radiation therapy

In patients who have undergone radiation therapy, MRI and MRSI may provide a target for biopsy and may help to determine the location, extent, and size of recurrence to improve treatment selection and planning. In one study [42] two radiologists used MRI to evaluate prostate cancer recurrence after radiation treatment in 45 patients scheduled for salvage prostatectomy. They achieved sensitivity/specificity values of 76%/73% and 55%/65% for tumor detection by quadrant, 86%/84% and 64%/76% for extracapsular extension, and 58%/96% and 42%/96% for seminal vesicle invasion – values similar to those found in studies of untreated patients [42]. Furthermore, in a small preliminary study that also used step-section pathology as the standard of reference, MRI and MRSI had higher sensitivities (68% and 77%, respectively) than DRE (16%) and TRUS-guided biopsy (48%) for the detection of recurrence after radiation therapy, although MRSI had lower specificity (78%) than the three other modalities, each of which had a specificity greater than 90% [43].

In a study of nine patients who underwent salvage prostatectomy, investigators compared the locations and volumes of prostate cancer lesions on pre-radiation-therapy MRI, post-radiation therapy MRI, and step-section pathology maps. They found that in every patient, clinically significant local recurrence occurred at the site of the original primary tumor [44]. These results provide support for the concept of boosting the radiation dose to the primary tumor using imaging guidance; they also suggest that the use of MRI before and after radiation treatment to identify and monitor the site of the primary tumor might facilitate detection of cancer recurrence at an earlier stage, when it is more likely to be treatable by salvage prostatectomy [44].

Detection of local recurrence after radical prostatectomy

Magnetic resonance imaging has demonstrated the capacity to detect local recurrence in many patients with a rising PSA but no palpable tumor in the prostatic fossa [45, 46]. Magnetic resonance imaging may show local recurrences in the perianastomotic and retrovesical regions [47]. In addition, MRI has demonstrated that 30% of local recurrences may occur at other sites in the pelvis, for example in retained seminal vesicles or at the lateral or anterior surgical margins [45]. While MRI can detect recurrent cancer that is not palpable, confirmation of MRI abnormalities by needle biopsy is recommended before therapeutic intervention (e.g., boost dose of salvage irradiation to nodules or addition of androgen-deprivation therapy to salvage radiation therapy). One limiting feature of MRI-detected local recurrence, especially if impalpable, is the difficulty of ultrasound-guided biopsy of abnormalities identified on MRI, as many suspected lesions will not be visible sonographically.

Imaging in the detection of advanced disease

Pre-treatment detection of metastases

The technetium bone scan is a widely available and sensitive method for diagnosing the initial spread of cancer to bone, particularly for osteoblastic metastases. However, it should be reserved for symptomatic patients and for those with high-risk disease, as the incidence of bone metastasis in men with clinically localized prostate cancer at diagnosis is low. The National Comprehensive Cancer Network (NCCN) recommends bone scans for asymptomatic patients with a life expectancy greater than 5 years only if the PSA is above 20 ng/ml, the Gleason score is at least 8, or the clinical stage is T3 or T4 [48]. The American College of Radiology recommends bone scans for patients with a PSA above 10 ng/ml [49] and a Gleason score greater than 6 (the same threshold used at our institution).

In prostate cancer, lymph node metastasis is even less common than bone metastasis. The NCCN guidelines recommend using CT or MRI only in patients with a nomogram-indicated probability of lymph node metastasis greater than 20%. As noted earlier, CT and MRI both have limited accuracy in the detection of lymph node metastases, but MRI does have the advantage of allowing the prostate and the pelvic lymph nodes to be assessed in a single examination.

Recent studies have demonstrated that MRI after administration of ultrasmall superparamagnetic iron oxide (USPIO) particles has high sensitivity and specificity (both above 90%) in the detection of prostate cancer lymph node metastases; it allows the identification of small metastatic lymph nodes (<5 mm), as well as the differentiation between benign reactive and malignant enlarged nodes [50, 51, 52]. Although this technique is extremely promising, it has not yet received regulatory approval in the United States. Furthermore, it is somewhat cumbersome, requiring contrast to be administered to the patient the day before imaging. Therefore, it has been suggested that standard MRI, in conjunction with the standard staging nomogram, could be used to determine whether imaging with USPIO particles is warranted [41].

Post-treatment detection of metastases

When recurrence is suspected, imaging plays an essential role in evaluating a patient for metastatic disease. With a rising PSA, the first investigation ordered to search for metastases is a bone scan. However, the bone scan is rarely positive until PSA values are high, around 30 ng/ml [53]. Recently, a highly discriminating nomogram was developed for predicting the probability of a positive bone scan after biochemical failure and before the initiation of hormone therapy. The nomogram, which is based on commonly available data (including pathologic findings from the analysis of the surgical specimen and post-operative PSA data), predicted bone scan results with a concordance index of 0.93. Although the nomogram does not apply to patients treated with hormone therapy, it may prove useful for selecting patients according to their risk for a positive bone scan and reducing the total number of scans ordered [54].

If bone scan findings are indeterminate, further imaging may allow clarification. Some studies have suggested that in cases where bone scan findings are questionable, MRI should be used as a supplementary form of imaging [55, 56]. Bone marrow MRI has been shown to be more sensitive and specific than bone scanning for the detection of bone metastases and to reveal them at an earlier stage [57]. In a recent study of 66 patients with high-risk prostate cancer, the sensitivity and specificity of one-step MRI of the axial skeleton (100% and 88%, respectively) were markedly higher than those of bone scanning (46% and 32%, respectively) for detecting bone metastases, and this changed treatment planning in a substantial proportion (22%) of patients [58]. Further research is needed to determine the diagnostic value and cost-effectiveness of one-step MRI relative to other modern imaging modalities in the assessment of bone metastases.

In patients with aggressive disease, ^{18}F-2-fluoro-D-deoxyglucose (^{18}F-FDG) PET/CT may allow precise localization of bone metastases, facilitating new treatment options such as bony ablation [59].

Computed tomography and/or FDG-PET (or FDG-PET/CT) may be used to search for nodal disease after treatment, especially in aggressive and/or hormone-refractory disease; however, as there have been no randomized clinical trials comparing the efficacy of FDG-PET/CT to that of CT in this setting, evidence-based recommendations cannot be made. Because a staging lymphadenectomy is usually performed during radical prostatectomy, assessment for nodal disease with cross-sectional imaging in surgical patients is focused on common iliac and retroperitoneal nodes; in patients treated with radiation therapy, cross-sectional imaging of the pelvis is standard. Limited data suggest that, unlike CT, FDG-PET can also demonstrate tumor in the prostate bed [60]. As with conventional imaging modalities, the detection of metastases with FDG-PET increases with higher PSA levels [59]. In a study of 91 patients with PSA relapse after radical prostatectomy, FDG-PET detected locally recurrent or systemic cancer in only 28 patients (31%) [60]; it appeared to be most useful in patients with PSA > 2.4 ng/ml or a PSA doubling time >1.3 ng/ml per year. Still, nearly all disease sites detected by CT or bone scanning were also detected by FDG-PET. The authors therefore suggested that the combination of FDG-PET (to detect systemic disease) and body MRI (to detect local recurrence) might provide a valuable imaging algorithm in appropriately selected patients with PSA relapse [60].

Preliminary results suggest that PET with ^{11}C-choline or ^{11}C-acetate may allow better detection of nodal disease than FDG-PET [60]. The rapid 10-min uptake and plateau of agents labeled with ^{11}C within prostate cancer allows whole-body PET/CT imaging (with decay correction) and results in less interference from the bladder [61]. However, because ^{11}C has a short half-life of approximately 20 min, its use requires a local cyclotron and is therefore not a widely available option.

Another tracer under development is ^{11}C-methionine, which differentiates tumor from normal tissue due to elevated protein synthesis [62]. Patients who receive ^{11}C-methionine and FDG scans on the same day may demonstrate metastases that are positive by both tracers, or that are positive by ^{11}C-methionine only or FDG only [63]. These differences appear to indicate changes that occur in tumor biology as the tumor adapts to specific sanctuary sites. The use of PET with multiple radiotracers that answer different questions is likely to play an important role in the future of metabolic prostate cancer imaging.

Monoclonal antibody imaging with the prostate-specific membrane antigen (PSMA) antibody ^{111}In-capromab pendetide (also known as ProstaScint®) is another modality used to detect soft-tissue metastases in high-risk patients who are being considered for local salvage therapy. In studies comparing capromab to CT and MRI, capromab proved capable of detecting some small soft-tissue metastases (5–10 mm in size) that could not be detected by the other two modalities. However, the overall sensitivity of capromab for soft-tissue metastases was only 50%–62%; it missed a fair number of metastases that were detected by CT or MRI and it yielded false-positive or false-negative results in approximately one-third of patients studied [64]. Furthermore, capromab demonstrated low sensitivity for detecting bone metastases, which usually occur before lymph node metastases [64]. For these reasons, its use is controversial. A new antibody, J591, is currently undergoing experimental investigation and appears more promising for the detection of both bone and soft-tissue metastases [64]. Further refinements in the procedures for performing and interpreting capromab scans may also increase its accuracy in advanced prostate cancer.

Follow-up of systemic therapy

Both bone scanning and CT are heavily used to assess response to systemic treatment for bone metastases, but they have substantial limitations. On bone scanning, uptake usually decreases after chemotherapy/hormone therapy or radiotherapy if a response is obtained. However, in prostate cancer patients, a "flare" phenomenon may be observed, where uptake initially increases after chemotherapy or hormone therapy, peaking at 6 weeks after treatment as bone turnover increases as part of the healing process [65, 66]. Thus care must be taken to avoid mistaking apparent new lesions for areas of new metastatic disease, when subtle changes were in fact present in prior studies. Computed tomography cannot be used to differentiate healing bone from progressive disease, but it can play a role in the assessment of more aggressive lytic lesions with potential for pathologic fracture. Bone marrow MRI or FDG-PET (or FDG-PET/CT) is better than bone scanning or CT for distinguishing between active bony metastasis and healing bone [67]. In addition, FDG-PET or FDF-PET/CT allows quantitative assessment of tumor response not only in terms of tumor volume and size, but also in terms of the degree of metabolic activity.

^{18}F-Fluorodihydrotestosterone (FDHT) PET may have potential for predicting and assessing the impact of androgen receptor blocking therapies in patients with metastatic prostate cancer. Recent studies have found a mismatch between FDG-PET and FDHT-PET findings in patients with metastatic disease that appeared to suggest variations in the androgen dependence of different disease sites [68, 69].

In patients with androgen-independent prostate cancer, calculation of the bone scan index (BSI) allows quantitative assessment of bone involvement [70, 71]. The BSI estimates the fraction of the skeleton that is involved by tumor and the regional distribution of bone metastases [71]. It may be useful for stratifying patients entering treatment protocols and for assessing the response to treatment, particularly in clinical trials of agents for which PSA changes do not accurately reflect clinical outcomes [70, 71].

It appears that FDG-PET may be a promising modality for the assessment of response to chemotherapy. A preliminary study [72] found that in patients undergoing antimicrotubule chemotherapy for castrate metastatic prostate cancer, the change in the average maximum standardized uptake (SUVmaxavg) value on FDG-PET scans indicated treatment effects usually described by a combination of PSA, bone scan and soft-tissue imaging. FDG-PET optimally distinguished between progressors and non-progressors when progression was defined as a more than 33% increase in SUVmaxavg or the appearance of a new lesion [72].

Conclusion

Prostate cancer is a heterogeneous disease with numerous treatment options and widely varying outcomes. While imaging cannot provide a definitive answer to every question that arises in the management of the disease, it has an essential role to play in reducing uncertainty and allowing more effective and evidence-based care. Magnetic resonance imaging and PET may be the most powerful weapons in the imaging arsenal. Not only does conventional MRI offer detailed anatomic assessment of the prostate and surrounding structures, but MRSI and PET allow assessment of disease biology. As more radiologists become familiar with MRI techniques and as research with new PET tracers continues, imaging can be expected to permit increasingly precise discrimination between high- and low-risk disease, more appropriate treatment selection, and more accurate assessment of treatment response.

REFERENCES

1. J. C. Presti, Jr., J. J. Chang, V. Bhargava, *et al.*, The optimal systematic prostate biopsy scheme should include 8 rather than 6 biopsies: results of a prospective clinical trial. *J Urol*, **163** (2000), 163–7.

2. K. Roehl, J. Antenor, W. Catalona, Serial biopsy results in prostate cancer screening study. *J Urol*, **167** (2002), 2435–9.

3. T. M. Koppie, F. J. Bianco, Jr., K. Kuroiwa, *et al.*, The clinical features of anterior prostate cancers. *BJU Int*, **98** (2006), 1167–71.

4. D. Beyersdorff, M. Taupitz, B. Winkelmann, *et al.*, Patients with a history of elevated prostate-specific antigen levels and negative transrectal US-guided quadrant or sextant biopsy results: value of MR imaging. *Radiology*, **224** (2002), 701–6.

5. M. Mullerad, H. Hricak, K. Kuroiwa, *et al.*, Comparison of endorectal magnetic resonance imaging, guided prostate biopsy and digital rectal examination in the preoperative anatomical localization of prostate cancer. *J Urol*, **174** (2005), 2158–63.

6. H. Hricak, S. White, D. Vigneron, *et al.*, Carcinoma of the prostate gland: MR imaging with pelvic phased array coil versus integrated endorectal-pelvic phased-array coils. *Radiology*, **193** (1994), 703–9.

7. O. Akin, E. Sala, C. S. Moskowitz, *et al.*, Transition zone prostate cancers: features, detection, localization, and staging at endorectal MR imaging. *Radiology*, **239** (2006), 784–92.

8. M. Schnall, H. M. Pollack, Magnetic resonance imaging of the prostate. *Urol Radiol*, **12** (1990), 109–14.

9. I. Kaplan, N. E. Oldenburg, P. Meskell, *et al.*, Real time MRI-ultrasound image guided stereotactic prostate biopsy. *Magn Reson Imaging*, **20** (2002), 295–9.

10. M. R. Cooperberg, D. P. Lubeck, M. V. Meng, *et al.*, The changing face of low-risk prostate cancer: trends in clinical presentation and primary management. *J Clin Oncol*, **22** (2004), 2141–9.

11. G. Draisma, R. Boer, S. J. Otto, *et al.*, Lead times and overdetection due to prostate-specific antigen screening: estimates from the European Randomized Study of Screening for Prostate Cancer. *J Natl Cancer Inst*, **95** (2003), 868–78.

12. R. Etzioni, D. F. Penson, J. M. Legler, *et al.*, Overdiagnosis due to prostate-specific antigen screening: lessons from U.S. prostate cancer incidence trends. *J Natl Cancer Inst*, **94** (2002), 981–90.

13. M. I. Patel, D. T. DeConcini, E. Lopez-Corona, *et al.*, An analysis of men with clinically localized prostate cancer who deferred definitive therapy. *J Urol*, **171** (2004), 1520–4.

14. M. W. Kattan, J. A. Eastham, A. M. Stapleton, *et al.*, A preoperative nomogram for disease recurrence following radical prostatectomy for prostate cancer. *J Natl Cancer Inst*, **90** (1998), 766–71.

15. M. W. Kattan, A. M. Stapleton, T. M. Wheeler, *et al.*, Evaluation of a nomogram used to predict the pathologic stage of clinically localized prostate carcinoma. *Cancer*, **79** (1997), 528–37.

16. A. J. Stephenson, P. T. Scardino, J. A. Eastham, *et al.*, Preoperative nomogram predicting the 10-year probability of prostate cancer recurrence after radical prostatectomy. *J Natl Cancer Inst*, **98** (2006), 715–17.

17. H. B. Carter, J. Sauvageot, P. C. Walsh, *et al.*, Prospective evaluation of men with stage T1C adenocarcinoma of the prostate. *J Urol*, **157** (1997), 2206–9.

18. J. I. Epstein, D. W. Chan, L. J. Sokoll, *et al.*, Nonpalpable stage T1c prostate cancer: prediction of insignificant disease using free/total prostate specific antigen levels and needle biopsy findings. *J Urol*, **160** (1998), 2407.

19. J. I. Epstein, H. Sanderson, H. B. Carter, *et al.*, Utility of saturation biopsy to predict insignificant cancer at radical prostatectomy. *Urology*, **66** (2005), 356–60.

20. J. I. Epstein, P. C. Walsh, M. Carmichael, *et al.*, Pathologic and clinical findings to predict tumor extent of nonpalpable (stage T1c) prostate cancer. *JAMA*, **271** (1994), 368–74.

21. Y. Goto, M. Ohori, A. Arakawa, *et al.*, Distinguishing clinically important from unimportant prostate cancers before treatment: value of systematic biopsies. *J Urol*, **156** (1996), 1059–63.

22. M. W. Kattan, J. A. Eastham, T. M. Wheeler, *et al.*, Counseling men with prostate cancer: a nomogram for predicting the presence of small, moderately differentiated, confined tumors. *J Urol*, **170** (2003), 1792–7.

23. A. W. Partin, M. W. Kattan, E. N. Subong, *et al.*, Combination of prostate-specific antigen, clinical stage, and Gleason score to predict pathological stage of localized prostate cancer. A multi-institutional update. *JAMA*, **277** (1997), 1445–51.

24. A. Shukla-Dave, H. Hricak, M. W. Kattan, *et al.*, The utility of magnetic resonance imaging and spectroscopy for predicting insignificant prostate cancer: an initial analysis. *BJU Int*, **99** (2007), 786–93.

25. F. V. Coakley, J. Kurhanewicz, Y. Lu, *et al.*, Prostate cancer tumor volume: measurement with endorectal MR and MR spectroscopic imaging. *Radiology*, **223** (2002), 91–7.

26. H. Hricak, MR imaging and MR spectroscopic imaging in the pre-treatment evaluation of prostate cancer. *Br J Radiol*, **78** (2005), S103–S111.

27. K. K. Yu, J. Scheidler, H. Hricak, *et al.*, Prostate cancer: prediction of extracapsular extension with endorectal MR imaging and three-dimensional proton MR spectroscopic imaging. *Radiology*, **213** (1999), 481–8.

28. F. Cornud, T. Flam, L. Chauveinc, *et al.*, Extraprostatic spread of clinically localized prostate cancer: factors predictive of pT3 tumor and of positive endorectal MR imaging examination results. *Radiology*, **224** (2002), 203–10.

29. M. R. Engelbrecht, G. J. Jager, R. J. Laheij, *et al.*, Local staging of prostate cancer using magnetic resonance imaging: a meta-analysis. *Eur Radiol*, **12** (2002), 2294–302.

30. F. May, T. Treumann, P. Dettmar, *et al.*, Limited value of endorectal magnetic resonance imaging and transrectal ultrasonography in the staging of clinically localized prostate cancer. *BJU Int*, **87** (2001), 66–9.

31. M. Mullerad, H. Hricak, L. Wang, *et al.*, Prostate cancer: detection of extracapsular extension by genitourinary and general body radiologists at MR imaging. *Radiology*, **232** (2004), 140–6.

32. E. K. Outwater, R. O. Petersen, E. S. Siegelman, *et al.*, Prostate carcinoma: assessment of diagnostic criteria for capsular penetration on endorectal coil MR images. *Radiology*, **193** (1994), 333–9.

33. M. D. Rifkin, E. A. Zerhouni, C. A. Gatsonis, *et al.*, Comparison of magnetic resonance imaging and ultrasonography in staging early prostate cancer. Results of a multi-institutional cooperative trial. *N Engl J Med*, **323** (1990), 621–6.

34. L. Wang, H. Hricak, M. W. Kattan, *et al.*, Prediction of prostate cancer organ-confined disease: the incremental value of endorectal coil magnetic resonance imaging to partin staging nomograms (2001 version). *Radiology*, **238** (2006), 597–603.

35. L. Wang, J. Zhang, L. H. Schwartz, *et al.*, Prediction of seminal vesicle invasion in prostate cancer: incremental value of adding endorectal MR imaging to the Kattan nomogram. *Radiology*, **242** (2007), 182–8.

36. L. Wang, M. Mullerad, H. N. Chen, *et al.*, Prostate cancer: incremental value of endorectal MR imaging findings for prediction of extracapsular extension. *Radiology*, **232** (2004), 133–9.

37. H. Hracik, L. Wang, D. C. Wei, *et al.*, The role of preoperative endorectal magnetic imaging in the decision regarding whether to preserve or resect neurovascular bundles during radical retropubic prostatectomy. *Cancer*, **100**:12 (2004), 2655–63.

38. J. A. Eastham, P. T. Scardino, Radical prostatectomy for clinical stage T1 and T2 prostate cancer. In: *Comprehensive Textbook of Genitourinary Oncology*, 2nd edn., eds. N. J. Vogelzand, P. T. Scardino, W. U. Shipley, *et al.* Philadelphia: Lippincott Williams & Wilkins, 2000; 722–38.

39. F. V. Coakley, S. Eberhardt, D. C. Wei, *et al.*, Blood loss during radical retropubic prostatectomy: relationship to morphologic features on preoperative endorectal magnetic resonance imaging. *Urology*, **59** (2002), 884–8.

40. F. V. Coakley, S. Eberhardt, M. W. Kattan, *et al.*, Urinary continence after radical retropubic prostatectomy: relationship with membranous urethral length on preoperative endorectal magnetic resonance imaging. *J Urol*, **168** (2002), 1032–5.

41. L. Wang, H. Hricak, M. W. Kattan, *et al.*, Combined endorectal and phased-array MRI in the prediction of pelvic lymph node metastasis in prostate cancer. *AJR Am J Roentgenol*, **186** (2006), 743–8.

42. E. Sala, S. C. Eberhardt, O. Akin, *et al.*, Endorectal MR imaging before salvage prostatectomy: tumor localization and staging. *Radiology*, **238** (2006), 176–83.

43. D. Pucar, A. Shukla-Dave, H. Hricak, *et al.*, Prostate cancer: correlation of MR imaging and MR spectroscopy with pathologic findings after radiation therapy-initial experience. *Radiology*, **236** (2005), 545–53.

44. D. Pucar, H. Hricak, A. Shukla-Dave, *et al.*, Clinically significant prostate cancer local recurrence after radiation therapy occurs at the site of primary tumor: magnetic resonance imaging and step-section pathology evidence. *Int J Radiat Oncol Biol Phys*, **69** (2007), 62–9.

45. T. Sella, L. H. Schwartz, P. W. Swindle, *et al.*, Suspected local recurrence after radical prostatectomy: endorectal coil MR imaging. *Radiology*, **231** (2004), 379–85.

46. J. M. Silverman, T. L. Krebs, MR imaging evaluation with a transrectal surface coil of local recurrence of prostatic cancer in men who have undergone radical prostatectomy. *AJR Am J Roentgenol*, **168** (1997), 379–85.

47. A. K. Leventis, S. F. Shariat, K. M. Slawin, Local recurrence after radical prostatectomy: correlation of US features with prostatic fossa biopsy findings. *Radiology*, **219** (2001), 432–9.

48. J. Mohler, R. J. Babaian, R. R. Bahnson, *et al.*, NCCN Clinical Practice Guidelines in Oncology Prostate Cancer, v 1.2007. In *National Comprehensive Cancer Network*, 2007.

49. E. S. Amis, Jr., L. R. Bigongiari, E. I. Bluth, *et al.*, Pretreatment staging of clinically localized prostate cancer. American College of Radiology. ACR Appropriateness Criteria. *Radiology*, **215** Suppl (2000), 703–8.

50. M. Fuchsjäger, A. Shukla-Dave, O. Akin, *et al.*, Prostate cancer imaging. *Acta Radiol*, **49**:1 (2008), 107–20.

51. M. G. Harisinghani, J. Barentsz, P. F. Hahn, *et al.*, Noninvasive detection of clinically occult lymph-node metastases in prostate cancer. *N Engl J Med*, **348**:25 (2003), 2491–9. Erratum in: *N Engl J Med*, **349**:10 (2003), 1010.

52. R. A. Heesakkers, J. J. Futterer, A. M. Hovels, *et al.*, Prostate cancer evaluated with ferumoxtran-10-enhanced T2*-weighted MR imaging at 1.5 and 3.0 T: early experience. *Radiology*, **239** (2006), 481–7.

53. M. L. Cher, F. J. Bianco, Jr., J. S. Lam, *et al.*, Limited role of radionuclide bone scintigraphy in patients with prostate specific antigen elevations after radical prostatectomy. *J Urol*, **160** (1998), 1387–91.

54. Z. A. Dotan, F. J. Bianco, Jr., F. Rabbani, *et al.*, Pattern of prostate-specific antigen (PSA) failure dictates the probability of a positive bone scan in patients with an increasing PSA after radical prostatectomy. *J Clin Oncol*, **23** (2005), 1962–8.

55. G. M. Freedman, W. G. Negendank, G. R. Hudes, *et al.*, Preliminary results of a bone marrow magnetic resonance imaging protocol for patients with high-risk prostate cancer. *Urology*, **54** (1999), 118–23.

56. D. I. Rosenthal, Radiologic diagnosis of bone metastases. *Cancer*, **80** (1997), 1595–607.

57. N. Ghanem, M. Uhl, I. Brink, *et al.*, Diagnostic value of MRI in comparison to scintigraphy, PET, MS-CT and PET/CT for the detection of metastases of bone. *Eur J Radiol*, **55**:1 (2005), 41–55.

58. F. E. Lecouvet, D. Geukens, A. Stainier, *et al.*, Magnetic resonance imaging of the axial skeleton for detecting bone metastases in patients with high-risk prostate cancer: diagnostic and cost-effectiveness and comparison with current detection strategies. *J Clin Oncol*, **25** (2007), 3281–7.

59. H. Hricak, P. L. Choyke, S. C. Eberhardt, *et al.*, Imaging prostate cancer: a multidisciplinary perspective. *Radiology*, **243** (2007), 28–53.

60. H. Schöder, K. Herrmann, M. Gönen, *et al.*, 2-[^{18}F]fluoro-2-deoxyglucose positron emission tomography for the detection of disease in patients with prostate-specific antigen relapse after radical prostatectomy. *Clin Cancer Res*, **11** (2005), 4761–9.

61. H. A. Macapinlac, J. L. Humm, T. Akhurst, *et al.*, Differential metabolism and pharmacokinetics of L-[1–^{11}C]-methionine and 2-[^{18}F]fluoro-2-deoxyglucose (FDG) in androgen independent prostate cancer. *Clin Positron Imaging*, **2** (1999), 173–81.

62. P. L. Jager, W. Vaalburg, J. Pruim, *et al.*, Radiolabeled amino acids: basic aspects and clinical applications in oncology. *J Nucl Med*, **42** (2001), 432–45.

63. R. Nunez, H. A. Macapinlac, H. W. Yeung, *et al.*, Combined ^{18}F-FDG and ^{11}C-methionine PET scans in patients with newly progressive metastatic prostate cancer. *J Nucl Med*, **43** (2002), 46–55.

64. N. H. Bander, Technology insight: monoclonal antibody imaging of prostate cancer. *Nat Clin Pract Urol*, **3** (2006), 216–25.

65. J. J. Pollen, K. S. Witztum, W. L. Ashburn, The flare phenomenon on radionuclide bone scan in metastatic prostate cancer. *AJR Am J Roentgenol*, **142** (1984), 773–6.

66. J. A. Schneider, C. R. Divgi, A. M. Scott, *et al.*, Flare on bone scintigraphy following Taxol chemotherapy for metastatic breast cancer. *J Nucl Med*, **35** (1994), 1748–52.

67. H. Yeung, H. Schoder, S. Larson, Utility of PET/CT for assessing equivocal PET lesions in oncology-initial experience [abstract]. *J Nucl Med*, **43** (2007), 32p.

68. F. Dehdashti, J. Picus, J. M. Michalski, *et al.*, Positron tomographic assessment of androgen receptors in prostatic carcinoma. *Eur J Nucl Med Mol Imaging*, **32** (2005), 344–50.

69. S. M. Larson, M. Morris, I. Gunther, *et al.*, Tumor localization of 16beta-^{18}F-fluoro-5alpha-dihydrotestosterone versus ^{18}F-FDG in patients with progressive, metastatic prostate cancer. *J Nucl Med*, **45** (2004), 366–73.

70. M. Imbriaco, S. M. Larson, H. W. Yeung, *et al.*, A new parameter for measuring metastatic bone involvement by prostate cancer: the Bone Scan Index. *Clin Cancer Res*, **4** (1998), 1765–72.

71. P. Sabbatini, S. M. Larson, A. Kremer, *et al.*, Prognostic significance of extent of disease in bone in patients with androgen-independent prostate cancer. *J Clin Oncol*, **17** (1999), 948–57.

72. M. J. Morris, T. Akhurst, S. M. Larson, *et al.*, Fluorodeoxyglucose positron emission tomography as an outcome measure for castrate metastatic prostate cancer treated with antimicrotubule chemotherapy. *Clin Cancer Res*, **11** (2005), 3210–16.

4

Surgical treatment of prostate cancer

Timothy A. Masterson and James A. Eastham

Introduction

Prostate cancer is the most common cancer and the second most common cause of cancer-related death of American men [1]. The American Cancer Society estimates that 186,320 new cases of prostate cancer will be diagnosed and that 28,660 men will die from this disease in the United States in 2008 [2]. The widespread use of prostate-specific antigen (PSA) for prostate cancer screening has led to a substantial decrease in stage at time of diagnosis. Data from the National Cancer Institute's Surveillance, Epidemiology, and End Results program reveal that 91% of diagnosed cancers in the period 1996–2002 were localized to the prostate [1], whereas only 80% are seen in series from previous years. The 5-year expected survival for prostate cancers diagnosed between 1996 and 2002 is 100%, up substantially from 76% between 1984 and 1986 [1]. With today's patients presenting at a younger age and with cancers at a lower stage and lower grade, the management of clinically localized prostate cancer has focused on decreasing the inherent morbidity and long-term consequences of specific therapies. Selecting the optimal therapeutic approach from an array of choices requires individualization of treatment plans based upon risk stratification, the effectiveness of the treatment, and the likelihood that a patient will experience a treatment-related complication.

Radical prostatectomy (RP) remains an excellent treatment option for men with clinically localized prostate cancer. Radical prostatectomy is an effective, curative procedure with surgical series suggesting freedom from cancer recurrence of 75% and cancer-specific survival in excess of 90% 15 years after treatment [3, 4, 5, 6]. In this chapter, we will address the surgical management of clinically localized prostate cancer, emphasizing the utility of imaging in both local staging and surgical planning after the initial diagnosis of prostate cancer, as well as the outcomes achieved.

Prostate Cancer, eds. Hedvig Hricak and Peter T. Scardino. Published by Cambridge University Press.
© Cambridge University Press 2009.

Pre-operative assessment

Limitations in clinical staging

Providing an accurate assessment of the extent of disease after the initial diagnosis of prostate cancer is crucial to optimizing cancer control while minimizing surgical morbidity for the patient. Pre-treatment serum PSA, biopsy Gleason grade, and clinical TNM stage serve as important prognostic parameters that are routinely used to stratify risk prior to definitive therapy [7]. Additional clinical parameters utilized to individualize management include patient age, and the burden of disease as assessed by systematic core needle prostate biopsy results [8, 9]. Nomograms incorporating a variety of clinical variables have been developed to more accurately predict the likelihood of organ-confined disease and risk of biochemical recurrence [8, 9, 10]. Nonetheless, there are several limitations in our ability to accurately characterize tumor location and extent.

Prostate-specific antigen is a serine protease produced principally by the epithelial cells lining the acini and ducts of the prostate gland, resulting in low serum concentrations under normal conditions. In the presence of a malignant tumor, disruption of the normal prostatic architecture occurs resulting in higher levels of circulating PSA. The degree of PSA elevation has been shown to serve as a surrogate for estimated tumor volume [11] and is an independent predictor of response to all forms of therapy, correlating with the risk of extracapsular extension (ECE), seminal vesicle involvement (SVI), and both regional and distant spread of disease [12]. However, the value of PSA within its most frequently encountered range of 4–10 ng/ml is limited in providing valuable staging information [13]. This is largely the result of the infectious, inflammatory, and benign processes within the prostate as well as certain medications, herbals, and hypogonadal states that are known to alter serum PSA concentrations within this range. Therefore, PSA must be interpreted carefully according to the patient's age, clinical presentation, and size of the gland.

Tumor aggressiveness is assessed by identifying the two most predominant architectural patterns identified within a given core needle biopsy. Described originally by Gleason, it is the most widely used and accepted grading system for prostate cancer and allows for assignment of an individual Gleason grade (scale from 1 to 5) and sum (total of the two most common Gleason grades; ranging from 2 to 10) [14]. A higher Gleason score is associated with more aggressive disease, a higher likelihood of adverse pathologic features, and an increased risk of biochemical progression after RP [15, 16]. Accurate pre-treatment grading assumes that representative samples from the prostate during biopsy have been provided. However, upgrading of cancers at the time of RP is reported to occur in nearly 30% of patients [15, 16, 17] and is more likely to occur in larger prostate volumes [16] and when fewer numbers of core biopsy samples are obtained [15]. In a study of prostate cancer patients undergoing RP with a pre-treatment Gleason score of 6, almost half were upgraded to a Gleason score of 7 on final pathologic review [16].

Tumor stage is defined according to the TNM staging classification for prostate cancer [18] and is utilized to predict both local and distant extent of disease. The clinical T stage for prostate cancer is primarily determined according to the presence or absence of palpable disease and its extent on digital rectal examination (DRE) in an attempt to differentiate between patients with organ-confined disease (stage T1–2) and those with locally advanced disease (i.e., presence of ECE or SVI). Digital rectal examination is limited by significant intra- and inter-observer variability rendering poor sensitivity for stratifying the clinical stage [19]. Furthermore, the presence of ECE is commonly microscopic and unappreciable by DRE. Similar to grading of prostate cancer, understaging of disease at the time of RP has been reported to occur in 24%–32% of cases in contemporary series [20, 21].

The importance of clinical understaging and undergrading of prostate cancer is significant, as an accurate assessment of stage directly affects the approach to primary therapy in an attempt to maximize cancer control. To improve our abilities to predict pathologic findings and outcomes of treatment, pre-operative nomograms incorporating PSA, clinical stage, Gleason grade on biopsy, and systematic prostate biopsy results have provided 5- and 10-year predictions for progression-free survival. Despite the utility of nomograms in pre-treatment planning, the lack of anatomic and molecular information incorporated into disease characterization limits our ability to provide the most accurate staging and prognostic information.

Role of imaging in pre-operative assessment

With the inherent limitations in clinical staging of prostate cancer, the incorporation of spatial information obtained from imaging may improve accuracy and further guide management. Transrectal ultrasonography (TRUS) has a well established role as a tool for guiding biopsy in the diagnosis of prostate cancer. Due to its ease of use, low cost and widespread availability, TRUS has also been evaluated in the local staging of prostate cancer. Despite its high specificity in the evaluation of ECE and SVI, TRUS is limited by poor contrast resolution resulting in low sensitivity and a tendency to understage prostate cancer [22]. Even with the advent of color and power Doppler to assist in identifying tumor vascularity [23], the accuracy of TRUS in local staging remains inadequate.

The role of endorectal magnetic resonance imaging (eMRI) in local staging of prostate cancer is controversial and has been hindered by significant inter-observer variability and high cost. Nevertheless, it provides an opportunity to fill the void in the anatomic and molecular characterization of prostate cancer, to improve the accuracy of local staging, and to enhance our ability to tailor treatment selection and planning in an attempt to ensure complete eradication of the cancer while mini-mizing treatment-related morbidity. Due to its high spatial and contrast resolution, eMRI is able to identify signal intensity changes in the peripheral zone of the prostate allowing for assessment of the location and extent of local disease (Figure 4.1) [24]. When compared to DRE and TRUS, eMRI contributes significant incremental value in terms of local prostate cancer staging [25]. Similarly, eMRI has been demonstrated to significantly enhance clinical variables in the pre-operative identification of ECE and SVI in men with prostate cancer when interpreted by dedicated genitourinary radiologists experienced in prostate imaging [26, 27]. In a recent study [28], when looking at the specificity, negative predictive value and positive predictive value of a measure's ability to evaluate the presence of ECE pre-operatively, eMRI outperformed clinical Gleason score, tumor stage, pre-operative PSA, the greatest percentage of cancer and the percentage of cancer-positive core specimens in all core biopsy specimens, and the presence of

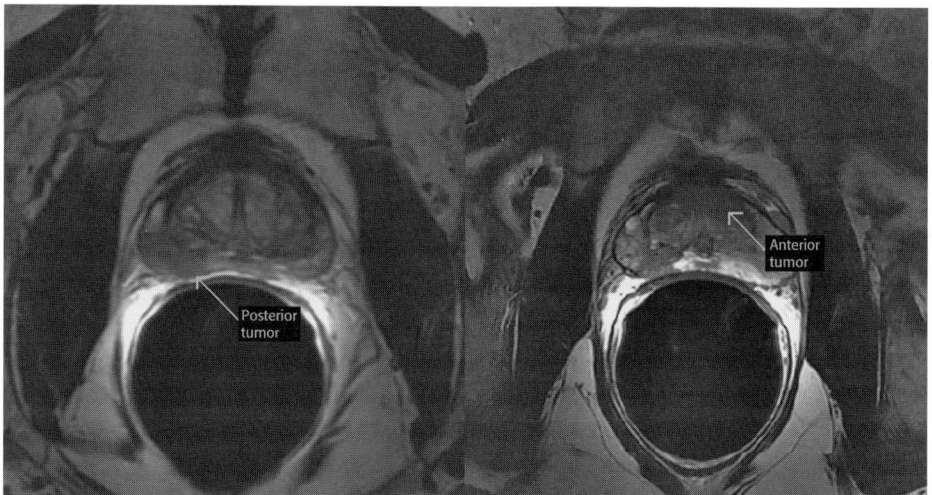

Figure 4.1. Endorectal-coil MRI images of peripheral zone (left) and anterior cancers.

perineural invasion (PNI) in a prostate needle biopsy sample. In terms of sensitivity, eMRI was second best only to clinical stage of tumor [28]. Endorectal MRI is similarly accurate in evaluating for the presence of SVI prior to RP [27]. The incorporation of eMRI findings into nomogram predictions for organ-confined disease and the presence of SVI improved the accuracy of both models [29]. Interestingly, the contribution of eMRI to staging nomograms in predicting organ-confined prostate cancer was significant in all risk categories [30].

Although the majority of prostate cancers originate within the peripheral zone, the transition zone harbors cancer in up to 25% of RP specimens [31]. Unlike the homogeneous high T2 signal intensity of the peripheral zone of the prostate, the normal T2 signal of the transition zone on MRI is quite heterogeneous, making characterization of tumors in this location difficult. The identification of lesions on eMRI with homogenous low T2 signal, ill-defined margins and lenticular shape has proved useful in evaluating for transition zone cancers (Figure 4.1), allowing for an improved ability to stage and characterize these cancers [32].

Magnetic resonance spectroscopic imaging (MRSI) allows for the assessment of tumor metabolism by displaying the relative concentrations of citrate, choline, creatine, and polyamines. Differences in concentrations of these chemical metabolites between normal and malignant prostate tissues allows for better tumor localization within the peripheral zone, increases the accuracy of detection of ECE by less-experienced readers and decreases inter-observer variability [33, 34]. Furthermore, correlations have been demonstrated between the metabolic signal pattern and pathologic Gleason score suggesting the potential for a non-invasive assessment of prostate cancer aggressiveness [35]. Nonetheless, future advances in molecular imaging to improve the predictive capabilities of MRSI will be required before clinical application in tumor characterization can be implemented.

Tailoring of surgical technique

Devising a surgical approach that minimizes treatment-related morbidity and maximally reduces time to recovery provides patients with the optimal treatment strategy. The success of RP is measured by both oncologic and functional outcomes including overall cancer control (i.e., freedom from post-operative biochemical recurrence and need for adjuvant therapies), post-operative rate of urinary continence, and return of erectile function (EF) [6, 36, 37]. Outcomes after RP are exquisitely sensitive to the fine details in the surgical technique. Increased surgeon experience and surgical modifications have been observed to improve surgical outcomes [38, 39]. Technical refinements have resulted in lower rates of positive surgical margins [5, 37, 40, 41, 42, 43], improved rates of both EF recovery [38, 44, 45] and urinary control [37, 46], less estimated blood loss [47, 48, 49], and shorter hospital stays [50]. The technique for open RP has been previously well described [51, 52, 53, 54, 55, 56]. In the following section, we review our method of pre-surgical planning and intra-operative decision-making to individualize surgical approach to each prostate cancer.

Extracapsular extension and positive surgical margins

Achieving a negative surgical margin (SM) serves as a pathologic surrogate for adequacy of complete tumor resection at time of RP. A positive SM has been proven to be associated with biochemical recurrence in 50% of men at 10 years after RP [43, 57]. The risk of a positive SM is influenced by the surgical approach and both the location and extent of disease (i.e., presence of ECE), with reported rates ranging from 6% to 41% in modern surgical series [4, 43, 58, 59]. The presence and location of ECE are difficult to predict using clinical parameters alone such as DRE, PSA kinetics, and TRUS-guided biopsy data. By improving pre-operative methods of identifying likely sites of ECE, surgical technique can be adjusted accordingly to reduce positive SM rates by allowing for a wider margin of resection in areas at risk and preservation of tissues uninvolved by cancer (Figure 4.2). The ability of eMRI to improve the predictive capabilities of clinical parameters and nomograms for the presence of ECE at the time of RP is significant [28, 30]. Based upon clinical and radiographic clues pre-operatively and intra-operative findings at the time of RP for the presence of ECE, adjustments of the approach to the apex, base, and posterior dissections of the prostate can be tailored accordingly. For instance, in men at high

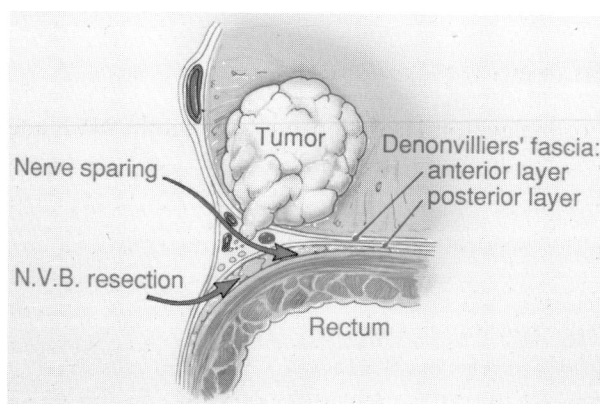

Figure 4.2. Prostate and surrounding anatomy demonstrating extracapsular extension of prostate cancer and variations in surgical approach to the neurovascular bundle (N.V.B.). See color plate section for full color version.

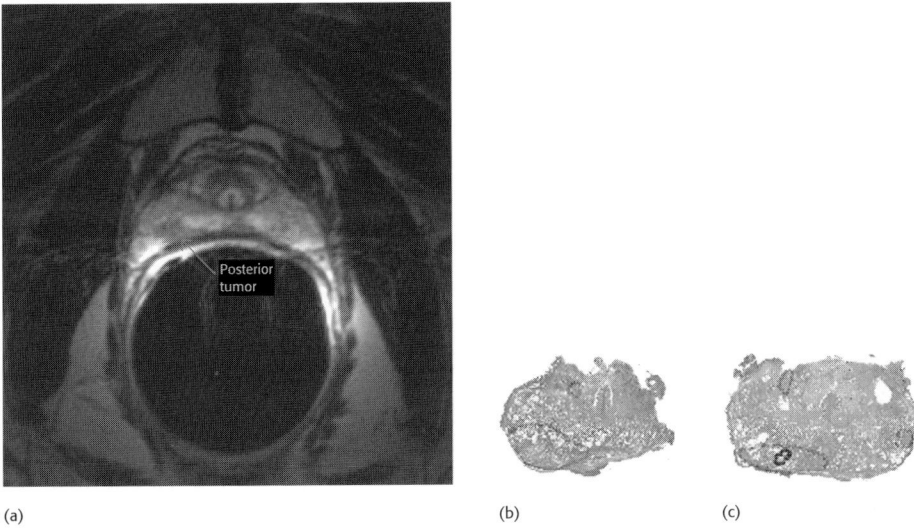

(a)   (b)   (c)

Figure 4.3. Endorectal MRI (a) demonstrating peripheral zone cancer with corresponding whole-mount tumor map (images b and c). A 65-year-old man with PSA 4.4 ng/ml, cT2a, Gleason 7 (4 + 3) prostatic adenocarcinoma in 3/14 cores with 40% involvement. Surgical planning assisted by endorectal MRI (a) demonstrated the right neurovascular bundle to be remote from the posteriorly located peripheral zone tumor. Neurovascular bundle preservation was performed bilaterally with negative surgical margins on final pathology (b, c). See color plate section for full color version.

risk for ECE posteriorly, knowing the location of the neurovascular bundle (NVB) relative to the area of disease can determine whether resection of the NVB is necessary to obtain a negative SM (Figure 4.3) [60]. Similarly, decisions regarding alterations of where the dorsal vein complex is divided and how the apex of the prostate is dissected can be made when anterior or transition zone tumors are suspected in order to improve local control (Figures 4.4, 4.5).

Erectile function recovery and neurovascular bundle preservation

Since the detailed description of the anatomic relationship between the NVB and capsule of the prostate by Walsh and Donker [61], modifications in RP surgical technique have been developed to reduce the long-term morbidity of erectile dysfunction (ED). The decision to preserve or resect the NVB responsible for EF is often difficult and based upon pre-operative clinical characteristics and intra-operative findings providing the surgeon with a crude assessment of risk for ECE and possible positive SM along the posterolateral aspect of the prostate (Figure 4.2). In a recent study, the impact of eMRI on the decision to preserve or resect the NVB

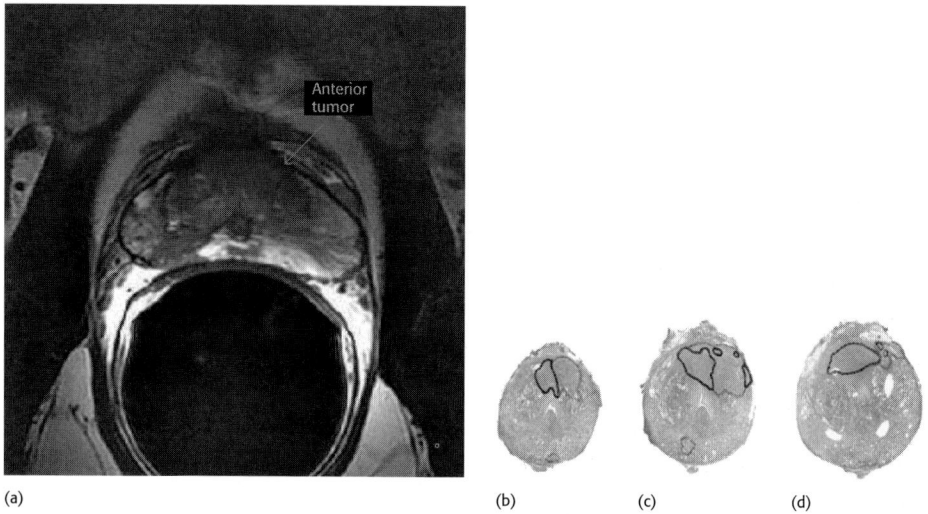

(a)   (b)   (c)   (d)

Figure 4.4. Endorectal MRI (a) demonstrating anterior cancer with corresponding whole-mount tumor map (b–d). A 55-year-old man with PSA of 7.4 ng/ml, cT1c Gleason 6 (3 + 3) prostatic adenocarcinoma in 1/6 cores with 5% involvement. Deferred therapy recommended as a good option, pending MRI and repeat biopsy. MRI showed a large anterior tumor. Patient underwent radical prostatectomy with bilateral nerve sparing. The pathology specimen confirmed the endorectal MRI findings. See color plate section for full color version.

was assessed in 135 patients [62]. The results demonstrated incremental benefit of eMRI in pre-operative decision-making as the risk of ECE increased. In high-risk patients (probability of organ-confined disease ≤25%), eMRI changed the approach to NVB preservation in nearly 80% of men, of which the change was appropriate 93% of the time. Additionally, eMRI correctly favored NVB preservation in 10 of 12 patients who were considered to have a high clinical probability of ECE. For low- and intermediate-risk patients, the strength of eMRI lies in its ability to predict the absence of tumor in the area of the NVB.

Urinary incontinence and apical dissection

Urinary incontinence remains one of the most troubling side-effects for patients after RP. Rates of urinary incontinence vary greatly after surgery and are multifactorial in nature. Results are influenced not only by surgical technique, but also how continence is defined, how data are collected (patient versus physician reporting), and the timing of assessment after RP. Nonetheless, an improved understanding of the pelvic floor anatomy and modifications in surgical approach to the

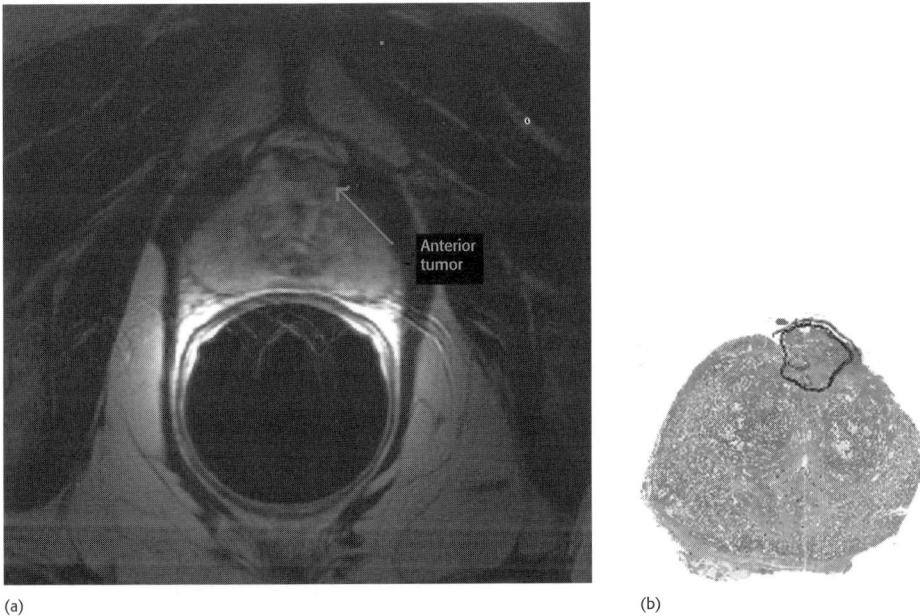

Figure 4.5. Endorectal MRI (a) demonstrating anterior cancer with corresponding whole-mount tumor map (b). A 67-year-old man with a rising PSA of 10.2 ng/ml, stage cT1c, TRUS prostate biopsy revealed Gleason sum 8 (4 + 4) prostatic adenocarcinoma in 1/14 cores with 10% involvement. Endorectal MRI (a) revealed a large anterior tumor with evidence of extracapsular extension. Surgical modifications allowed for a more distal division of the dorsal vein complex with bilateral neurovascular bundle preservation, surgical margins were negative on final pathology (b). See color plate section for full color version.

apical dissection of the prostate have resulted in improved rates of urinary control after RP [46].

Imaging of the pelvic floor musculature and urethral length has provided interesting results on the impact of urinary continence after RP. In a study evaluating membranous urethral length on eMRI, a pre-operative length >12 mm was associated with a statistically significant improvement in post-operative incontinence after RP (Figure 4.6) [63]. Not surprisingly, preliminary data from our institution suggest that preservation of urethral length during RP as determined on pre- and post-operative eMRI likely correlates with improved return of urinary continence. Therefore, by improving our ability to characterize the location and extent of disease near the apex of the prostate, modifications in the approach to the apical dissection can be made to allow for a more or less aggressive apical dissection in attempts to improve continence rates without compromising cancer control.

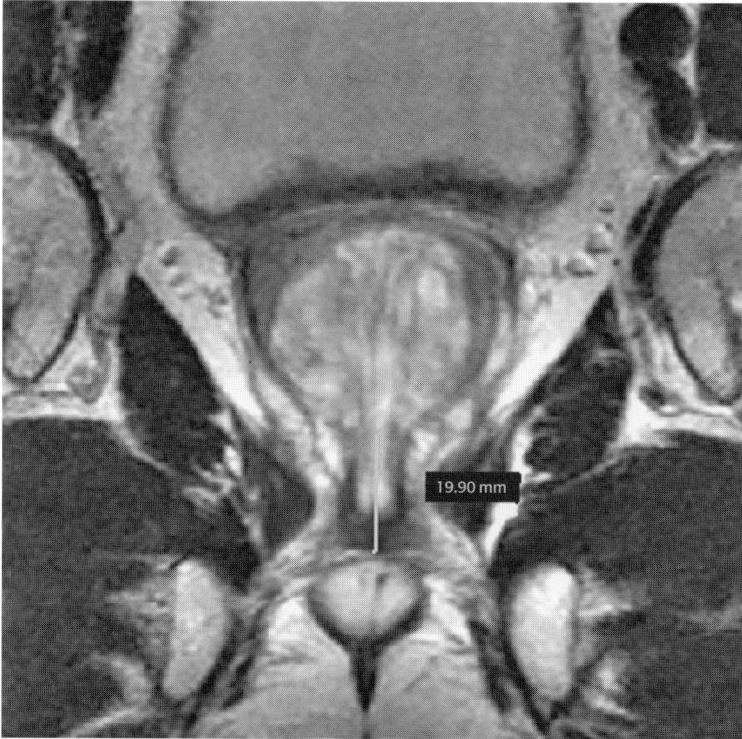

Figure 4.6. Membranous urethral length was measured on coronal images as distance from prostatic apex to entry of urethra into penile bulb.

Intra-operative blood loss

Blood loss associated with RP varies with approach (laparoscopic versus open) and technique (nerve sparing versus non-nerve sparing). In the past, blood loss was a substantial source of perioperative morbidity frequently requiring blood transfusion [64, 65]. With an improved understanding of the anatomy of the dorsal vein complex and periprostatic veins associated with the NVB, techniques have been developed to more effectively control these vessels earlier in the operation [47, 52, 65, 66]. With improved control over intra-operative hemorrhage, better visualization of the surgical field and attention to the fine details of the operation can be achieved. Recently, an assessment of the prominence of the apical periprostatic veins on eMRI has been positively associated with intra-operative blood loss and may assist in predicting men at risk for substantial intra-operative hemorrhage [67]. Although blood loss during RP is multifactorial, improved pre-operative assessment of venous anatomy may provide an opportunity for individually tailoring the surgical approach in order to minimize this complication in those at higher risk.

Surgical outcomes after radical prostatectomy

The goal of surgical extirpation of prostate cancer remains to ensure the best oncologic outcome (i.e., freedom from cancer recurrence) while minimizing the impact on quality of life after treatment. The individual risks for disease recurrence, urinary incontinence and erectile function after RP have been well described. Long-term cancer-specific survival ranges 82%–90% at 15 years for localized prostate cancer in large series at centers with a large amount of experience [6, 36, 37]. Biochemical, progression-free survival after RP at Johns Hopkins University and Memorial Sloan-Kettering Cancer Center at 15 years are 66% and 75%, respectively [4, 37]. Incidence of urinary continence after RP in large series is a consistent 93%, while recovery of erectile function ranges from 76% to 86% in men undergoing bilateral NVB preservation by 18–24 months [38, 44, 45]. Individually, these rates of functional recovery and oncologic control after RP are high. However, most important to the patient is the likelihood of returning to their baseline level of function while remaining cancer-free. In an analysis evaluating for incidence of achieving the "trifecta" of full recovery of EF and urinary continence without evidence of biochemical recurrence, 60% of patients at 24 months reached this goal [37]. Therefore, an optimal outcome after RP can be achieved in the majority of cases. Nevertheless, continued effort to improve upon our ability to more accurately stage prostate cancer and tailor our surgical approach is pivotal for improving upon these results for patients.

Conclusion

Radical prostatectomy is an effective and reliable means of eradicating localized prostate cancer resulting in long-term cancer control and freedom from recurrence. Nonetheless, through better pre-operative assessment of the extent and location of disease, functional outcomes of preservation of erectile function and urinary continence can be improved. Endorectal MRI offers an opportunity to facilitate our understanding of the spatial relationship of disease relative to the surrounding tissues allowing us to better tailor our surgical approach in an effort to improve oncologic and functional outcomes for our patients.

REFERENCES

1. A. Jemal, R. Siegel, E. Ward, *et al.*, Cancer statistics, 2007. *CA: Cancer J Clini*, **57**(1): (2007), 43–66.
2. A. Jemal, R. Siegal, E. Ward, *et al.*, Cancer statistics, 2008. *CA Cancer J Clin*, **58**:2 (2008), 71–96.
3. R. P. Gibbons, R. J. Correa, Jr., G. E. Brannen, *et al.*, Total prostatectomy for clinically localized prostatic cancer: long-term results. *J Urol*, **141**:3 (1989), 564–6.
4. M. Han, A. W. Partin, C. R. Pound, *et al.*, Long-term biochemical disease-free and cancer-specific survival following anatomic radical retropubic prostatectomy. The 15-year Johns Hopkins experience. *Urol Clin North Am*, **28**:3 (2001), 555–65.
5. G. W. Hull, F. Rabbani, F. Abbas, *et al.*, Cancer control with radical prostatectomy alone in 1,000 consecutive patients. *J Urol*, **167**:2 Pt 1 (2002), 528–34.
6. H. Zincke, J. E. Oesterling, M. L. Blute, *et al.*, Long-term (15 years) results after radical prostatectomy for clinically localized (stage T2c or lower) prostate cancer. *J Urol*, **152**:5 Pt 2 (1994), 1850–7.
7. A. V. D'Amico, A. Desjardin, A. Chung, *et al.*, Assessment of outcome prediction models for patients with localized prostate carcinoma managed with radical prostatectomy or external beam radiation therapy. *Cancer*, **82**:10 (1998), 1887–96.
8. M. W. Kattan, A. M. Stapleton, T. M. Wheeler, *et al.*, Evaluation of a nomogram used to predict the pathologic stage of clinically localized prostate carcinoma. *Cancer*, **79**:3 (1997), 528–37.
9. A. J. Stephenson, P. T. Scardino, J. A. Eastham, *et al.*, Preoperative nomogram predicting the 10-year probability of prostate cancer recurrence after radical prostatectomy. *J Natl Cancer Inst*, **98**:10 (2006), 715–17.
10. M. W. Kattan, J. A. Eastham, A. M. Stapleton, *et al.*, A preoperative nomogram for disease recurrence following radical prostatectomy for prostate cancer. *J Natl Cancer Inst*, **90**:10 (1998), 766–71.
11. T. A. Stamey, F. S. Freiha, J. E. McNeal, *et al.*, Localized prostate cancer. Relationship of tumor volume to clinical significance for treatment of prostate cancer. *Cancer*, **71**:3 Suppl (1993), 933–8.
12. J. E. Oesterling, S. K. Martin, E. J. Bergstralh, *et al.*, The use of prostate-specific antigen in staging patients with newly diagnosed prostate cancer. *JAMA*, **269**:1 (1993), 57–60.
13. P. Narayan, V. Gajendran, S. P. Taylor, *et al.*, The role of transrectal ultrasound-guided biopsy-based staging, preoperative serum prostate-specific antigen, and biopsy Gleason score in prediction of final pathologic diagnosis in prostate cancer. *Urology*, **46**:2 (1995), 205–12.
14. D. F. Gleason, Histologic grading and clinical staging of prostate carcinoma. In: *Urologic Pathology: The Prostate*, ed. M. Tannenbaum, Philadelphia: Lea and Febiger, 1977; 171–97.
15. S. J. Freedland, C. J. Kane, C. L. Amling, *et al.*, Upgrading and downgrading of prostate needle biopsy specimens: risk factors and clinical implications. *Urology*, **69**:3 (2007), 495–9.
16. J. H. Pinthus, M. Witkos, N. E. Fleshner, *et al.*, Prostate cancers scored as Gleason 6 on prostate biopsy are frequently Gleason 7 tumors at radical prostatectomy: implication on outcome. *J Urol*, **176**:3 (2006), 979–84; discussion 84.
17. F. K. Chun, A. Briganti, S. F. Shariat, *et al.*, Significant upgrading affects a third of men diagnosed with prostate cancer: predictive nomogram and internal validation. *BJU Int*, **98**:2 (2006), 329–34.
18. F. Greene, D. Page, I. Fleming, *et al.*, *American Joint Committee on Cancer Staging Manual*, 6th edn., New York: Springer, 2002.
19. E. Varenhorst, K. Berglund, O. Lofman, *et al.*, Inter-observer variation in assessment of the prostate by digital rectal examination. *Br J Urol*, **72**:2 (1993), 173–6.
20. G. D. Grossfeld, J. J. Chang, J. M. Broering, *et al.*, Under staging and under grading in a contemporary series of patients undergoing radical prostatectomy: results from the Cancer of the Prostate Strategic Urologic Research Endeavor database. *J Urol*, **165**:3 (2001), 851–6.
21. A. Sciarra, G. Voria, S. Monti, *et al.*, Clinical under-staging in patients with prostate adenocarcinoma

submitted to radical prostatectomy: predictive value of serum chromogranin A. *The Prostate*, **58**:4 (2004), 421–8.

22. F. May, T. Treumann, P. Dettmar, *et al.*, Limited value of endorectal magnetic resonance imaging and transrectal ultrasonography in the staging of clinically localized prostate cancer. *BJU Int*, **87**:1 (2001), 66–9.

23. J. P. Sedelaar, G. J. van Leenders, T. E. Goossen, *et al.*, Value of contrast ultrasonography in the detection of significant prostate cancer: correlation with radical prostatectomy specimens. *The Prostate*, **53**:3 (2002), 246–53.

24. M. D. Schnall, H. M. Pollack, Magnetic resonance imaging of the prostate gland. *Urol Radiol*, **12**:2 (1990), 109–14.

25. M. Mullerad, H. Hricak, K. Kuroiwa, *et al.*, Comparison of endorectal magnetic resonance imaging, guided prostate biopsy and digital rectal examination in the preoperative anatomical localization of prostate cancer. *J Urol*, **174**:6 (2005), 2158–63.

26. M. Mullerad, H. Hricak, L. Wang, *et al.*, Prostate cancer: detection of extracapsular extension by genitourinary and general body radiologists at MR imaging. *Radiology*, **232**:1 (2004), 140–6.

27. E. Sala, O. Akin, C. S. Moskowitz, *et al.*, Endorectal MR imaging in the evaluation of seminal vesicle invasion: diagnostic accuracy and multivariate feature analysis. *Radiology*, **238**:3 (2006), 929–37.

28. L. Wang, M. Mullerad, H. N. Chen, *et al.*, Prostate cancer: incremental value of endorectal MR imaging findings for prediction of extracapsular extension. *Radiology*, **232**:1 (2004), 133–9.

29. L. Wang, H. Hricak, M. W. Kattan, *et al.*, Prediction of seminal vesicle invasion in prostate cancer: incremental value of adding endorectal MR imaging to the Kattan nomogram. *Radiology*, **242**:1 (2007), 182–8.

30. L. Wang, H. Hricak, M. W. Kattan, *et al.*, Prediction of organ-confined prostate cancer: incremental value of MR imaging and MR spectroscopic imaging to staging nomograms. *Radiology*, **238**:2 (2006), 597–603.

31. J. E. McNeal, E. A. Redwine, F. S. Freiha, *et al.*, Zonal distribution of prostatic adenocarcinoma.

Correlation with histologic pattern and direction of spread. *Am J Surg Pathol*, **12**:12 (1988), 897–906.

32. O. Akin, E. Sala, C. S. Moskowitz, *et al.*, Transition zone prostate cancers: features, detection, localization, and staging at endorectal MR imaging. *Radiology*, **239**:3 (2006), 784–92.

33. J. Scheidler, H. Hricak, D. B. Vigneron, *et al.*, Prostate cancer: localization with three-dimensional proton MR spectroscopic imaging – clinicopathologic study. *Radiology*, **213**:2 (1999), 473–80.

34. K. K. Yu, J. Scheidler, H. Hricak, *et al.*, Prostate cancer: prediction of extracapsular extension with endorectal MR imaging and three-dimensional proton MR spectroscopic imaging. *Radiology*, **213**:2 (1999), 481–8.

35. K. L. Zakian, K. Sircar, H. Hricak, *et al.*, Correlation of proton MR spectroscopic imaging with Gleason score based on step-section pathologic analysis after radical prostatectomy. *Radiology*, **234**:3 (2005), 804–14.

36. M. Han, A. W. Partin, M. Zahurak, *et al.*, Biochemical (prostate specific antigen) recurrence probability following radical prostatectomy for clinically localized prostate cancer. *J Urol*, **169**:2 (2003), 517–23.

37. F. J. Bianco, Jr., P. T. Scardino, J. A. Eastham, Radical prostatectomy: long-term cancer control and recovery of sexual and urinary function ("trifecta"). *Urology*, **66**:5 Suppl (2005), 83–94.

38. S. D. Kundu, K. A. Roehl, S. E. Eggener, *et al.*, Potency, continence and complications in 3,477 consecutive radical retropubic prostatectomies. *J Urol*, **172**:6 Pt 1 (2004), 2227–31.

39. S. J. Kausik, M. L. Blute, T. J. Sebo, *et al.*, Prognostic significance of positive surgical margins in patients with extraprostatic carcinoma after radical prostatectomy. *Cancer*, **95**:6 (2002), 1215–19.

40. E. A. Klein, P. A. Kupelian, L. Tuason, *et al.*, Initial dissection of the lateral fascia reduces the positive margin rate in radical prostatectomy. *Urology*, **51**:5 (1998), 766–73.

41. J. A. Wieder, M. S. Soloway, Incidence, etiology, location, prevention and treatment of positive

surgical margins after radical prostatectomy for prostate cancer. *J Urol,* **160**:2 (1998), 299–315.

42. J. W. Saranchuk, M. W. Kattan, E. Elkin, *et al.,* Achieving optimal outcomes after radical prostatectomy. *J Clin Oncol,* **23**:18 (2005), 4146–51.

43. P. C. Walsh, P. Marschke, D. Ricker, *et al.,* Patient-reported urinary continence and sexual function after anatomic radical prostatectomy. *Urology,* **55**:1 (2000), 58–61.

44. C. Noh, A. Kshirsagar, J. L. Mohler, Outcomes after radical retropubic prostatectomy. *Urology,* **61**:2 (2003), 412–16.

45. M. S. Steiner, R. A. Morton, P. C. Walsh, Impact of anatomical radical prostatectomy on urinary continence. *J Urol,* **145**:3 (1991), 512–14; discussion 514–15.

46. J. R. Goad, P. T. Scardino, Modifications in the technique of radical retropubic prostatectomy to minimize blood loss. *Atlas Urol Clin North Am,* **2**: (1994), 65–80.

47. H. Lepor, A. M. Nieder, M. N. Ferrandino, Intraoperative and postoperative complications of radical retropubic prostatectomy in a consecutive series of 1,000 cases. *J Urol,* **166**:5 (2001), 1729–33.

48. M. Maffezzini, M. Seveso, G. Taverna, *et al.,* Evaluation of complications and results in a contemporary series of 300 consecutive radical retropubic prostatectomies with the anatomic approach at a single institution. *Urology,* **61**:5 (2003), 982–6.

49. B. D. Leibman, O. Dillioglugil, F. Abbas, *et al.,* Impact of a clinical pathway for radical retropubic prostatectomy. *Urology,* **52**:1 (1998), 94–9.

50. M. S. Chuang, R. C. O'Connor, B. A. Laven, *et al.,* Early release of the neurovascular bundles and optical loupe magnification lead to improved and earlier return of potency following radical retropubic prostatectomy. *J Urol,* **173**:2 (2005), 537–9.

51. J. A. Eastham, P. T. Scardino, Radical prostatectomy for clinical Stage T1 and T2 prostate cancer. In: *Comprehensive Textbook of Genitourinary Oncology,* 3rd edn., eds. N. J. Vogelzang, P. T. Scardino, W. U. Shipley, *et al.,* Philadelphia: Lippincott Williams & Wilkins, 2006; 166–89.

52. M. Graefen, J. Walz, H. Huland, Open retropubic nerve-sparing radical prostatectomy. *Eur Urol,* **49**:1 (2006), 38–48.

53. F. Montorsi, A. Salonia, N. Suardi, *et al.,* Improving the preservation of the urethral sphincter and neurovascular bundles during open radical retropubic prostatectomy. *Eur Urol,* **48**:6 (2005), 938–45.

54. R. P. Myers and A. Villers, Anatomic considerations in radical prostatectomy. In: *Prostate Cancer: Surgical Principles and Practice,* eds. R. Kirby, A. W. Partin, M. Feneley, *et al.,* London: Martin Dunitz Publishers Ltd, 2005.

55. P. C. Walsh, Anatomic radical prostatectomy: evolution of the surgical technique. *J Urol,* **160**:6 Pt 2 (1998), 2418–24.

56. L. Cheng, M. R. Darson, E. J. Bergstralh, *et al.,* Correlation of margin status and extraprostatic extension with progression of prostate carcinoma. *Cancer,* **86**:9 (1999), 1775–82.

57. M. L. Blute, D. G. Bostwick, T. M. Seay, *et al.,* Pathologic classification of prostate carcinoma: the impact of margin status. *Cancer,* **82**:5 (1998), 902–8.

58. M. Ohori, P. T. Scardino, Localized prostate cancer. *Curr Probl Surg,* **39**:9 (2002), 833–957.

59. P. Swindle, J. A. Eastham, M. Ohori, *et al.,* Do margins matter? The prognostic significance of positive surgical margins in radical prostatectomy specimens. *J Urol,* **174**:3 (2005), 903–7.

60. J. R. Hill, S. W. Fine, J. Zhang, *et al.,* Radical prostatectomy for clinical T3 disease: expanding indications while optimizing cancer control and quality of life. *Nat Cin Pract Urol,* **4**:8 (2007), 451–4.

61. P. C. Walsh, P. J. Donker, Impotence following radical prostatectomy: insight into etiology and prevention. *J Urol,* **128**:3 (1982), 492–7.

62. H. Hricak, L. Wang, D. C. Wei, *et al.,* The role of preoperative endorectal magnetic resonance imaging in the decision regarding whether to preserve or resect neurovascular bundles during radical retropubic prostatectomy. *Cancer,* **100**:12 (2004), 2655–63.

63. F. V. Coakley, S. Eberhardt, M. W. Kattan, *et al.,* Urinary continence after radical retropubic prostatectomy: relationship with membranous urethral

length on preoperative endorectal magnetic resonance imaging. *J Urol*, **168**:3 (2002), 1032–5.

64. C. A. Peters, P. C. Walsh, Blood transfusion and
anesthetic practices in radical retropubic prostatectomy. *J Urol*, **134**:1 (1985), 81–3.

65. W. G. Reiner, P. C. Walsh, An anatomical
approach to the surgical management of the dorsal
vein and Santorini's plexus during radical retropubic surgery. *J Urol*, **121**:2 (1979), 198–200.

66. R. P. Myers, Improving the exposure of the prostate
in radical retropubic prostatectomy: longitudinal
bunching of the deep venous plexus. *J Urol*, **142**:5
(1989), 1282–4.

67. F. V. Coakley, S. Eberhardt, D. C. Wei, *et al.*, Blood
loss during radical retropubic prostatectomy: relationship to morphologic features on preoperative
endorectal magnetic resonance imaging. *Urology*,
59:6 (2002), 884–8.

5

Radiation therapy

Marisa A. Kollmeier and Michael J. Zelefsky

Introduction

Radiation therapy has played a significant role in the management of prostate cancer for over half a century. High-energy megavoltage linear accelerators developed in the 1950s provided deeper penetration of tumoricidal dose, superficial tissue sparing and hence lower morbidity profiles than earlier models. The introduction of the CT scanner and complex computer-based treatment planning software in the 1980s improved three-dimensional target localization and enhanced accuracy. Subsequently, intensity-modulated treatment planning capabilities enabled highly conformal dose escalation for improved outcomes without added toxicity. New image-guidance techniques have further refined treatment delivery by compensating for internal organ variability. Concurrent with vast improvements in external beam radiation therapy, modern brachytherapy methods, facilitated by dynamic imaging, have become sophisticated and popular techniques for primary as well as salvage therapies. In addition, refinement of prognostic factors, particularly prostate-specific antigen (PSA), and contemporary imaging for staging have substantially improved patient selection for individualized therapy.

Today, modern radiotherapeutic approaches rely on accurate staging, precise imaging, and prognostic prediction, as well as technical advances in dose delivery and normal tissue protection.

Imaging for patient selection and radiation treatment planning

An accurate staging assessment prior to definitive therapy is critical in order to maximize cure rates. Prognostic risk factors including American Joint Commission on Cancer (AJCC) stage, Gleason score and pre-treatment PSA assess the risk of

Prostate Cancer, eds. Hedvig Hricak and Peter T. Scardino. Published by Cambridge University Press.
© Cambridge University Press 2009.

disease beyond the prostate, predict the yield of diagnostic studies, and guide radiotherapeutic decision-making.

Pelvic imaging to detect adenopathy and assess local disease extent may be accomplished with either CT or MRI. Pelvic CT primarily detects nodal enlargement, however the sensitivity in detecting small-volume disease is low. Although routinely obtained, current National Comprehensive Cancer Network (NCCN) guidelines recommend a staging CT scan only for T3–T4 disease or T1–T2 disease with a risk of lymph node involvement of >20% [1]. Magnetic resonance imaging, particularly using an endorectal coil, has the advantage of better soft-tissue plane resolution and hence better evaluation of extracapsular penetration and seminal vesicle involvement as compared with CT [2, 3] (Figure 5.1). In addition, detailed prostate anatomy is obtained, which is essential for individualized treatment decision-making. For example, the use of cytoreductive hormone therapy for large prostate volumes may help reduce radiation fields, minimize normal tissue dose, and reduce toxicity [4]. Hormone therapy may be used prior to brachytherapy for similar reasons. Image-based evaluation of a prior transurethral resection of the prostate (TURP) defect may assist in determining the feasibility and application of brachytherapy. Magnetic resonance imaging may also improve accuracy in prostate contouring on treatment-planning software, particularly in defining the apex, which is critical for

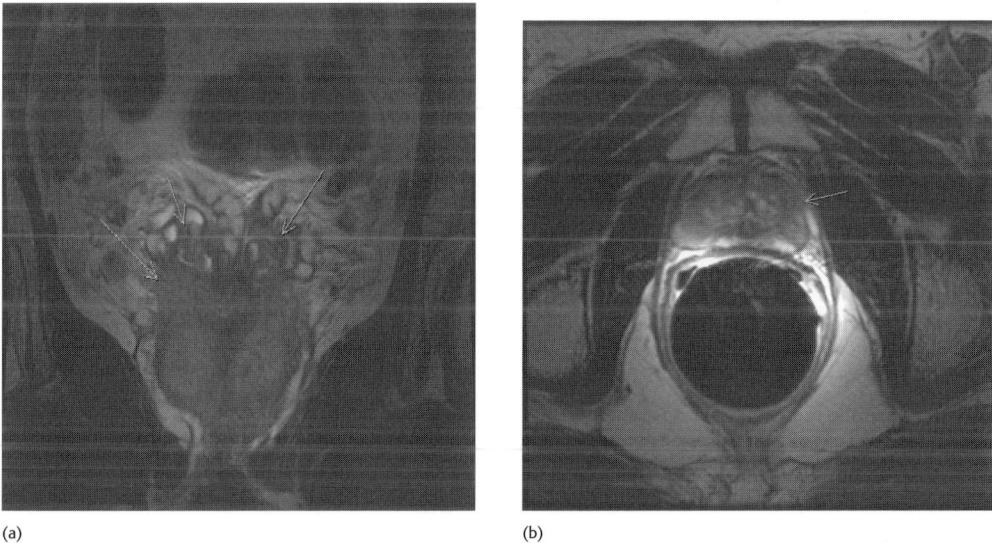

(a)   (b)

Figure 5.1. a Coronal T2-weighted MRI image demonstrating seminal vesicle invasion and extracapsular extension. b Axial T2-weighted MRI image showing extracapsular extension.

optimal dose coverage and difficult to visualize on treatment-planning CT scans. Magnetic resonance spectroscopic imaging (MRSI), as a functional imaging study, can clarify intraprostatic disease extent by measuring differential metabolite ratios within subregions of the prostate. The addition of spectroscopy not only enhances tumor localization in the peripheral zone, where most tumors develop, but also in the transition zone which is often difficult to assess clinically and pathologically [5]. Indeed, MRSI may also correlate with Gleason grade, which may be useful for guiding biopsies or radiation-therapy planning [6, 7].

Positron emission tomography (PET), as a functional imaging modality, has gained renewed interest in the area of prostate cancer [8]. Previously, noise caused by ^{18}F-2-fluoro-D-deoxyglucose (FDG) excretion into the bladder obscured imaging of the prostate; however with new iterative image reconstruction this can be minimized. Also, new tracers, such as ^{11}C-methionine and ^{18}F-fluorohydrotestosterone, may be able to distinguish inflammatory changes from prostate cancer, one of the major limitations of PET imaging. This may be particularly useful as part of the workup for patients with suspected local or regionally recurrent disease following primary therapy [9, 10]. Whether PET will replace radionuclide bone scanning, commonly used to detect osseous metastases for high-risk patients (PSA >10 ng/ml, T3–4, or node-positive disease), is unknown and it is not currently integrated into the standard staging evaluation.

Prognostic risk stratification

The appropriate selection of patients for local therapy is largely based on prognostic risk. For patients with clinically localized disease, risk stratification using a combination of clinical AJCC stage, Gleason score, and PSA variables allows prediction of subclinical extraprostatic disease, i.e., extracapsular disease extension (ECE), seminal vesicle involvement (SVI), and lymph node involvement (LNI). Based on a highly selected, large surgical series, predictive tables were developed to estimate pathologic organ-confined versus non-organ-confined disease and these have been recently updated to reflect stage migration in the PSA era [11, 12]. In general, an increased risk of non-organ-confined disease occurs with increases in any single prognostic factor. For example, a man with non-palpable Gleason-8 disease with a pre-treatment PSA of 8 ng/ml would have a 51% likelihood of organ-confined prostate cancer as compared with 81% for a man with the same variables but a Gleason score of 6. Based on the original tables developed by Partin *et al.* Roach *et al.* described simple equations (Table 5.1) that may be used to estimate the risk of

Table 5.1. Roach formulas [13, 14, 15]

Risk	Formula
extracapsular involvement	$\frac{1}{2}$ PSA + (Gleason − 3) × 10
% seminal vesicle involvement	PSA + (Gleason − 6) × 10
% lymph node involvement	$\frac{2}{3}$ PSA + (Gleason − 6) × 10

Table 5.2. National Comprehensive Cancer Network risk group definitions for clinically staged patients [1]

	Low	Intermediate[a]	High	Very high
Clinical stage	T1–T2a	T2b–T2c	T3a	T3b–T4
		or	or	or
Gleason score	2–6	7	8–10	
		or	or	
PSA (ng/ml)	<10	10–20	>20	Node positive

[a] Patients with multiple adverse factors may be shifted into the high-risk category.

ECE, LNI, and SVI [13, 14, 15]. These equations have been validated and used as entry criteria in randomized trials, e.g., RTOG 94–13 [16, 17]; however, they have not been updated and may overestimate risk.

Several risk group definitions for clinically staged patients have been proposed and criteria established by D'Amico *et al.* and those defined by the NCCN (Table 5.2) are the most widely used [1, 18]. Although useful at predicting pathologic stage, some question has arisen regarding their ability to predict outcome for individual patients [19]. Predictive nomograms have therefore been developed to predict outcomes following definitive therapy using algorithms based on continuous variables. Kattan *et al.* have established nomograms based on pre-operative PSA, Gleason score, and AJCC stage to predict PSA-failure-free survival post-operatively and similar nomograms are available for external beam radiation and brachytherapy [20, 21, 22].

Several additional prognostic factors have been described as predictive of disease extent and outcome after primary therapy [23, 24, 25, 26, 27, 28, 29, 30]. The percentage of positive biopsy cores has been shown to reflect tumor volume and pathologic stage at radical prostatectomy as well as to predict biochemical failure and disease-specific survival following radical prostatectomy and primary radiotherapy [23, 24, 25, 26, 27]. In an analysis by D'Amico *et al.* the stratification of percentage positive biopsies (less than 34%, 34%–50%, and greater than 50%) proved a clinically significant factor predicting PSA-failure-free survival following external beam radiotherapy [27]. Specifically, intermediate-risk patients with <34% positive cores had similar outcomes compared to low-risk patients and, conversely, those with >50% positive cores had biochemical failure rates comparable to those of high-risk patients. This stratification may be useful for selecting intermediate-risk patients for monotherapy or more aggressive multi-modality regimens.

The prognostic significance of pre-treatment PSA kinetics has been recently demonstrated [28, 29, 30, 31]. In a large series of men undergoing radiation therapy for clinically localized disease, a PSA rate of change of >2 ng/ml per year prior to diagnosis was shown to be significantly associated with a shorter time to prostate cancer-specific mortality [31]. In a large surgical series, PSA doubling times of >24 months were manifest by almost all men with organ-confined disease and only half of patients with non-organ-confined disease [28]. In addition, patients with relatively high stage and high grade disease were more likely to have more rapid PSA doubling times compared to patients with lower stage and lower grade disease.

Definitions of biochemical outcome

Outcome measures following surgery differ from those following radiation therapy, thus creating difficulties comparing efficacy. Following radical prostatectomy, treatment failure is noted as a detectable PSA, variably defined as ranging from greater than 0.2 ng/ml to 0.4 ng/ml [32, 33]. Following radiotherapy, failure definitions can be more ambiguous as prostate tissue remains intact. In 1997, the American Society of Therapeutic Radiology and Oncology (ASTRO) established a definition of PSA relapse as three consecutive rises, obtained at intervals of 3–4 months apart, following a post-radiation nadir level [34]. A minimum of 24 months of observation was recommended with the date of failure calculated at the midpoint between the nadir and the first rise (i.e., backdated). Three consecutive rises was selected to exclude patients experiencing a "PSA bounce" or brief, benign rise in PSA followed by a subsequent decline. Despite a step forward in defining failure after radiation therapy, serious concerns arose regarding biases imposed upon survival estimates which, when using this definition, worsen with shorter follow-up. The ASTRO definition was also inappropriately applied to patients treated with brachytherapy, hormone therapy, and non-radiation therapies rather than exclusively in external beam radiation patients for whom it was developed.

Thus in 2005 a second conference convened in Phoenix, Arizona and a new definition was recommended addressing some of these concerns [35]. The Phoenix definition (also known as the Houston definition or "nadir +2" definition) is defined as a rise by ≥ 2 ng/ml above a nadir PSA after external beam radiation therapy with or without hormone therapy. A level of 2 ng/ml was selected as up to 30% of patients may have a nadir >1.0 ng/ml after external radiation [36]. In addition, the date of failure is determined as the date "at call" (i.e., not backdated). It is likely that, as more reliable aspects of PSA kinetics and molecular markers are identified, the definition of failure following radiation therapy will continue to evolve.

Choice of local therapy

Two major therapeutic modalities for clinically localized prostate cancer include radical prostatectomy and radiotherapy. Radiotherapeutic options include external beam radiotherapy or brachytherapy either as monotherapy or combined modalities. Due to accrual difficulties, rapidly improving technology in both surgical and radiation oncology fields as well as the long follow-up necessary to demonstrate comparable survival benefits, there have been no randomized studies to date directly comparing these therapies. Two large-scale trials – Surgical Prostatectomy vs. Interstitial Radiation Intervention phase III trial (SPIRIT, ACOSOG Z0070 NCIC PR10) and the Medical Research Council PR06 trial, both randomizing men with clinically localized prostate cancer to radical prostatectomy, radiotherapy or watchful waiting – did not meet accrual expectations and were closed prematurely [37, 38]. A similar phase III UK trial (*Prostate Testing for Cancer Treatment, ProtecT*) has completed patient accrual; however, results will not be available for some time [39].

Many large single- and multi-institutional studies have reported comparable 10- to 15-year disease-free and overall survival outcomes with surgery and radiotherapy for patients with clinically localized prostate cancer [40, 41, 42, 43]. A retrospective series of 2991 patients treated with radical prostatectomy, low-dose (<72 Gy) external beam radiotherapy, high-dose (72 Gy) external beam radiotherapy (EBRT), permanent seed brachytherapy (BRT) or combined brachytherapy and external radiation for stage T1–T2 prostate cancer suggested similar 5-year outcomes with all approaches, except for low-dose EBRT [42]. For many patients with organ-confined disease, the choice for treatment lies in weighing quality-of-life aspects of therapy, i.e., toxicities, and individual patient preference. For patients with more locally advanced disease, aggressive combination therapies including

hormonal ablation therapy, high-dose EBRT and/or combined interstitial implantation and EBRT may be more comprehensive and deliver more potent biologic
doses within the tumor.

External beam radiation therapy

Developments in image-based computer treatment planning, delivery and verification have marked a new era in the evolution of modern radiation therapy.
Conventional two-dimensional planning techniques limited dose delivery to
65–70 Gy, currently considered inadequate for local disease control [44, 45].
Three-dimensional imaging technology and complex radiation dose calculation
algorithms have allowed for substantial improvements in tumor localization and
dose distributions. Volumetric dose calculations provide a more detailed and
precise estimation of actual dose to specific tissue allowing the construction of
dose-volume histograms (DVHs), which have been correlated with toxicity outcomes. Computed tomography/magnetic resonance imaging fusion allows integration of precise visualization of prostate and tumor anatomy into treatment planning
software. Furthermore, the development of intensity-modulated radiation therapy
has further improved dose conformality and has effectively reduced the incidence
of normal tissue toxicity. Now, image-guided technologies provide dynamic
three-dimensional information and verification of targeting precision.

Intensity-modulated radiation therapy

Intensity-modulated radiation therapy (IMRT) is a technological advance that
allows the intensity of the radiation beam to be modulated in each of many small
pixels or beamlets within the target allowing more intense dose delivery to tumor
targets and a less intense dose to non-targets. A major advantage of this technique is
that it allows the planner to specify multiple dosimetric goals and the planning
software will design a customized plan to meet these goals, i.e., "inverse planning."
Treatment planning based on inverse planning and iterative computer-based optimization allows the generation of optimal beam number/angles with varying
intensity based on individualized three-dimensional (3D) targets. This provides
more control over the shaping of dose distributions; for example, the creation of a
concavity adjacent to a critical structure with a steep dose gradient (Figure 5.2).
Perhaps most importantly, IMRT has permitted dose escalation to previously
unattainable levels without increased acute or late toxicity [46, 47].

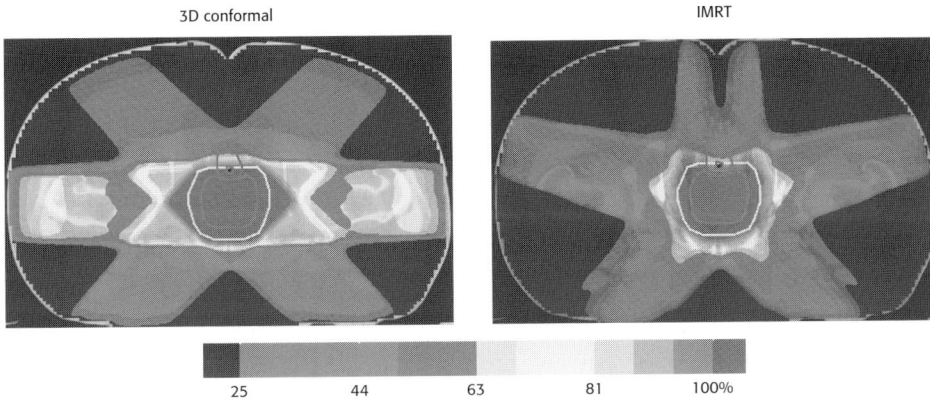

3D conformal · IMRT

25   44   63   81   100%

Figure 5.2. Three-dimensional (left) and intensity-modulated radiation therapy (IMRT) (right) treatment plan comparison demonstrating improved conformality of dose using IMRT (dose colorwash representation). See color plate section for full color version.

Dose escalation

The association between higher radiation dose and improved biochemical outcome has been established from multiple retrospective series [42, 44, 46, 47, 48, 49, 50, 51]. One of the largest series establishing a benefit of dose escalation was reported by Memorial Sloan-Kettering Cancer Center. Zelefsky *et al.* in a series of 2047 patients with favorable-, intermediate-, and high-risk prostate cancer were treated with systematic dose escalation from 64.8 Gy to 86.4 Gy using 3D conformal radiotherapy or IMRT [48, 49]. With a median follow-up of 6.6 years, intermediate- and high-risk patients were noted to have significantly improved biochemical-free and distant-metastasis-free survival with escalated radiation dose. For patients with favorable risk features, a significant correlation of outcome with dose was not demonstrated; although longer follow-up for indolent disease may be necessary. When comparing IMRT and 3D conformal approaches, a significantly reduced incidence of gastrointestinal (GI) toxicities of grade 2 or higher was noted with IMRT (13% to 5%) [50].

Multiple randomized trials have been published establishing the role of dose-escalated external beam radiotherapy and are summarized in Table 5.3 [52, 53, 54, 55, 56]. One of the first randomized trials establishing a clinical benefit from dose escalation was conducted at M. D. Anderson Cancer Center randomizing 305 clinically localized prostate cancer patients to 70 Gy versus 78 Gy in 2-Gy daily fractions [53]. Although biochemical outcomes were improved in the 78-Gy arm, this came at a cost of higher late rectal toxicity (26% vs. 12%, $p = 0.001$) which was

Table 5.3. Phase III external beam radiation therapy dose-escalation studies

Reference	n	Eligibility	Study design	Hormone therapy	Results
Shipley et al. [52]	201	T3–4, Nx –2	50.4 Gy → 25.2 GyE boost vs. 16.8 GyE boost	None	Improved LC in high Gleason subgroup only (5 year LC 94% vs. 64%, $p = 0.0014$)
Pollack et al. [53]	305	T1–T3, Nx –0	70 Gy vs. 78 Gy	None	Improved BCF failure in high-dose arm (6 years 70% vs. 64% $p = 0.03$); benefit limited to subgroup with PSA > 10
Zietman et al. [54]	393	T1b–T2b, N0, PSA^a < 15	19.8 GyE* vs. 28.8 GyE → 50.4 Gy	None	Improved BC in high-dose arm (5 years bFFF, 80.4% vs. 61.4% $p = $ <0.001) for both low- and high-risk groups
Peeters et al. [55]	669	T1b–T4, PSA < 60 (T1b-c, PSA ≤ 4 excluded)	68 Gy vs. 78 Gy	Yes	Improved BCF in high-dose arm (5 years FFF 64% vs. 54% $p = 0.01$)
Dearnaley et al. [56]	843	T1b–T3a, N0, PSA < 50	64 Gy vs. 74 Gy	Yes	Improved bFFF in high-dose arm (5 years bFFF 71% vs. 60% HR 0.67, $p = 0.0007$)

Abbreviations: BC, biochemical control; BCF, biochemical and clinical failure; bFFF, biochemical freedom from failure; FFF, freedom from failure; Gy, Gray; GyE, Gray equivalents; LC, local control; PSA, prostate-specific antigen.
*photon + proton beams.
^{a} PSA values are in ng/ml.

directly correlated with dose-volume effects. A more recent multicenter Dutch trial randomized 664 patients with T1b–T4 prostate cancer with a PSA ≤60 ng/ml to 68 Gy versus 78 Gy using 3D conformal therapy [55]. Overall in the high-dose arm, the 5-year PSA failure-free survival was significantly higher (64% vs. 53%, $p = 0.02$); however, when subset analyses were performed the benefit was limited to intermediate- and high-risk patients. A non-significant increase (32% vs. 27%, $p = 0.2$) in grade ≥2 late GI toxicity was noted in the high-dose arm. The largest randomized dose escalation trial, MRC RT01, has recently been reported demonstrating that escalating dose from 64 Gy to 74 Gy using 3D conformal therapy improved biochemical outcomes in all prognostic groups with a small increase in late GI toxicity in the high-dose arm [56]. A large, ongoing Radiation Therapy Oncology Group (RTOG) trial (RTOG-0126) comparing high-dose (79.2 Gy) with standard-dose (70.2 Gy) therapy with an accrual goal of over 1500 patients is ongoing to address whether these biochemical and clinical outcomes correspond to survival benefits.

The classic approach to conformal radiotherapy planning has been based on homogeneous dose distributions within targets; however, with IMRT, heterogeneous dose delivery is achievable. This may be particularly beneficial for delivering higher doses to specific tumor-bearing regions in the prostate, and lower doses to normal tissue. With better definition of these subvolumes, an opportunity arises for defining intraprostatic lesions as boost targets with potentially better tumor control [57, 58]. The ability of MRI/MRSI to delineate the internal prostate anatomy, prostate margins, and extent of local disease makes this technique feasible. As radiation dose calculations rely on differential electron density of tissue based on Hounsfield units, MR/CT fusion capabilities provide a mechanism for superimposing these images and precisely delineating specific radiation targets. Pucar *et al.* have reported on the importance of pre-treatment MRI-detected lesions and confirmed via pathologic analysis confirmation at salvage prostatectomy that post-radiotherapy recurrence typically occurs in the original location of the dominant lesion [59]. The addition of functional spectroscopic imaging may also be able to distinguish high-grade or hypoxic (i.e., radioresistant) subclones that require higher tumoricidal doses. Differential doses can be simultaneously prescribed allowing specified dose escalation to these high-risk tumor-bearing regions (i.e., "dose painting") (Figure 5.3). Using this method, doses of 94.5 Gy have been delivered to focal subregions with promising preliminary tolerance outcomes [60].

As dose escalation continues, daily target localization becomes critical as small degrees of patient set-up or internal prostate motion can significantly affect

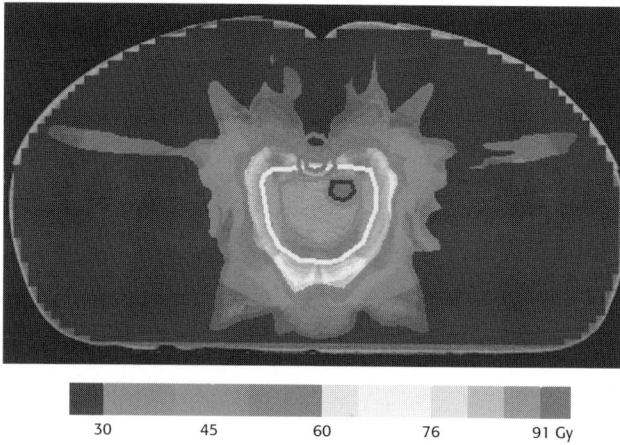

Figure 5.3. Dose painting IMRT treatment plan. Note dominant intraprostatic lesion outlined in blue receiving 91 Gy. See color plate section for full color version.

normal and target tissue coverage. Recently, image-guided techniques have been improving the tracking of these fluctuations further improving precise radiation dose delivery.

Image-guided radiation therapy

The accurate delivery of radiotherapy relies on identifying the precise relationship of the target and radiation beams. The prostate, as an internal organ, can move with daily alterations in bowel and bladder filling. In addition, small changes in daily patient set-up, particularly when reduced planning margins are used, may cause a geographic "miss" and, despite careful immobilization, are difficult to control. Image guidance tracks these alterations and provides an opportunity to make critical corrections. Currently, ultrasound-guided tracking systems and radio-opaque marker placement are widely available. Small radio-opaque gold seeds, or fiducial markers, can be placed into the prostate transrectally in a simple office procedure prior to simulation. Using two-dimensional kilovoltage imaging, these markers can be easily visualized daily and matched with simulation radiographs, and critical corrections can be made on a daily basis prior to the delivery of each fraction (Figure 5.4). In addition, their spatial arrangement can be monitored providing crucial information about prostate interfraction motion and volume changes.

More recently, online cone-beam computed tomography (CBCT) imaging has become available to generate a 3D view of the target while the patient is in the treatment position. These images can be fused and aligned, based on bony anatomy

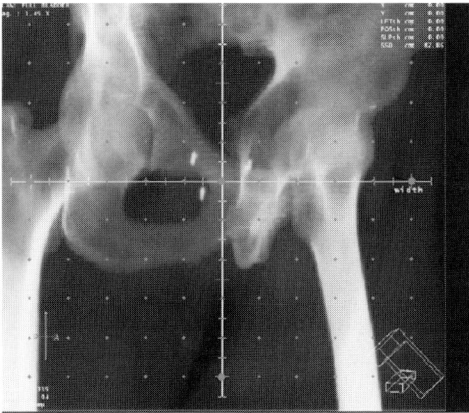 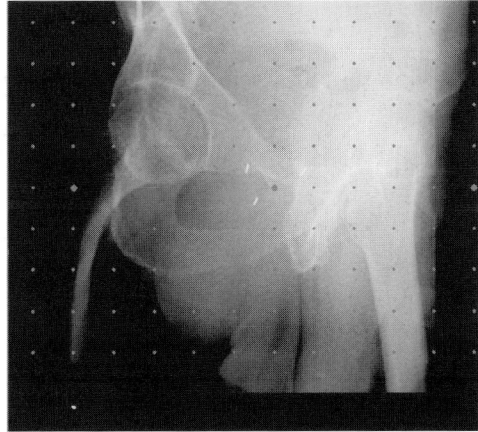

(a)   (b)

Figure 5.4. (a) Digitally reconstructed radiograph (DRR) depicting prostate fiducial markers in place.
(b) Portal image taken prior to treatment delivery with patient in treatment position.

or fiducial marker location, with planning CT scans for daily patient alignment. Two-dimensional detectors mounted on linear accelerators are capable of producing kilovoltage CBCTs by rotating a small beam using a large field of view and single revolution [61]. The images generated have inferior image quality compared to diagnostic scans; however, precise anatomically based alignment can be achieved. Megavoltage CBCTs are produced in a similar fashion by gantry rotations of the treatment beam [62]. Using a megavoltage beam, a relatively high dose (in the range of 6–10 cGy) is often necessary to obtain adequate soft-tissue contrast for verification purposes [63]. Depending on the frequency of imaging, this dose could be significant and require incorporation into treatment plans. Helical tomotherapy is a rotational delivery technique that replaces the traditional treatment beam with a CT ring and a megavoltage beam source [64]. Treatments are delivered with both the gantry and the treatment table in continuous, simultaneous motion thus allowing 360° treatment delivery in addition to onboard megavoltage-CT-verification capability. In addition to pre- and post-treatment scans, megavoltage CTs (MVCTs) can be obtained during radiation delivery allowing real-time anatomic verification of dose delivery to targets. Another potential role of image-guided therapy is to modify the treatment fields to account for positional variations, i.e., adaptive radiotherapy. Whether these verification strategies allow a reduction in treatment margin or improved clinical efficacy is unknown but will undoubtedly be an area of significant interest in future studies.

Hypofractionation

Radiation-induced cell death has been described according to the linear-quadratic model such that the dose response to a fractionated course of radiation correlates to the α/β specific for that tissue. In general, the α/β is high for early-responding tissue such as mucosa and low for late-responding cell lines such as nerve tissue, which may be important for optimal fractionation regimens. Recent evidence has been accumulating that the biology of prostate cancer may favor a low α/β, implying a favorable therapeutic benefit from delivery of a higher daily dose in an overall shorter treatment time, i.e., hypofractionated radiotherapy [65, 66]. Kupelian *et al.* reported excellent long-term biochemical control using 70 Gy at 2.5 Gy fractions daily with minimal late genitourinary or gastrointestinal toxicity [67]. Preliminary data are now available from two randomized phase III trials comparing hypofractionation and conventional fractionation regimens. An Australian trial included 217 men with clinically localized prostate cancer randomized to receive 64 Gy in 2 Gy/day versus 55 Gy in 2.75 Gy/day using two-dimensional treatment planning [68]. At a median follow-up of 43.5 months, there was no difference in biochemical outcome (85.5% vs. 86.2%, respectively); however, a higher rate of rectal toxicity (42% vs. 27%, $p<0.05$) was noted in the hypofractionation arm, perhaps related to the use of conventional treatment planning techniques. A Canadian trial included 936 early-stage patients randomized to receive 66 Gy in 2 Gy/day versus 52.5 Gy in 2.63 Gy/day using three-dimensional treatment planning [69]. With a median follow-up of 5.7 years, a non-significant increase in biochemical and clinical failure (59.95% vs. 52.95%) was seen in the hypofractionation arm. A small (5%) but significant increase in acute genitourinary and GI toxicity was noted in the hypofractionation arm without a difference in late toxicity. The interpretation of these trials is limited given the relatively low doses compared to current standards, older treatment planning techniques and larger field margins used. RTOG 04–15, an ongoing trial comparing a hypofractionation (70 Gy in 2.5 Gy/d) regimen and higher dose conventional (73.8 Gy in 1.8 Gy/day) fractionation, may help clarify any benefit of using this approach.

Acute and late toxicity after external beam radiotherapy

Acute irritative urinary symptoms, related to urethritis, prostatitis, and cystitis, are common. Urinary outlet symptoms, i.e., weak stream, straining, and incomplete emptying, may be related to prostate edema. Tools to assess the severity of lower urinary tract symptoms such as the RTOG grading system and International Prostate Symptom Score (IPSS) (or American Urologic Symptom Score) question-naire are useful for individual patient monitoring as well as morbidity reporting [70, 71]. Short-term use of α-adrenergic blockade, anti-spasmodics and/or anti-inflammatory medications are often sufficient to manage these early symptoms, which typically appear gradually during radiotherapy and resolve within weeks to months after completion of treatment. Approximately 10% of patients will require use of prolonged medication for urinary symptom control. Chronic urinary complications are rare; however, urethral stricture and bladder neck contracture may occur. The risk of late grade 3 urinary complications was 0.6% in a recent high-dose IMRT series [47]. Urinary incontinence is rare except in patients who have had prior transurethral resection of the prostate (TURP) [72].

Acute bowel toxicity is usually mild and may include proctalgia, tenesmus, mucus discharge, and increased bowel frequency, likely related to dose-volume effects. Small bowel may be included in radiation fields when pelvic lymphatics are targeted, which may increase toxicity; however, this can be mini-mized using IMRT techniques [73]. Chronic radiation proctitis may occur within the first 2 years or after and is caused by rectal mucosa telangiectatic changes, which may produce rectal bleeding [74, 75]. In the Memorial Sloan-Kettering Cancer Center experience using high-dose IMRT, grade 2 or grade 3 rectal bleeding was seen in only 3% and <1%, respectively [47]. This is in striking comparison to a 15%–25% rate of grade 2 or greater rectal bleeding using 3D conformal techniques. Serious long-term bowel complications, i.e., rectal ulceration, incontinence, and stricture are rare (<1%).

Erectile dysfunction (ED) may affect 36%–59% of patients after external beam radiotherapy [76, 77]. The assessment of sexual dysfunction, however, is complex and fraught by inaccuracies due to limitations and variations in the definition of ED and in assessment tools. Confounding factors involved in male sexual health include medical co-morbidities (i.e., diabetes, atherosclerosis), medications, and age, which may compromise baseline erectile function. The International Index of Erectile Function (IIEF) is a validated patient questionnaire commonly used to assess baseline and post-treatment sexual dysfunction. The true etiology of post-radiation ED remains controversial; however, it likely involves damage to local vasculature of the penile corporal structures and neurovascular bundles [78, 79, 80]. Erectile dysfunction medications, i.e., sildenafil citrate, are commonly used to improve sexual function following therapy and are currently being investigated in a prophylactic setting.

Brachytherapy

Brachytherapy refers to placement of radioactive sources at a close distance from or within target tissue. Typical radioisotopes deposit radiation energy at short distances from the source and are particularly useful in conformal approaches. Brachytherapy techniques have been revolutionized with image guidance in order to optimize source placement, which is critical for normal tissue sparing and dose escalation strategies in the primary setting and for post-radiation local recurrence.

Modern permanent (LDR) brachytherapy

Low-dose-rate (LDR) brachytherapy consists of the permanent insertion of radioactive seeds into the prostate. Due to the relatively short half-lives, ^{125}I ($t_{1/2} = 60$ days) and ^{103}Pd ($t_{1/2} = 17$ days) are ideal for permanent implants. Newer sources with shorter half-lives, such as ^{131}Cs ($t_{1/2} = 9.7$ days), are currently being evaluated. To date, no clear evidence exists demonstrating that one isotope is better than the others, although one comparative trial preliminarily reported no significant differences yet observed in outcome between ^{125}I and ^{103}Pd [81].

The technique of LDR brachytherapy relies on optimal visualization of the prostate. The most common technique utilizes a transrectal ultrasound probe to visualize the prostate gland in transverse and sagittal dimensions. The probe is mounted on a stabilization apparatus affixed to the operating room table and a template grid is attached. Ultrasound imaging allows guidance of needles placed through perineal skin into the prostate tissue (Figure 5.5). In the real-time intra-operative planning approach, ultrasound images are obtained every 5 mm from the base of the prostate through the apex and these images are captured into a treatment-planning computer. The path of the urethra may be visualized on ultrasound via a urinary catheter with aerated gel. Target and normal tissue contours are defined and source and dose distributions are optimized immediately prior to seed insertion (Figure 5.6).

The goal for dosimetric coverage using brachytherapy techniques, as for external beam approaches, is for comprehensive coverage of the prostate. For further optimization, knowledge of tumor-bearing regions within the prostate may be useful. Regions of interest identified by MRI/MRSI allow specific attention to these locations on ultrasound to ensure adequate coverage and, potentially, dose escalation. In addition, MRI/US image fusion technology allows the superimposition of images to directly correlate these areas. Zelefsky *et al.* evaluated the feasibility of dose escalation to MRS-defined intraprostatic lesions

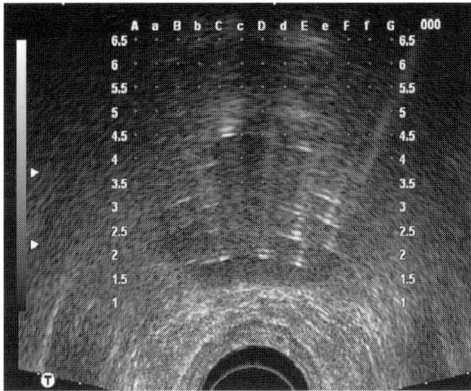

(a)

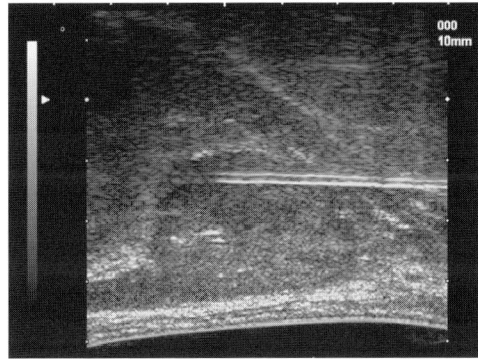

(b)

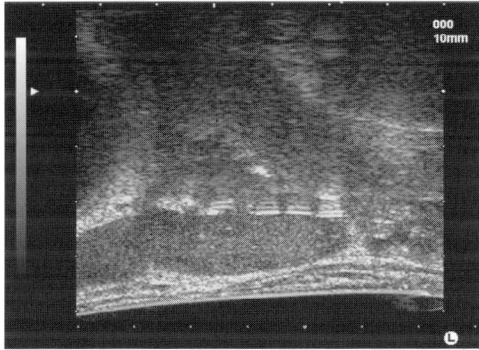

(c)

Figure 5.5. (a) Axial ultrasound image demonstrating needles in place within the prostate. (b) Longitudinal view. (c) Radioactive seeds implanted within the prostate gland.

via intra-operative image fusion in patients undergoing ^{125}I monotherapy [82]. The prescription dose to the entire prostate was 144 Gy and a range of 139% to 192% of prescription was deliverable to the MRS-identified lesion while maintaining low urethral doses. DiBiase *et al.* conducted a similar study designed to increase dose to MRS-defined volumes to 130% of prescription (145 Gy using ^{125}I) [83]. With only short follow-up, this series confirmed the feasibility of the technique without sacrificing morbidity.

Additional techniques for imaging in brachytherapy include use of CT or MRI guidance in place of ultrasound. Due to their difficulty in practical application, i.e., operating room constraints, these modalities are available only at a limited number of institutions. Further refinements of image-guided, dynamic, dose-escalated brachytherapy and its impact on clinical, biochemical, and toxicity outcomes are of significant interest.

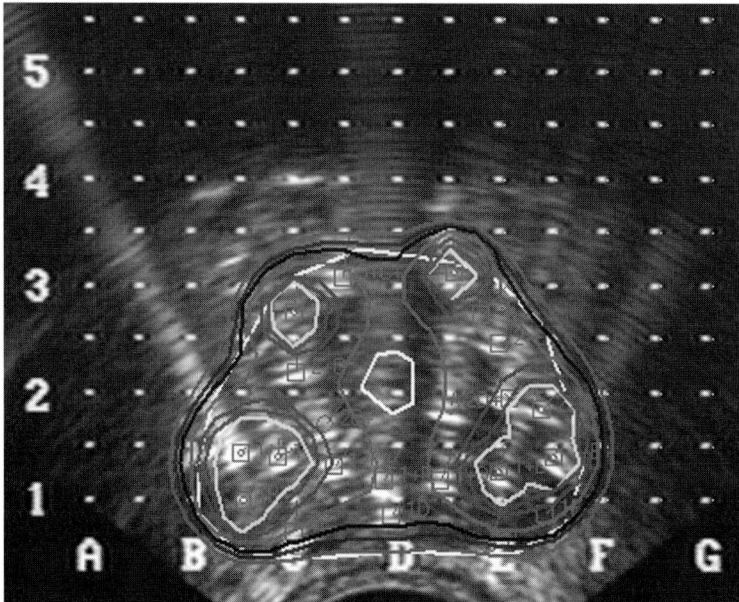

Figure 5.6. Intra-operative axial ultrasound image demonstrating conformal dose distribution achievable with optimized treatment planning. Green line represents the 100% prescription dose; light blue line represents 150% prescription dose. See color plate section for full color version.

Dose

The precise dose necessary to eradicate prostate cancer with permanent brachytherapy has not been firmly established; therefore, current prescription doses have evolved from retrospective data. Early data confirmed excellent local control rates based on DRE and biopsy follow-up using a prescribed dose of 160 Gy [84]. Subsequently, in the PSA era, biochemical outcomes continue to confirm an important relationship between implant dose and quality [85, 86, 87]. Dosimetric measures of quality are often reported as D_{90}, i.e., dose to 90% of the prostate gland, or V_{100}, i.e., volume receiving 100% of the prescription dose. A recent multi-institutional analysis of over 1800 patients treated with ^{125}I brachytherapy for clinically localized disease demonstrated a significantly improved 8-year PSA relapse-free survival with D_{90} of ≥130 Gy as compared with lower doses (93% vs. 76% $p<0.001$) [87]. Currently, the American Brachytherapy Society recommends prescription doses of 145 Gy using ^{125}I or 125 Gy when using [103]Pd for monotherapy [88, 89].

Due to differences in the radiobiologic properties of various isotopes and treatment modalities as well as the difficulty inherent in comparing treatment regimens, i.e., combination implant and external beam radiation, the concept of biologic effective dose (BED) may be more relevant. Using BED values, Stock *et al.* were able to demonstrate a significant dose–response relationship between increasing BED and higher biochemical control and negative biopsy rates [90]. Ten-year freedom from PSA failure rates increased from 46% to 92% as BED values increased from <100 to >200 using BED increments of 20. Using these same BED groupings, post-treatment positive biopsy rates dropped from 24% to 3%.

Temporary (HDR) brachytherapy

High-dose-rate (HDR) brachytherapy involves the temporary placement of a highly active radioactive source (^{192}Ir) within the tissue. The procedure involves placing, via a transperineal approach, blind-ended catheters through a template that is then sutured to the perineum in a short operative procedure (Figure 5.7). A CT scan is obtained to document the location and position of the catheters and a computer-optimized plan is designed to determine the optimal position and duration of the source within each catheter. In this manner, various dose distributions can be

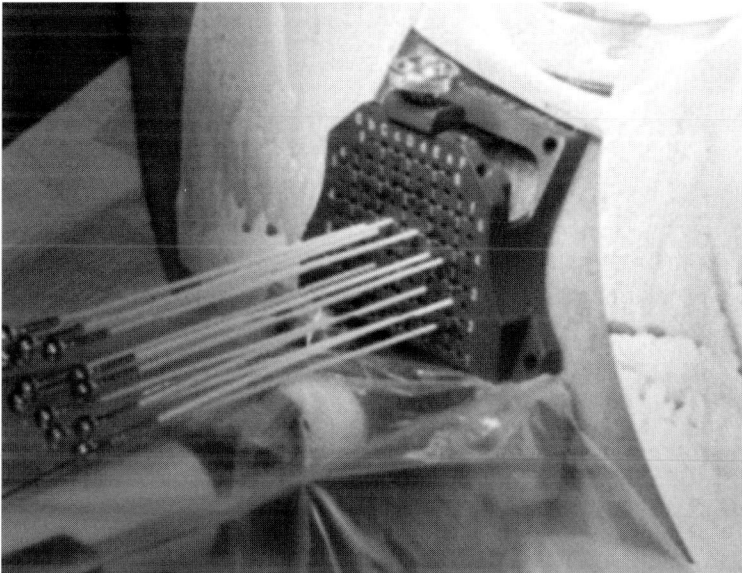

Figure 5.7. HDR catheters and perineal template in place. See color plate section for full color version.

analyzed and the optimal plan selected for therapy. Due to the high energy of this isotope, a remote afterloading technique is necessary where the source is controlled remotely via a computer-operated guidewire with minimal radiation exposure to personnel. A typical treatment plan consists of several treatments delivered at least 6 h apart over 2 days.

There are several potential advantages to HDR brachytherapy. Firstly, given the potential sensitivity of prostate cancer cells to fractionation (i.e., low α/β ratio), the influence of dose rate may be important. Since large dose fraction sizes are used with HDR, tumor control may be superior compared with LDR techniques. A second major advantage of HDR is the afterloading technique, which allows for careful shaping of dose prior to treatment delivery. Because permanent radioactive seeds may shift within or outside of prostate tissue, control over actual dose delivery is improved with HDR. Also, radiation safety considerations for staff and the patient are minimized.

In general, patients selected for HDR brachytherapy have relatively unfavorable prognostic factors and, hence, it has been used predominantly as a boost in combination with external beam radiation therapy [91, 92, 93, 94, 95]. Recently, increasing interest in HDR monotherapy for early and intermediate-risk patients has developed [96, 97, 98]. A recent phase II study using 9.5 Gy delivered twice daily over 2 days for favorable-risk patients demonstrated excellent dosimetric coverage and favorable toxicity [98]. In one study with a median follow-up of 35 months, biochemical control rates appear equivalent to LDR approaches [96].

Morbidity after brachytherapy

Image-guided techniques have significantly reduced acute and long-term toxicities associated with brachytherapy. Acute genitourinary symptoms are common and similar to those from external beam radiotherapy; however, they have a more rapid onset and may be more intense [99]. Perioperative acute urinary retention (AUR) may occur and is likely due to patient- or treatment-related factors, rather than dose. The risk of temporary catheterization is 5%–22% with only 2%–3% requiring prolonged catheterization [96, 97]. Pre-implant factors which may confer a higher risk include prostate volume >50 ml, pre-implant hormone use, pre-existing lower urinary tract symptoms, and variations in brachytherapy technique [100, 101, 102, 103]. Attempts to correlate AUR with urethral dosimetry have been inconclusive to date [104]. Late grade 3 or 4 urinary toxicities are infrequent, 7% and 1% respectively. Urinary incontinence is rare except in patients who have had TURP post-brachytherapy

[105]. Radiation proctitis, usually limited to RTOG grade 1–2, occurs in approximately 2%–10% of patients and has been correlated with dose – volume relationships, dose rate, and addition of external beam [106, 107, 108]. Recent evidence suggests that genetic factors may also play a role in the development and severity of radiation proctitis [109]. The risk of impotency has been reported as 10%–50% in reported series and largely influenced by factors such as pre-treatment erectile function, confounding co-morbidities and dose to erectile tissue [110, 110, 112]. Post-brachytherapy ED may also be effectively managed with ED medication, with previously potent patients achieving the best outcomes [113]. In addition, earlier post-treatment ED therapy may have an impact on long-term erectile function [114].

Combined modality approaches

Failure following definitive radiotherapy stems from either systemic micrometastases or inadequate local control due to insufficient dose or dosimetric coverage. For intermediate- and high-risk patients, there are concerns that brachytherapy alone may not adequately encompass periprostatic disease extension and thus a combination approach may be more comprehensive [115]. In addition to better dose coverage, a higher intraprostatic dose is achievable with a combination approach than with either modality alone, facilitating dose escalation. Combined approaches typically include brachytherapy (temporary or permanent), external beam radiation therapy and/or hormone therapy to escalate dose, and more comprehensively address potential sites of disease.

Brachytherapy combined with external beam radiation

Several single-institution retrospective analyses have shown excellent outcomes using combined modality therapy with only modest effects on morbidity [92, 95, 116, 117, 118, 119, 120, 121]. Stock *et al.* reported excellent 5-year freedom from PSA failure rates in a cohort of 132 high-risk patients treated with 9 months of androgen suppression, permanent LDR brachytherapy and external beam radiation therapy [118]: 85% of patients with Gleason 7 disease and 76% of patients with Gleason 8–10 disease were biochemically free from failure at 5 years. In addition, pathologically confirmed local control rates were excellent. A summary of selected retrospective analyses utilizing brachytherapy and external beam radiation is summarized in Table 5.4.

Recently, two randomized trials have been reported comparing external beam radiation therapy with or without an HDR brachytherapy boost [122, 123]. Sathya *et al.* reported a randomized trial including 51 T2–T3 patients treated with external

Table 5.4. Retrospective series using combined brachytherapy and external beam radiation

Study	n	Eligibility	Treatment	Hormone therapy	Median follow-up	Results
Critz and Levinson [116]	1469	T1–T2, pN0	LDR-BT→EBRT	No	6 years (min 5 years)	[a]10 year DFS – low-risk 93%, intermediate-risk 80%, high-risk 61%
Ragde et al. [117]	231	≥T2b, ≥Gl 7, PSA ≥15	EBRT→LDR-BT	No	60 months	[b]8 years bFFF 65%; 8 years LC 91%
Sylvester et al. [119]	232	T1–T3	EBRT→LDR-BT	No	63 months	[c]10 years BRFS – low-risk 85%, intermediate-risk 77%, high-risk 45%
Stock et al. [118]	132	T2c–T3 or Gl 8–10 or PSA > 20	LDR-BT→EBRT	NAAC	50 months	[d]5 years bFFF 86%. Better outcome for low-grade, neg SV biopsy
Dattoli et al. [120]	243	T2c–T3 ± Gl 7 – 10 ± PSA > 10	EBRT→LDR-BT	NA or A	9.5 years	14 years bFFF – intermediate-risk 87%, high-risk 72%; LC 100%. Better outcome for low-grade, low PSA
Singh et al. [121]	95	T1–T2	EBRT→LDR-BT	NAAC	38 months (min 24 months)	[d]5 years BFFS 86%
Phan et al. [95]	309	T1–T3	HDR-BT→EBRT (75%)	NAAC	59 months	[d]5 years BC – low-risk 98%; intermediate-risk 90%; high-risk 78%
Vargas et al. [92]	197	≥T2b, ≥Gl 7, PSA ≥10	EBRT + HDR-BT (concurrently)	No	4.9 years	5 years DFS 84.8%; HDR dose escalation improved biochemical and overall survival

Abbreviations: A, adjuvant; BC, biochemical control; bFFF, biochemical freedom from failure; bFFS, biochemical failure-free survival; BRFS, biochemical recurrence-free survival; DFS, disease-free survival; EBRT, external beam radiation therapy; Gl, Gleason score; HDR-BT, high-dose-rate brachytherapy; LDR-BT, low-dose-rate brachytherapy; NA, neoadjuvant; NAAC, neoadjuvant and concurrent.

[a]Failure = PSA > 0.2 ng/ml.
[b]Failure = PSA > 1 ng/ml.
[c]Failure = two consecutive rises; initiation of hormone therapy.
[d]Failure = ASTRO definition.

radiation therapy of 66 Gy in 33 fractions versus an HDR implant (35 Gy in 2 fractions) followed by additional external radiation of 40 Gy in 20 fractions [122]. With a median follow-up of 8.2 years, reduced biochemical or clinical failure rates were noted in the combination arm (29% vs. 61%, $p = 0.0024$) in addition to a decreased post-radiation positive biopsy rate (24% vs. 51% $p = 0.015$). Hoskin *et al.* reported results of 220 patients with clinically localized prostate cancer randomized to external radiation therapy of 55 Gy in 20 fractions versus 35.75 Gy in 13 fractions followed by an HDR brachytherapy boost for an additional 17 Gy in 2 fractions [123]. At a median follow-up of 30 months, a significant improvement in PSA relapse-free survival was noted in the combination arm for all prognostic risk groups.

Androgen suppression

Hormonal ablation therapy is an extremely effective systemic therapy for prostate cancer and commonly used in combined modality regimens [124]. A luteinizing-hormone-releasing hormone (LHRH) agonist with or without an anti-androgen is used with the goal of suppressing testosterone to castrate levels, thereby reducing androgen-sensitive local and, potentially, micrometastatic tumor clones. In the neoadjuvant setting, prostate volumes are often decreased by 20%–30% from baseline [125]. Cytoreduction allows for a smaller radiation target and less normal tissue exposure, which is particularly useful for large prostate volumes. In addition, evidence points to a synergistic benefit with radiotherapy leading to enhanced tumor cell kill and reduction of hypoxia [126].

Multiple randomized trials have been reported demonstrating improved outcomes when radiation therapy is combined with hormone therapy in certain patient populations and are summarized in Table 5.5 [127, 128, 129, 130, 131, 132, 133, 134, 135, 136]. In particular, bulky, locally advanced and unfavorable-risk patients appear to derive the most significant benefit. Hormone therapy should be initiated prior to and concurrent with radiation therapy for optimal effect. Long-term adjuvant hormone ablation following radiation therapy has also shown an overall survival benefit in the RTOG and European Organisation for Research and Treatment of Cancer (EORTC) series [127, 128]. A recent meta-analysis confirmed significantly improved clinical and biochemical disease-free survival using neoadjuvant hormone therapy prior to radiation therapy in addition to an overall survival benefit using adjuvant therapy [137]. The optimal duration of therapy and whether dose-escalated therapies reduce the need for hormone therapy remain unknown.

Table 5.5. Phase III randomized trials of combined radiotherapy and hormone therapy

Study	n	Eligibility	Study design	Results
EORTC 22863 [127]	415	T3–4 or T1–2 WHO 3	RT vs. RT + HAT (3 years)	Improved LC, DFS and OS with HAT
RTOG 85-31 [128]	977	T3 or T1–2, N+ or pT3 and (+) margin or (+) seminal vesicles	RT vs. RT + HAT (indefinite)	Improved LC, DFS and OS with HAT for Gleason 8–10
RTOG 86-10 [129]	456	Bulky T2b, T3–4, N+	RT vs. RT +HAT (4 months)	Improved OS with HAT for Gleason <7
RTOG 92-02 [130]	1554	T2c–T4; PSA[a] <150, N+	4 months HAT →RT vs. 4 months HAT →RT + HAT (2 years)	Improved DFS and OS for adjuvant HAT for Gleason 8–10
RTOG 94-13 [131]	1323	T2c–T4, Gleason ≥6, or node (+) risk >15%, PSA < 100	2 × 2 factorial: 4 months HAT→RT-WP vs. 4 months HAT →RT-PO vs. RT-WP→4 months HAT vs. RT-PO→4 months HAT	Improved PFS with neoadjuvant HAT and RT-WP
L-101 [132]	161	T2–T3	RT alone vs. 3 months HAT→RT vs. 5 months HAT →RT + 5 months HAT	Improved biochemical control with HAT
L-200 [132]	325	T2–T3	5 months HAT→RT vs. 5 months HAT→RT + 5 months HAT	No difference
D'Amico et al. [133]	206	T1b–T2b, Gleason ≥7, PSA 10–40	RT vs. 3 months HAT →RT+3 months HAT	Improved PFS, CSS, OS with HAT
Gransfors et al. [134]	91	T1–T4, pN0–3, WHO 1–3	RT vs. orchiectomy→RT	Improved PFS and OS with orchiectomy for N+
CUOG [135]	378	All	3 months vs. 8 months HAT →RT	No difference
TROG 96-01 [136]	818	T2b–T4, N0	3 months vs. 6 months HAT →RT	Improved biochemical control, LC, DFS, CSS with 6 months HAT

Abbreviations: CSS, cause-specific survival; DFS, disease-free survival; HAT, hormone ablation therapy; LC, local control; OS, overall survival; PFS, progression-free survival; RT, radiation therapy; RT-PO, radiation therapy to prostate only; RT-WP, radiation therapy to whole pelvis and prostate.
[a] Note PSA values given in ng/ml.

Adjuvant and salvage radiation therapy

Approximately 30%–50% of patients following radical prostatectomy with adverse pathologic features, i.e., extracapsular extension, seminal vesicle invasion, or positive surgical margins, will ultimately develop PSA recurrence [138, 139]. Adjuvant therapy, as opposed to salvage therapy, is given before evidence of recurrence is found, as a preventive measure. Three large randomized trials evaluating the role of adjuvant radiation therapy have been reported [140, 141, 142]. The Southwest Oncology Group trial (SWOG) 8794 randomized 374 patients with adverse pathology at radical prostatectomy to immediate post-operative radiotherapy (60–64 Gy) or observation and found significant reductions in the risk of biochemical, local, and distant recurrence at 10 years with the use of adjuvant radiotherapy [140]. EORTC 22911 included 1005 node-negative patients following radical prostatectomy with one or more adverse pathologic risk factors (i.e., capsule perforation, positive surgical margins or seminal vesicle invasion) [141]. Similarly, patients were randomized to immediate or deferred radiotherapy (60 Gy), and at a median follow-up of 5 years improved biochemical progression-free survival (74% vs. 52.6%, $p<0.0001$) and decreased local-regional failure (15.4% vs. 5.4%, $p<0.0001$) were noted for irradiated patients. Unfortunately, many in the control arm of this study did not receive early salvage therapy, important for optimal outcome, but had clinically evident relapse. The preliminary results of the third phase III trial have been reported with similar results [142]. Despite encouraging results, a survival benefit of adjuvant radiotherapy has not been demonstrated.

Salvage radiotherapy is used in the setting of biochemical and/or clinically localized relapse. Recently reported long-term PSA remission rates range from 35% to 50% [143, 144, 145]. Optimal candidates include patients without detectable metastases, risk factors for locally persistent disease (i.e., extensive extracapsular extension, positive surgical margins) and/or radiographic evidence of local recurrence. Magnetic resonance imaging is particularly useful in the post-operative setting to identify gross local recurrence and direct biopsies for pathologic confirmation (Figure 5.8). In addition, these images provide the critical information needed to precisely define target volumes and allow for dose escalation with potentially improved PSA remission rates.

Multiple retrospective studies have defined prognostic factors for response to salvage therapy including: initially undetectable post-operative PSA, low pre-salvage PSA ≤1–2.5 ng/ml, PSA doubling time of ≥10 months, Gleason ≤7, no seminal vesicle invasion, positive surgical margins, and salvage radiation dose of >65 Gy [143, 144, 145]. In 1999, the ASTRO consensus panel recommended that

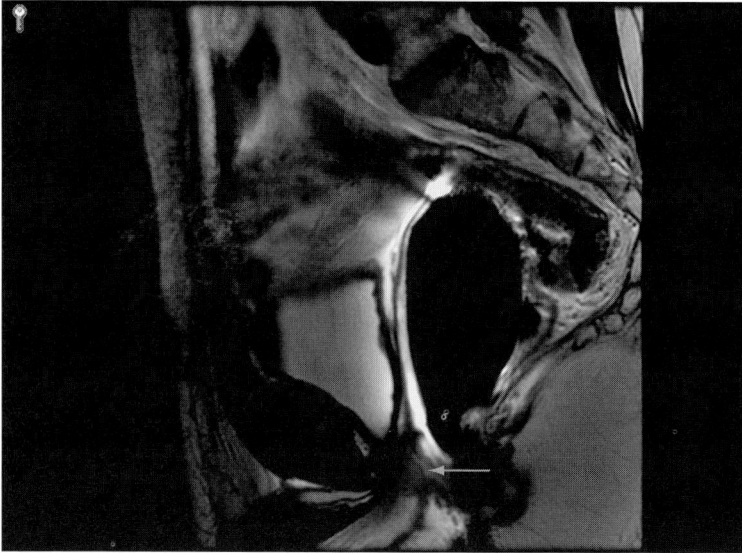

Figure 5.8. Sagittal T2-weighted MRI showing vesicourethral local recurrence (yellow arrow) following radical prostatectomy.

salvage radiotherapy should be delivered when PSA<1.5 ng/ml and that "the highest dose of radiation therapy that can be given without morbidity is justifiable" which should be ≥64 Gy [146]. Generally, doses of 65–72 Gy have been used with acceptable morbidity when employing intensity-modulated radiation therapy. With image-guided approaches, the feasibility and toxicity of dose escalation for clinical, local-disease recurrence will be actively studied.

Currently, it is unknown what additive role hormonal ablation may have in the salvage setting. RTOG 96-01 is an ongoing phase III trial investigating the role of concurrent hormone therapy in patients with biochemically recurrent disease following radical prostatectomy. An ongoing MRC/NCIC phase III trial (RADICALS) is evaluating the timing of adjuvant compared with salvage radiotherapy in addition to the use and duration of concurrent/adjuvant hormone therapy.

Salvage brachytherapy

Among men with PSA failure after definitive radiotherapy, many will harbor occult metastatic disease; however, a significant number of patients will have local recurrence only, which may be cured with aggressive local therapy [147, 148]. Although it is difficult to differentiate these patients, local-only failures tend to have long intervals until PSA failure (>2–3 years), long PSA doubling times (≥8–12 months), and lower risk factors at primary diagnosis [138, 145, 147, 149]. Due to the normal-tissue-sparing advantages of brachytherapy, increasing interest in salvage HDR and LDR is developing. Single-institution reports have been reporting excellent early results with favorable morbidity as compared with salvage surgery or local ablative therapies [150, 151, 152]. Undoubtedly, future studies will be necessary to confirm these findings.

Conclusion

The integration of radiographic and radiotherapeutic strategies to stage, select, and treat patients with clinically localized prostate cancer has provided a major step forward in treatment of this disease. Patient selection for integrated modalities continues to improve with better imaging technologies. Image-guided treatment planning and dose-escalation strategies have improved clinical outcomes while simultaneously minimizing toxicity. Alternative fractionation regimens and/or high-dose-rate brachytherapy may prove beneficial with further clarity of the radiobiologic behavior of prostate cancer. Future directions in prostate radiotherapy will use higher doses to more precise intraprostatic targets as defined by advanced imaging.

REFERENCES

Introduction/Imaging for patient selection

1. National Comprehensive Cancer Network. Prostate cancer. In: *National Comprehensive Cancer Network Clinical Practice Guidelines in Oncology*, version 1.2008. Jenkinstown, PA: National Comprehensive Cancer Network, March 2008. Available from: http://www.nccn.org/ (accessed May 2 2008).

2. J. Schiedler, H. Hricak, D. B. Vigneron, *et al.*, Prostate cancer: prediction of extracapsular extension with endorectal MR imaging and three dimensional proton MR spectroscopic imaging. *Radiology*, **213**:2 (1999), 481–8.

3. E. Sala, O. Akin, C. S. Moskowitz, *et al.*, Endorectal MR imaging in the evaluation of seminal vesicle invasion: diagnostic accuracy and multivariate feature analysis. *Radiology*, **238**:3 (2006), 929–37.

4. M. J. Zelefsky, A. Harrison, Neoadjuvant androgen ablation prior to radiotherapy for prostate cancer: reducing the potential morbidity of therapy. *Urology*, **49**:3A Suppl (1997), 38–45.

5. O. Akin, E. Sala, C. S. Moskowitz, *et al.*, Transition zone prostate cancer: metabolic characteristics at ^{1}H MR spectroscopic imaging – initial results. *Radiology*, **239**:3 (2006), 784–92.

6. K. L. Zakian, K. Sircar, H. Hricak, *et al.*, Correlation of proton MR spectroscopic imaging with Gleason score based on step-section pathologic analysis after radical prostatectomy. *Radiology*, **234**:3 (2005), 804–14.

7. T. Mizowaki, G. N. Cohen, A. Y. Fung, *et al.*, Towards integrating functional imaging in the

treatment of prostate cancer with radiation: the registration of the MR spectroscopy imaging to ultrasound/CT images and its implementation in treatment planning. *Int J Radiat Oncol Biol Phys*, **54**:5 (2003), 1558–64.

8. P. L. Jager, W. Vaalburg, J. Prium, *et al.*, Radio-labeled amino acids: basic aspects and clinical applications in oncology. *J Nucl Med*, **42** (2001), 432–45.

9. L. Rinnab, F. M. Mottaghy, N. M. Blumstein, *et al.*, Evaluation of [^11^C]-choline positron-emission/

computed tomography in patients with increasing prostate-specific antigen levels after primary treatment for prostate cancer. *BJU Int*, **100**:4 (2007), 786–93.

10. H. Vees, F. Buchegger, S. Albrecht, *et al.*, ^18^F-choline and/or ^11^C-acetate positron emission tomography: detection of residual or progressive subclinical disease at very low prostate-specific antigen values (<1 ng/ml) after radical prostatectomy. *BJU Int*, **99**:6 (2007), 1415–20.

Prognostic risk stratification

11. A. W. Partin, M. W. Kattan, E. N. Subong, *et al.*, Combination of prostate-specific antigen, clinical stage, and Gleason score to predict pathological stage of localized prostate cancer. A multi-institutional update. *JAMA*, **277** (1997), 1445–51.

12. A. W. Partin, L. A. Mangold, D. M. Lamm, *et al.*, Contemporary update of prostate cancer staging nomograms (Partin tables) for the new millennium. *Urology*, **58** (2001), 843–8.

13. M. Roach 3rd, A. Chen, J. Song, *et al.*, Pretreatment prostate-specific antigen and Gleason score predict the risk of extracapsular extension and the risk of failure following radiotherapy in patients with clinically localized prostate cancer. *Semin Urol Oncol*, **18**:2 (2000), 108–14.

14. A. Diaz, M. Roach 3rd, C. Marquez, *et al.*, Indication for and the significance of seminal vesicle irradiation during 3D conformal radiotherapy for localized prostate cancer. *Int J Radiat Oncol Biol Phys*, **30**:2 (1994), 323–9.

15. M. Roach 3rd, C. Marquez, H. S. You, *et al.*, Predicting the risk of lymph node involvement using the pre-treatment prostate specific antigen and Gleason score in men with clinically localized prostate cancer. *Int J Radiat Oncol Biol Phys*, **28**:1 (1994), 33–7.

16. M. Medica, M. Giglio, F. Germinale, *et al.*, Roach's mathematical equations in predicting pathologic stage in men with clinically localized prostate cancer. *Tumori*, **87** (2001), 130.

17. M. Roach, M. DeSilvio, C. Lawton, *et al.*, Phase III trial comparing whole-pelvic versus prostate-only

radiotherapy and neoadjuvant versus adjuvant combined androgen suppression: Radiation Therapy Oncology Group 9413. *J Clin Oncol*, **21**:10 (2003), 1904–11.

18. A. V. D'Amico, R. Whittington, S. B. Malkowicz, Biochemical outcome after radical prostatectomy, external beam radiation therapy, or interstitial radiation therapy for clinically localized prostate cancer. *JAMA*, **280** (1998), 969–74.

19. A. J. Stephenson, M. W. Kattan. Nomograms for prostate cancer. *BJU Int*, **8**:1 (2006), 39–46.

20. M. W. Kattan, J. A. Eastham, A. M. F. Eastham, *et al.*, A preoperative nomogram for disease recurrence following radical prostatectomy for prostate cancer. *J Natl Cancer Inst*, **90** (1998), 766–71.

21. M. W. Kattan, L. Potters, J. C. Blasko, *et al.*, Pretreatment nomogram for predicting freedom from recurrence after permanent prostate brachytherapy in prostate cancer. *Urology*, **58** (2001), 393–9.

22. M. J. Zelefsky, M. W. Kattan, P. Fearn, *et al.*, Pretreatment nomogram predicting ten-year biochemical outcome of three-dimensional conformal radiotherapy and intensity-modulated radiotherapy for prostate cancer. *Urology*, **70**:2 (2007), 283–7.

23. P. A. Peller, D. C. Young, D. P. Marmaduke, *et al.*, Sextant prostate biopsies. A histopathologic correlation with radical prostatectomy specimens. *Cancer*, **75** (1995), 530–9.

24. I. F. San Francisco, M. M. Regan, A. F. Olumi, *et al.*, Percent of cores positive for cancer is a better preoperative predictor of cancer recurrence after

radical prostatectomy than prostate specific antigen. *J Urol*, **171** (2004), 1492–9.

25. A. C. Spalding, S. Daignault, H. M. Sandler, *et al.*,
    Percent positive biopsy cores as a prognostic factor
    for prostate cancer treated with external beam
    radiation. *Urology*, **69**:5 (2007), 936–40.

26. L. L. Kestin, N. S. Goldstein, F. A. Vicini, *et al.*,
    Percentage of positive biopsy cores as a predictor
    of clinical outcome in prostate cancer treated with
    radiotherapy. *J Urol*, **168**:5 (2002), 1994–9.

27. A. V. D'Amico, D. Schultz, B. Silver, *et al.*, The
    clinical utility of the percent of positive prostate
    biopsies in predicting biochemical outcome follow-
    ing external beam radiation therapy for patients
    with clinically localized prostate cancer. *Int J
    Radiat Oncol Biol Phys*, **49**:3 (2001), 679–84.

28. A. V. D'Amico, M. H. Chen, K. A. Roehl, *et al.*,
    Preoperative PSA velocity and the risk of death
    from prostate cancer after radical prostatectomy.
    N Engl J Med, **351**:2 (2004), 125–35.

29. D. A. Patel, J. C. Presti, Jr., J. E. McNeal, *et al.*,
    Preoperative PSA velocity is an independent prog-
    nostic factor for relapse after radical prostatectomy.
    J Clin Oncol, **23** (2005), 6157–62.

30. D. Palma, S. Tyldesley, P. Blood, *et al.*, Pretreat-
    ment PSA velocity as a predictor of disease out-
    come following radical radiation therapy. *Int J
    Radiat Oncol Biol Phys* **67**:5 (2007), 1425–9.

31. A. V. D'Amico, A. A. Renshaw, B. Sussman, *et al.*,
    Pretreatment PSA velocity and risk of death from
    prostate cancer following external beam radiation
    therapy. *JAMA*, **294** (2005), 440–7.

Definitions of biochemical outcome

32. A. J Stephenson, M. W. Kattan, J. A. Eastham, *et al.*,
    Defining biochemical recurrence of prostate cancer
    after radical prostatectomy: a proposal for a stan-
    dardized definition. *J Clin Oncol*, **24** (2006), 3973.

33. A. J. Stephenson, S. F. Shariat, M. J. Zelefsky, *et al.*,
    Salvage radiotherapy for recurrent prostate cancer
    after radical prostatectomy. *JAMA*, **291** (2004), 1325.

34. American Society for Therapeutic Radiology and
    Oncology Consensus Panel. Consensus statement:
    guidelines for PSA following radiation therapy. *Int
    J Radiat Oncol Biol Phys*, **37** (1997), 1035–41.

35. M. Roach 3rd, G. Hanks, H. Thames, Jr., *et al.*,
    Defining biochemical failure following radiotherapy
    with or without hormonal therapy in men with clini-
    cally localized prostate cancer: recommendations of
    the RTOG-ASTRO Phoenix Consensus Conference.
    Int J Radiat Oncol Biol Phys, **65** (2006), 965–74.

36. M. K. Buyyounouski, A. L. Hanlon, E. M. Horwitz,
    et al., Biochemical failure and the temporal kinetics
    of prostate-specific antigen after radiation therapy
    and hormone therapy. *Int J Radiat Oncol Biol Phys*,
    61:5 (2005), 1291–8.

Choice of local therapy

37. K. Wallace, N. Fleshner, M. Jewett, *et al.*, Impact of
    a multi-disciplinary patient education session on
    accrual to a difficult clinical trial: the Toronto
    experience with the surgical prostatectomy versus
    interstitial radiation intervention trial. *J Clin Oncol*,
    24:25 (2006), 4158–62.

38. PR06 Collaborators. Early closure of a randomized
    controlled trial of three treatment approaches to
    early localised prostate cancer: the MRC PR06 trial.
    BJU Int, **94** (2004), 1400–1.

39. N. Mills, J. Donovan, M. Smith, *et al.*, Perceptions
    of equipoise are crucial to trial participation: a

qualitative study of men in the ProtecT study.
    Control Clin Trials, **24** (2003), 272–82.

40. M. J. Zelefsky, D. A. Kuban, L. B. Levy, *et al.*, Multi-
    institutional analysis of long term outcome for
    stages T1-T2 prostate cancer treatment with per-
    manent seed implantation. *Int J Radiat Oncol Biol
    Phys*, **67**:2 (2007), 327–33.

41. P. A. Kupelian, M. Elshaikh, C. A. Reddy, *et al.*,
    Comparison of the efficacy of local therapies for
    localized prostate cancer in the prostate-specific
    antigen era: a large single institution experience
    with radical prostatectomy and external beam

radiation therapy. *J Clin Oncol*, **20**:16 (2002), 3376–85.

42. P. A. Kupelian, L. Potters, D. Khuntia, *et al.*, Radical prostatectomy, external beam radiotherapy <72 Gy, external beam radiotherapy ≥72 Gy, permanent seed implantation, or combined seeds/ external beam radiotherapy for stage T1-T2

prostate cancer. *Int J Radiat Oncol Biol Phys*, **58**:1 (2004), 25–33.

43. S. G. Fletcher, S. M. Mills, M. E. Smolkin, *et al.*, Case-matched comparison of contemporary radiation therapy to surgery in patients with locally advanced prostate cancer. *Int J Radiat Oncol Biol Phys*, **66**:4 (2006), 1092–9.

External beam radiation therapy

44. G. E. Hanks, A. L. Hanlon, T. E. Schultheiss, *et al.*, Dose escalation with 3D conformal treatment: five year outcomes, treatment optimization and future directions. *Int J Radiat Oncol Biol Phys*, **41** (1998), 501.

45. C. A. Perez, H. K. Lee, A. Georgiou, *et al.*, Technical and tumor-related factors affecting outcome of definitive irradiation for clinically localized carcinoma of the prostate. *Int J Radiat Oncol Biol Phys*, **26** (1993), 581.

46. M. J. Zelefsky, H. Chan, M. Hunt, *et al.*, Long term outcome of high dose intensity modulated radiation therapy for patients with clinically localized prostate cancer. *J Urol*, **176** (2006), 1415–19.

47. O. Cahlon, M. J. Zelefsky, A. Shippy, *et al.*, Ultra-high dose (86.4 Gy) IMRT for localized prostate cancer: toxicity and biochemical outcomes. *Int J Radiat Oncol Biol Phys* 2007 Dec 28 (Epub ahead of print).

48. M. J. Zelefsky, Y. Yamada, Z. Fuks, *et al.*, Long-term results of conformal radiotherapy for prostate cancer: impact of dose escalation on biochemical tumor control and distant metastasis-free survival outcomes. *Int J Radiat Oncol Biol Phys*, 2008 Feb 13 (Epub ahead of print).

49. M. J. Zelefsky, Z. Fuks, M. Hunt, *et al.*, High dose radiation delivered by intensity-modulated conformal radiotherapy improves outcome of localized prostate cancer. *J Urol*, **166** (2001), 876–81.

50. M. J. Zelefsky, E. J. Levin, M. Hunt, *et al.*, Incidence of late rectal and urinary toxicities after three-dimensional conformal radiotherapy and intensity-modulated radiotherapy for localized prostate cancer. *Int J Radiat Oncol Biol Phys*, **70**:4 (2008), 1124–9.

51. P. A. Kupelian, J. C. Buchsbaum, C. A. Reddy, *et al.*, Radiation dose-response in patients with favorable, localized prostate cancer (stage T1-T2, biopsy Gleason ≤6, and pretreatment prostate-specific antigen ≤10). *Int J Radiat Oncol Biol Phys*, **50**:3 (2001), 621–5.

52. W. U. Shipley, L. J. Werhey, J. E. Munzenrider, *et al.*, Advanced prostate cancer: the results of a randomized comparative trial of high dose irradiation boosting with conformal protons compared with conventional dose irradiation using photons alone. *Int J Radiat Oncol Biol Phys*, **32** (1995), 3–12.

53. A. Pollack, G. K. Zagars, G. Starkschall, *et al.*, Prostate cancer radiation dose response: results of the M. D. Anderson phase III randomized trial. *Int J Radiat Oncol Biol Phys*, **53** (2002), 1097–105.

54. A. L. Zietman, M. L. DeSilvio, J. D. Slater, *et al.*, Comparison of conventional-dose vs high-dose conformal radiation therapy in clinically localized adenocarcinoma of the prostate: a randomized controlled trial. *JAMA*, **294** (2005), 1233–9.

55. S. T. H. Peeters, W. D. Heemsbergen, P. C. M. Koper, *et al.*, Dose-response in radiotherapy for localized prostate cancer: results of the Dutch multicenter randomized phase III trial comparing 68 Gy of radiotherapy with 78 Gy. *J Clin Oncol*, **24** (2006), 1990–6.

56. D. P. Dearnaley, M. R. Sydes, J. D. Graham, *et al.*, Escalated-dose versus standard-dose conformal radiotherapy in prostate cancer: first results from the MRC RT01 randomised controlled trial. *Lancet Oncol*, **8**:6 (2007), 475–87.

57. B. Pickett, E. Vigenault, J. Kurthanewicz, *et al.*, Static field intensity modulation to treat a dominant intraprostatic lesion to 90 Gy compared to seven field 3-dimensional radiotherapy. *Int J Radiat Oncol Biol Phys*, **45** (1999), 857–65.

58. G. DeMeerleer, G. Villiers, S. Bral, *et al.*, The magnetic resonance detected intraprostatic lesion in
prostate cancer: planning and delivery of intensity-
modulated radiotherapy. *Radiother Oncol*, **75**:3
(2005), 325–33.
59. D. Pucar, H. Hricak, A Shukla-Dave, *et al.*,
Clinically significant prostate cancer local recurrence
after radiation therapy occurs at the site of primary

tumor: magnetic resonance imaging and step-section
pathology evidence. *Int J Radiat Oncol Biol Phys*,
69:1 (2007), 62–9.
60. A. K. Singh, P. Guion, N. Sears-Crouse, *et al.*,
Simultaneous integrated boost of biopsy proven,
MRI defined dominant intra-prostatic lesions to
95 Gy with IMRT: early results of a phase I NCI
study. *Radiat Oncol*, **2** (2007), 36.

Image-guided radiation therapy

61. D. A. Jaffray, J. H. Siewerdsen, J. W. Wong, *et al.*,
Flat-panel cone-beam computed tomography for
image-guided radiation therapy. *Int J Radiat Oncol
Biol Phys*, **53** (2002), 1337–49.
62. J. Pouliot, A. Bani-Hashemi, J. Chen, *et al.*, Low
dose megavoltage cone-beam CT for radiation therapy. *Int J Radiat Oncol Biol Phys*, **61** (2005), 552–60.

63. O. Gayou, D. S. Parda, M. Johnson, *et al.*, Patient
dose and image quality from mega-voltage computed
tomography imaging. *Med Phys* **34** (2007), 499–506.
64. K. M. Langen, Y. Zhang, R. D. Andrews, *et al.*,
Initial experience with megavoltage (MV) CT guidance for daily prostate alignments. *J Radiat Oncol
Biol Phys*, **62**:5 (2005), 1517–24.

Hypofractionation

65. J. F. Fowler, The radiobiology of prostate cancer
including new aspects of fractionated radiotherapy.
Acta Oncol, **44**:3 (2005), 265–76.
66. S. G. Williams, J. M. Taylor, N. Lium *et al.*, Use of
individual fraction size data from 3756 patients to
directly determine the α/β ratio of prostate cancer.
Int J Radiat Biol Oncol Phys, **68** (2007), 24–33.
67. P. A. Kupelian, V. V. Thakkar, D. Khuntia, *et al.*,
Hypofractionated intensity-modulated radiotherapy (70 Gy at 2.5 Gy per fraction) for localized

prostate cancer: long-term outcome. *Int J Radiat
Oncol Biol Phys*, **63**:5 (2005), 1463–8.
68. E. E. Yeoh, R. H. Holloway, R. J. Fraser, *et al.*,
Hypofractionated versus conventionally fractionated radiation therapy for prostate carcinoma:
updated results of a phase III randomized trial.
Int J Radiat Biol Oncol Phys, **66** (2006), 1072–83.
69. H. Lukka, C. Hayter, J. A. Julian, *et al.*, Randomized
trial comparing two fractionation schedules for
patients with localized prostate cancer. *J Clin
Oncol*, **23** (2005), 6132–8.

Acute/late toxicity

70. Radiation Therapy Oncology Group. Acute
Radiation Morbidity Scoring Criteria. Available at:
http://rtog.org/members/toxicity/acute.html#genito
(accessed May 2, 2008).
71. H. M. Scarpero, J. Fiske, X. Xue, *et al.*, American
Urological Association Symptom Index for lower
urinary tract symptoms in women: correlation with
degree of bother and impact on quality of life.
Urology, **61** (2003), 1118–22.
72. A. S. Sandhu, M. J. Zelefsky, H. J. Lee, *et al.*,
Long term urinary toxicity after 3-dimensional

conformal radiotherapy for prostate cancer in
patients with prior history of transurethral resection. *Int J Radiat Oncol Biol Phys*, **48**:3 (2000),
643–7.
73. A. W. Su, A. B. Jani, Chronic genitourinary and
gastrointestinal toxicity of prostate cancer
patients undergoing pelvic radiotherapy with
intensity-modulated versus 4-field technique.
Am J Clin Oncol, **30**:3 (2007), 215–19.
74. P. C. O'Brien, Radiation injury of the rectum.
Radiother Oncol, **60** (2001), 1–14.

75. J. W. Hopewell, W. Calvo, R. Jaenke, *et al.*, Microvasculature and radiation damage. *Recent Results Cancer Res*, **130** (1993), 1–16.

76. G. J. van der Wielen, W. L. van Putten, L. Incrocci, Sexual function after three-dimensional conformal radiotherapy for prostate cancer: results from a dose-escalation trial. *Int J Radiat Oncol Biol Phys*, **68** (2007), 479–84.

77. S. L. Turner, K. Adams, C. A. Bull, *et al.*, Sexual dysfunction after radical radiation therapy for prostate cancer: a prospective evaluation. *Urology*, **54** (1999), 124–9.

78. J. P. Mulhall, P. Yonover, A. Sethi, *et al.*, Radiation exposure to the corporeal bodies during 3-dimensional conformal radiation therapy for prostate cancer. *J Urol*, **167** (2002), 539–42.

79. S. A. Mangar, M. R. Sydes, H. L. Tucker, *et al.*, Evaluating the relationship between erectile dysfunction and dose received by the penile bulb: using data from a randomized controlled trial of conformal radiation therapy in prostate cancer (MRC RT01, ISRCTN47772397). *Radother Oncol*, **80** (2006), 355–62.

80. M. J. Zelefsky, J. F. Eid, Elucidating the etiology of erectile dysfunction after definitive therapy for prostatic cancer. *Int J Radiat Oncol Biol Phys*, **40** (1998), 129–33.

Brachytherapy

81. K. Wallner, G. Merrick, L. True, *et al.*, ^{125}I versus [103]Pd for low-risk prostate cancer: preliminary PSA outcomes from a prospective randomized multicenter trial. *Int J Radiat Oncol Biol Phys*, **57** (2003), 1297–303.

82. M. J. Zelefsky, G. Cohen, K. L. Zakian, *et al.*, Intraoperative conformal optimization for transperineal prostate implantation using magnetic resonance spectroscopic imaging. *Cancer J*, **6**:4 (2000), 249–55.

83. S. J. DiBiase, K. Hosseinzadeh, R. P. Gullapalli, *et al.*, Magnetic resonance spectroscopic imaging-guided brachytherapy for localized prostate cancer. *Int J Radiat Oncol Biol Phys*, **52**:2 (2002), 429–38.

84. P. Grimm, Clinical results of prostate brachytherapy. Radiological Society of North America Annual Meeting, Chicago 1998.

85. R. G. Stock, N. N. Stone, A. Tabert, *et al.*, A dose response study for I-125 prostate implants. *Int J Radiat Oncol Biol Phys*, **41**:1 (1998), 101–8.

86. M. A. Kollmeier, R. G. Stock, N. Stone, Biochemical outcomes after prostate brachytherapy with 5-year minimal follow-up. Importance of patient selection and implant quality. *Int J Radiat Oncol Biol Phys*, **57** (2003), 645–53.

87. M. J. Zelefsky, D. A. Kuban, L. B. Levy, *et al.*, Multi-institutional analysis of long-term outcome for stages T1-T2 prostate cancer treated with permanent seed implantation. *Int J Radiat Oncol Biol Phys*, **67** (2007), 327–33.

88. S. Nag, D. Beyer, J. Friedland, *et al.*, American Brachytherapy Society (ABS) recommendations for transperineal permanent brachytherapy of prostate cancer. *Int J Radiat Oncol Biol Phys*, **44** (1999), 789–99.

89. M. J. Rivard, W. M. Butler, P. M. Devlin, *et al.*, American Brachytherapy Society (ABS) recommends no change for prostate permanent implant dose prescriptions using iodine-125 or palladium-103. *Brachytherapy*, **6**:1 (2007), 34–7.

90. R. G. Stock, N. N. Stone, J. A. Cesaretti, *et al.*, Biologically effective dose values for prostate brachytherapy: effect on PSA failure and posttreatment biopsy results. *Int J Radiat Oncol Biol Phys*, **64**:2 (2005), 527–33.

HDR

91. A. M. Syed, A. Puthawala, A. Sharma, *et al.*, High-dose-rate brachytherapy in the treatment of carcinoma of the prostate. *Cancer Control*, **8** (2001), 511–21.

92. C. E. Vargas, A. A. Martinez, T. P. Boike, *et al.*, High dose irradiation for prostate cancer via a high-dose-rate brachytherapy boost: results of a

phase I to II study. *Int J Radiat Oncol Biol Phys*, **66**:2 (2006), 416–23.

93. R. M. Galalae, A. A. Martinez, T. Mate, *et al.*, Long-term outcome by risk factors using conformal high-dose-rate brachytherapy (HDR-BT) boost with or without neoadjuvant androgen suppression for localized prostate cancer. *Int J Radiat Oncol Biol Phys*, **58**:4 (2004), 1048–55.

94. G. Kovacs, R. Galalae, Fractionated perineal high-dose-rate temporary brachytherapy combined with external beam radiation in the treatment of localized prostate cancer: is lymph node sampling necessary? *Cancer Radiother*, **7** (2003), 100–6.

95. T. P. Phan, A. M. Syed, A. Puthawala, *et al.*, High dose rate brachytherapy as a boost for the treatment of localized prostate cancer. *J Urol*, **177** (2007), 123–7.

96. I. S. Grills, A. A. Martinez, M. Hollander, *et al.*, High dose rate brachytherapy as prostate cancer monotherapy reduces toxicity compared to low dose rate palladium seeds. *J Urol*, **171**:3 (2004), 1098–104.

97. T. Martin, D. Baltas, R. Kurek, *et al.*, 3-D conformal HDR brachytherapy as monotherapy for localized prostate cancer. A pilot study. *Strahlenther Onkol*, **280** (2004), 225–32.

98. A. A. Martinez, I. Pataki, G. Edmundson, *et al.*, Phase II prospective study of the use of conformal high-dose-rate brachytherapy as monotherapy for the treatment of favorable stage prostate cancer: a feasibility report. *Int J Radiat Oncol Biol Phys*, **49** (2001), 61–9.

Morbidity

99. D. Y. Gelblum, L. Potters, R. Ashley, *et al.*, Urinary morbidity following ultrasound-guided transperineal prostate seed implantation. *Int J Radiat Oncol Biol Phys*, **45** (1999), 59.

100. M. D. Terk, R. G. Stock, N. N. Stone, Identification of patients at increased risk for prolonged urinary retention following radioactive seed implantation of the prostate. *J Urol*, **160** (1998), 1379–82.

101. N. Lee, C. Wuu, R. Brody, *et al.*, Factors predicting for postimplantation urinary retention after permanent prostate brachytherapy. *Int J Radiat Oncol Biol Phys*, **48** (2000), 1457–60.

102. M. D. Thomas, R. Cormack, C. M. Tempany, *et al.*, Identifying the predictors of acute urinary retention following magnetic-resonance-guided prostate brachytherapy. *Int J Radiat Oncol Biol Phys*, **47** (2000), 905–8.

103. J. Crook, M. McLean, C. Catton, *et al.*, Factors influencing risk of acute urinary retention after TRUS-guided permanent prostate seed implantation. *Int J Radiat Oncol Biol Phys*, **52** (2002), 453–60.

104. M. Neill, G. Studer, L. Le, *et al.*, The nature and extent of urinary morbidity in relation to prostate brachytherapy urethral dosimetry. *Brachytherapy*, **6**:3 (2007), 173–9.

105. M. A. Kollmeier, R. G. Stock, J. Cesaretti, *et al.*, Urinary morbidity and incontinence following transurethral resection of the prostate after brachytherapy. *J Urol*, **173** (2005), 808–12.

106. K. M. Snyder, R. G. Stock, S. M. Hong, *et al.*, Defining the risk of developing grade 2 proctitis following ^{125}I prostate brachytherapy using a rectal dose–volume histogram analysis. *Int J Radiat Oncol Biol Phys*, **50** (2001), 335–41.

107. B. H. Han, K. E. Wallner, Dosimetric and radiographic correlates to prostate brachytherapy-related rectal complications. *Int J Cancer*, **96** (2001), 372–8.

108. F. M. Waterman, A. P. Dicker, Probability of late rectal morbidity in ^{125}I prostate brachytherapy. *Int J Radiat Oncol Biol Phys*, **55** (2003), 342–53.

109. J. A. Cesaretti, R. G. Stock, D. P. Atencio, *et al.*, A genetically determined dose-volume histogram predicts for rectal bleeding among patients treated with prostate brachytherapy. *Int J Radiat Oncol Biol Phys*, **68**:5 (2007), 1410–16.

110. Y. Yamada, S. Bhatia, M. Zaider, *et al.*, Favorable clinical outcomes of three-dimensional computer-optimized high-dose-rate prostate brachytherapy in the management of localized prostate cancer. *Brachytherapy*, **5**:3 (2006), 157–64.

111. G. Tsui, C. Gillan, G. Pond, *et al.*, Posttreatment complications of early stage prostate cancer patients: brachytherapy versus three-dimensional conformal radiation therapy. *Cancer J*, **11**:2 (2005), 122–32.

112. G. S. Merrick, W. M. Butler, K. E. Wallner, *et al.*, Erectile function after prostate brachytherapy. *Int J Radiat Oncol Biol Phys*, **62**:2 (2005), 437–47.

113. N. N. Stone, R. G. Stock, Long-term urinary, sexual, and rectal morbidity in patients treated with iodine-125 prostate brachytherapy followed up for a minimum of 5 years. *Urology*, **69**:2 (2007), 338–42.

114. M. Ohebshalom, M. Parker, P. Guhring, *et al.*, The efficacy of sildenafil citrate following radiation therapy for prostate cancer: temporal considerations. *J Urol*, **174**:1 (2005), 258–62.

Combined modality

115. B. J. Davis, T. M. Pisansky, T. M. Wilson, *et al.*, The radial distance of extraprostatic extension of prostate carcinoma: implications for prostate brachytherapy. *Cancer*, **85** (1999), 2630–7.

116. F. A. Critz, K. Levinson, 10-year disease-free survival after simultaneous irradiation for prostate cancer with a focus on calculation methodology. *J Urol*, **172**:6 Pt 1 (2004), 2232–8.

117. H. Ragde, J. C. Blasko, P. D. Grimm, *et al.*, Brachytherapy for clinically localized prostate cancer: results at 7- and 8-year followup. *Semin Surg Oncol*, **13** (1997), 438–43.

118. R. G. Stock, O. Cahlon, J. A. Cesaretti, *et al.*, Combined modality treatment in the management of high risk prostate cancer. *Int J Radiat Oncol Biol Phys*, **59** (2004), 1352–9.

119. J. E. Sylvester, J. C. Blasko, P. D. Grimm, *et al.*, Ten-year biochemical relapse-free survival after external beam radiation and brachytherapy for localized prostate cancer: the Seattle experience. *Int J Radiat Oncol Biol Phys*, **57** (2003), 944–52.

120. M. Dattoli, K. Wallner, L. True, *et al.*, Long term outcomes after treatment with brachytherapy and supplemental conformal radiation for prostate cancer patients having intermediate and high-risk features. *Cancer*, **110**:3 (2007), 551–5.

121. A. M. Singh, G. Gagnon, B. Colliins, *et al.*, Combined external beam radiotherapy and Pd-103 brachytherapy boost improves biochemical failure-free survival in patients with clinically localized prostate cancer: results from a matched pair analysis. *The Prostate*, **62** (2005), 54–60.

122. J. R. Sathya, I. R. Davis, J. A. Julian, *et al.*, Randomized trial comparing iridium implant plus external-beam radiation therapy alone in node-negative locally advanced cancer of the prostate. *J Clin Oncol*, **23**:6 (2005), 1192–9.

123. P. J. Hoskin, K. Motohashi, P. Bownes, *et al.*, High dose rate brachytherapy in combination with external beam radiation therapy in the radical treatment of prostate cancer: initial results of a randomized phase three trial. *Radiother Oncol*, **84** (2007), 114–20.

Hormone therapy

124. M. R. Cooperberg, G. D. Grossfeld, D. P. Lubeck, *et al.*, National practice patterns and time trends in androgen ablation for localized prostate cancer. *J Natl Cancer Inst*, **95** (2003), 981–9.

125. M. B. Garnick, W. R. Fair, D. Botswick, *et al.*, Overview consensus statement. Fifth International Conference on Neoadjuvant Hormonal Therapy for Prostate Cancer. *Mol Urol*, **4**:3 (2000), 89–92.

126. A. L. Zietman, E. A. Prince, B. M. Nafoor, *et al.*, Androgen deprivation and radiation therapy: sequencing studies using the Shionogi in vivo tumor system. *Int J Radiat Oncol Biol Phys*, **38** (1997), 1067.

127. M. Bolla, L. Collette, L. Blank, *et al.*, Long term results with immediate androgen suppression and external irradiation in patients with locally advanced prostate cancer (an EORTC study): a phase III randomized trial. *Lancet*, **360** (2002), 103–8.

128. M. V. Pilepich, K. Winter, C. A. Lawton, *et al.*, Androgen suppression adjuvant to definitive

radiotherapy in prostate carcinoma – long-term results of phase III RTOG 85–31. *Int J Radiat Oncol Biol Phys*, **61**:5 (2005), 1285–90.

129. M. V. Pilepich, K. Winter, M. J. John, *et al.*, Phase III Radiation Therapy Oncology Group (RTOG) 86–10 of androgen deprivation adjuvant to definitive radiotherapy in locally advanced carcinoma of the prostate. *Int J Radiat Oncol Biol Phys*, **50**:5 (2001), 1243–52.

130. G. E. Hanks, T. F. Pajak, A. Porter, *et al.*, Phase III trial of long-term adjuvant androgen deprivation after neoadjuvant hormonal cytoreduction and radiotherapy in locally advanced carcinoma of the prostate: the Radiation Therapy Oncology Group Protocol 92-02. *J Clin Oncol*, **21**:21 (2003), 3972–8.

131. C. A. Lawton, M. DeSilvio, M. Roach, *et al.*, An update of the phase III trial comparing whole pelvic to prostate only radiotherapy and neoadjuvant to adjuvant total androgen suppression: updated analysis of RTOG 94–13, with emphasis on unexpected hormone/radiation interactions. *Int J Radiat Oncol Biol Phys*, **69**:3 (2007), 646–55.

132. J. Laverdiére, A. Nabid, L. D. De Bedoya, *et al.*, The efficacy and sequencing of a short course of androgen suppression on freedom from biochemical failure when administered with radiation

therapy for T2-T3 prostate cancer. *J Urol*, **171**:3 (2004), 1137–40.

133. A. V. D'Amico, J. Manola, M. Loffredo, *et al.*, 6-month androgen suppression plus radiation therapy vs radiation therapy alone for patients with clinically localized prostate cancer. *JAMA*, **292**:7 (2004), 821–7.

134. T. Gransfors, H. Modig, J. Damber, *et al.*, Long-term followup of a randomized study of locally advanced prostate cancer treated with combined orchiectomy and external radiotherapy versus radiotherapy alone. *J Urol*, **176** (2006), 544–7.

135. L. H. Klotz, S. L. Goldenberg, M. Jewett, *et al.*, CUOG randomized trial of neoadjuvant androgen ablation before radical prostatectomy: 36-month post-treatment PSA results. *Urology*, **53**:4 (1999), 757–63.

136. J. W. Denham, A. Steigler, D. S. Lamb, *et al.*, Short term androgen deprivation and radiotherapy for locally advanced prostate cancer: results from the Trans-Tasman Radiation Oncology Group 96.01 randomised controlled trial. *Lancet Oncol*, **6** (2005), 841–50.

137. S. Kumar, M. Shelley, C. Harrison, *et al.*, Neoadjuvant and adjuvant hormone therapy for localized and locally advanced prostate cancer. *Cochrane Database Syst Rev*, **4** (2006), CD006019.

Adjuvant and salvage

138. G. W. Hull, F. Rabbani, F. Abbas, *et al.*, Cancer control with radical prostatectomy alone in 1000 consecutive patients. *J Urol*, **167** (2002), 528–34.

139. C. R. Pound, A. W. Partin, M. A. Eisenberger, *et al.*, Natural history of progression after PSA elevation following radical prostatectomy. *JAMA*, **281**:17 (1999), 1591–7.

140. G. P. Swanson, M. A. Hussey, C. M. Tangen, *et al.*, Predominant treatment failure in postprostatectomy patients is local: analysis of patterns of treatment failure in SWOG 8794. *J Clin Oncol*, **25**:16 (2007), 2225–9.

141. M. Bolla, H. van Poppel, L. Collette, *et al.*, Postoperative radiotherapy after radical prostatectomy: a

randomised controlled trial (EORTC 22911). *Lancet*, **366** (2005), 571–8.

142. I. M. Thompson, Jr., C. M. Tangen, J Paradelo, *et al.*, Adjuvant radiotherapy for pathologically advanced prostate cancer: a randomized clinical trial. *JAMA*, **296** (2006), 2329–35.

143. S. J. Buskirk, T. M. Pisansky, S. E. Schild, *et al.*, Salvage radiotherapy for isolated prostate specific antigen increase after radical prostatectomy: evaluation of prognostic factors and creation of a prognostic scoring system. *J Urol*, **176** (2005), 985–90.

144. S. B. Hayes, A. E. Pollack, Parameters for treatment decisions for salvage radiation therapy. *J Clin Oncol*, **23** (2005), 8204–11.

145. A. K. Lee, A. C. D'Amico, Utility of prostate-specific antigen kinetics in addition to clinical factors in the selection of patients for salvage local therapy. *J Clin Oncol*, **23** (2005), 8192–7.

146. J. D. Cox, M. J. Gallagher, E. H. Hammond, *et al.*, Consensus statements on radiation therapy of prostate cancer: guidelines for prostate re-biopsy after radiation and for radiation therapy with rising prostate-specific antigen levels after radical prostatectomy. American Society for Therapeutic Radiology and Oncology Consensus Panel. *J Clin Oncol*, **17**:4 (1999), 1155.

147. W. R. Lee, G. E. Hanks, A. Hanlon, Increasing prostate-specific antigen profile following definitive radiation therapy for localized prostate cancer: clinical observations. *J Clin Oncol*, **15** (1997), 230–8.

148. F. J. Bianco, Jr., P. T. Scardino, A. J. Stephenson, *et al.*, Long-term oncologic results of salvage radical prostatectomy for locally recurrent prostate cancer after radiotherapy. *Int J Radiat Oncol Biol Phys*, **62** (2005), 448–53.

149. P. L. Nguyen, A. V. D'Amico, A. K. Lee, *et al.*, Patient selection, cancer control, and complications after salvage local therapy for postradiation prostate-specific antigen failure: a systematic review of the literature. *Cancer*, **110** (2007), 1417–28.

150. P. L. Nguyen, M. H. Chen, A. V. D'Amico, *et al.*, Magnetic resonance image-guided salvage brachytherapy after radiation in select men who initially presented with favorable-risk cancer: a prospective phase 2 study. *Cancer*, **110**:7 (2007), 1485–92.

151. K. Lo, R. G. Stock, N. N. Salvage, Prostate brachytherapy following radiotherapy failure. *Int J Radiat Oncol Biol Phys*, **63**:2 Suppl (2005), S290–S291.

152. B. Lee, K. Shinohara, V. Weinberg, *et al.*, Feasibility of high-dose-rate brachytherapy salvage for local prostate cancer recurrence after radiotherapy: the University of California-San Francisco experience. *Int J Radiat Oncol Biol Phys*, **67** (2007), 1106–12.

6

Systemic therapy

Lawrence H. Schwartz and Michael J. Morris

Introduction

In 2005, approximately 128 000 American men were newly diagnosed with recurrent or advanced prostate cancer. For the vast majority of these men, hormonal therapy is the most common first line of treatment [1, 2]. This first-line hormonal treatment is typically surgical or medical castration, which is known as androgen-deprivation therapy. Most patients show a response to androgen-deprivation therapy as manifested by a drop in prostate-specific antigen and/or symptomatic improvement. Ultimately, all patients on androgen-lowering therapy eventually fail this treatment, with the re-emergence of castration-resistant tumors. These tumors may still be susceptible to secondary hormonal therapies that block androgen receptors, decrease the adrenal production of androgens, or increase circulating estrogens. Like androgen-deprivation therapy, secondary hormonal therapies improve symptoms and induce variable decreases in prostate-specific antigen, but they also have not been shown to provide a survival advantage. These patients will ultimately progress despite an initial success with such hormonal maneuvers.

Clinical states model of prostate cancer

The clinical states model of prostate cancer developed at Memorial Sloan-Kettering Cancer Center defines milestones for assessing prognosis and defining therapeutic objectives and outcomes in patients with advanced prostate cancer (Figure 6.1) [3]. The "clinical states" relevant to this review include:
- **Rising PSA after primary therapy**. Those in this state include patients with a rising prostate-specific antigen (PSA) after definitive therapy. It can be reached

Prostate Cancer, eds. Hedvig Hricak and Peter T. Scardino. Published by Cambridge University Press.
© Cambridge University Press 2009.

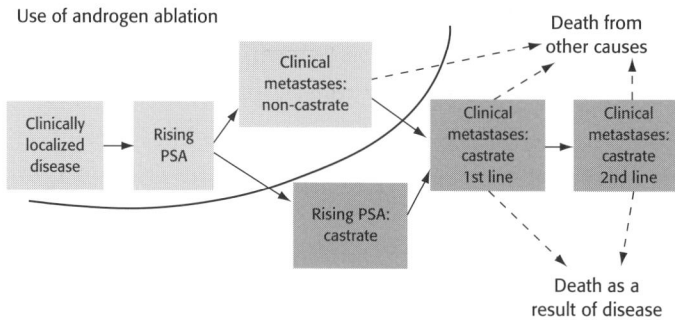

Figure 6.1. Clinical states model of prostate cancer. The clinical states model for prostate cancer outlines the conditions for assessing prognosis and redefining therapeutic options. (Reproduced by permission from H. I. Scher and C. L. Sawyers, Biology of progressive, castration-resistant prostate cancer: directed therapies targeting the androgen-receptor signaling axis. *J Clin Oncol*, 23:32 (2005), 8253–61.)

after radical prostatectomy, radiation therapy, or both surgery and radiation, with or without prior hormone exposure. For these patients, therapy is directed toward preventing progression to the point at which the disease becomes detectable or symptomatic. This is because the state of clinically detectable metastases represents the point at which the probability of death from disease increases significantly, and therefore the patient must confront the morbidity and mortality from the disease more directly. However, in this state, an important distinction is "failure." Defined by a rise in PSA, this does not signify that the patient is destined to die of prostate cancer.

Prostate-specific antigen kinetics

Prostate-specific antigen kinetics can identify patients with a rising PSA after surgery or radiation therapy who are at high risk for metastatic disease and prostate-cancer-specific mortality. In a prospective study of 148 patients with a rising PSA after primary therapy and a PSA doubling time of less than 12 months enrolled on clinical protocols testing alternatives to castration, tumor characteristics at the time of diagnosis, including T stage, Gleason grade, PSA at the time of enrolment on the trial, and PSA doubling time following relapse, were predictive of metastatic progression [8]. Other retrospective analyses have confirmed the prognostic significance of a rapid PSA doubling time of less than 12 months in the rising PSA state [4, 9, 10].

- **Non-castrate metastatic disease (detectable tumor on imaging studies)**. Some patients are diagnosed with metastatic disease, others develop it after a rising PSA, and, in some cases, metastases develop without a rise in PSA. Regardless of the path or the time to clinically detectable metastases, once these patients are identified, the disease has progressed to the point at which the overwhelming cause of death is their prostate cancer and not co-morbid conditions. Even so, the therapeutic objectives for this cohort of patients may vary depending on the extent of disease (single versus diffuse metastases, nodal versus bone spread), on whether the patient is symptomatic, and what the symptoms actually are. Once the transition to clinical metastatic disease has occurred, different factors (related to the above) than those identified for the state of a rising PSA may predict for death from disease.

- **Metastatic disease after castration**. As is the case in other states, patients who are progressing after castration also have a range of prognoses. It is known that the molecular profile of a castration-resistant metastatic lesion differs from that of a non-castrate tumor in the primary site. Once again, by considering the disease in the context of states, any clinical, historical or biologic factor can be evaluated in the context of the history of the disease and its place, or not, in the management defined. This shows the importance of "resetting the clock" as the disease evolves in the individual patient.

The challenge is to target patients for treatment before metastasis, so that the risk of death from prostate cancer does not exceed that from death of other causes [4].

Androgen-deprivation therapy

Androgen-deprivation therapy consists of either medical or surgical intervention. It has long been the standard of care for patients with metastatic disease. The advantages of androgen-deprivation therapy were first seen in a large study conducted by the Veterans Administration research group in the 1960s. In the end, all patients in the placebo arm had crossed over to the treatment arm due to the overwhelming palliative benefits observed with androgen-deprivation therapy [5]. In 1997, another study performed in the United Kingdom demonstrated that androgen-deprivation therapy significantly reduces morbidity associated with metastatic disease such as spinal cord compression, ureteral obstruction, and bone pain [6]. Treatment options to induce androgen depletion include orchiectomy or drugs that lower serum testosterone (such as gonadotropin-releasing hormone (GnRH) analogs and estrogens) alone or with non-steroidal anti-androgens (flutamide, bicalutamide and nilutamide). Tumor flare can occur due to paradoxical increases in testosterone during some initial treatments with GnRH agonists [11]. As such, anti-androgens are sometimes used to block this response, particularly in patients with bone disease or possible spinal cord compromise/involvement as seen on imaging. Continuous combined androgen blockade with a GnRH analog and anti-androgen has at best a modest survival advantage over GnRH analog monotherapy in some meta-analyses [12, 13].

Androgen-deprivation therapy is associated with numerous side-effects, including hot flashes, decreased libido, mood changes, metabolic changes, and osteopenia, and increased risk of bone fracture [15]. Another possible side-effect is the risk of bone fracture in patients treated with androgen-deprivation therapy. The increased risk for fracture with androgen-deprivation therapy is significant, even when the data are adjusted for age and stage of the cancer.

Timing of hormone therapy

For patients with a rising PSA after primary treatment with or without evidence of metastases and a non-castrate level of serum testosterone, hormone therapy has been used to slow the progression of disease. The timing of treatment is controversial since a biochemical PSA relapse can precede the physical manifestation of disease by a median of 8 years [4]. Any survival advantage that may arise from early treatment needs to be assessed in light of the potential side-effects of therapy, which can include gynecomastia, weight gain, impotency, a decline in skeletal muscle mass, fatigue, hot flashes, changes in personality, depression, anemia, and loss of bone density over time [7]. Prostate-specific antigen kinetics have been used to predict patients at high risk for cancer-specific mortality who might benefit from early treatment of their disease [8, 9, 10].

Continuous versus intermittent hormone therapy

Intermittent androgen-deprivation therapy has been examined in an effort to delay the development of castration resistance and minimize toxicity. This is a cyclic process whereby androgen-depletion therapy is stopped and then resumed when tumor regrowth reaches a pre-determined level. Pre-clinical models suggest that this approach may prolong the time of sensitivity to changes in androgen levels and reduce the number of cells showing a castration-resistant phenotype [16, 17]. Building on phase II data [18], there are currently several ongoing large-scale phase III trials addressing whether intermittent hormone therapy is superior, equivalent, or inferior to more traditional continuous treatment [19, 20]. As a result, this approach remains experimental at this time and guidelines for starting and stopping treatment are not yet established.

Secondary hormonal interventions

Additional hormonal manipulations for patients who progress through castrating therapy include the use of anti-androgens, ketoconazole, and estrogens. Some patients on long-term hormone therapy experience a decline in PSA following discontinuation of an anti-androgen. This "anti-androgen withdrawal" response can occur in up to 30% of patients and can be associated with alterations of the androgen receptor (AR) [21, 22, 23, 24]. Ultimately, after failure of the anti-androgen withdrawal, androgen-independent cancers are still susceptible to secondary hormonal treatments, which are often able to induce PSA and radiographic responses, and may even provide symptomatic clinical improvement. None of these agents has been shown to lengthen survival, however, and each is associated with mild to moderate toxicities that have the potential to have a negative impact on quality of life. A study of 78 patients treated with ketoconazole therapy identified variables that are predictive of duration of response to treatment and also overall survival [25]. In a proportional hazards model, log of baseline PSA, duration of androgen-deprivation therapy, and percentage PSA decrease on ketoconazole were predictive of response duration, whereas log of baseline PSA, bone scan stage, and percentage PSA decrease were significant predictors of survival. Interestingly, when broken down into quartiles, a PSA response of 75%–100% was predictive of longer survival when compared to the other quartiles, while a response of 50%–74% was not. This may suggest a better overall prognosis for patients who have large biochemical responses to ketoconazole therapy. Importantly, this study provides predictive and prognostic information to patients who are reaching an increasingly uncertain point in their disease course.

Chemotherapy

Patients with progression of disease despite castrate levels of testosterone are candidates for cytotoxic chemotherapy. Until 2004, mitoxantrone and prednisone were approved for the treatment of prostate cancer on the basis of improvement in quality of life but no significant improvement in overall survival [28, 29, 30]. More recently, two randomized clinical trials (Southwest Oncology Group 9916 and TAX327) have demonstrated a 2-3-month survival and quality-of-life benefit for patients treated with docetaxel and prednisone on an every-21st-day schedule [31, 32].

Unfortunately this approach is not curative and there is controversy over the optimal timing and duration of administration.

Targeted therapy: androgen receptor signaling axis

Recent clinical observations, molecular profiling studies, and laboratory work support the concept of androgen receptor signaling as a mechanism of oncogenic growth even in patients with castration-resistant disease [33, 34, 35, 36, 37]. Thus, novel AR targeting therapies are focused on inhibiting ligand, AR activation, and the AR protein itself. For example, abivaterone is an irreversible inhibitor of 17α-hydroxyluse/C17,20 lyase, thereby blocking androgen synthesis, and is presently in phase III trials. Novel anti-androgens, designed to maximize antagonistic and minimize agonistic actions, are also in testing at present. In addition, Hsp90 chaperone inhibitors (17AAG, DMAG) that induce protein degradation and histone deacetylase inhibitors (SAHA, LBH589) are strategies being tested to target the AR protein itself.

Palliative therapy

Radioactive isotopes such as samarium-153 and strontium-89 provide palliation of symptomatic bone disease. Again, however, there has been no definitive proven improvement in survival and the isotopes have been associated with treatment-related myelotoxicity [38]. With samarium-153, a single dose of 1.0 mCi/kg of 37 MBq/kg ^{153}Sm-EDTMP provided relief from the pain associated with bony metastases. Pain relief was observed within 1 week of administration and persisted until at least week 16 in the majority of patients who did respond to this therapy [39]. With strontium-89, as many as 80% of selected patients with painful osteoblastic bony metastases from prostate or breast cancer may experience some pain relief following its administration. In addition, as many as 10% or more may become pain free. The duration of clinical response may average 3–6 months in some cases [40]. Zoledronic acid is a bisphosphonate, which has been shown to reduce the frequency of skeletal events in hormone-refractory prostate cancer patients with bone metastases. In a placebo-controlled study of 643 men, patients treated with zoledronic acid had a lower incidence of skeletal-related events than did those in the placebo group, regardless of the skeletal-related events prior to entry into the study [41].

Summary

Metastatic prostate cancer represents a challenge for the oncologist and other treating physicians. There is a need to accurately define when treatment intervention should begin and what the appropriate regimen is. While classic androgen-deprivation therapy remains a mainstay for treatment, there are modifications and other options such as taxane-based chemotherapy and zoledromic acid that are increasingly being utilized, to reduce the morbidity and mortality of this disease. Novel targeted therapies offer the promise of even more effective treatments in the future.

REFERENCES

1. American Cancer Society. Cancer Facts and Figures 2005. Atlanta, GA: American Cancer Society; 2005.

2. J. F. Ward, J. W. Moul, Treating the biochemical recurrence of prostate cancer after definitive primary therapy. *Clin Prostate Cancer*, **4** (2005), 38–44.

3. H. I. Scher, G. Heller, Clinical states in prostate cancer: towards a dynamic model of disease progression. *Urology*, **55** (2000), 323–7.

4. C. R. Pound, A. W. Partin, M. A. Eisenberger, *et al.*, Natural history of progression to metastases and death from prostate cancer in men with PSA recurrence following radical prostatectomy. *JAMA*, **281** (1999), 1591–7.

5. D. P. Byar, Proceedings: The Veterans Administration Cooperative Urological Research Group's studies of cancer of the prostate. *Cancer*, **32**:5 (1973), 1126–30.

6. The Medical Research Council Prostate Cancer Working Party Investigators Group, Immediate versus deferred treatment for advanced prostatic cancer: initial results of the Medical Research Council trial. *Br J Urol*, **79** (1997), 235–46.

7. J. M. Holzbeierlein, E. P. Castle, J. B. Thrasher, Complications of androgen-deprivation therapy for prostate cancer. *Clin Prostate Cancer*, **2** (2003), 147–52.

8. S. F. Slovin, A. S. Wilton, G. Heller, *et al.*, Time to detectable metastatic disease in patients with rising prostate-specific antigen values following surgery or radiation therapy. *Clin Cancer Res*, **11** (2005), 8669–73.

9. M. J. Zelefsky, L. Ben-Porat, H. I. Scher, *et al.*, Outcome predictors for the increasing PSA state after definitive external-beam radiotherapy for prostate cancer. *J Clin Oncol*, **23** (2005), 826–31.

10. A. J. Stewart, H. I. Scher, M. H. Chen, *et al.*, Prostate-specific antigen nadir and cancer specific mortality following antigen failure. *J Clin Oncol*, **23** (2005), 6556–60.

11. J. Waxman, A. Man, W. F. Hendry, *et al.*, Importance of early tumour exacerbation in patients treated with long acting analogues of gonadotrophin releasing hormone for advanced prostatic cancer. *Br Med J*, **291** (1985), 1387–8.

12. J. F. Caubet, T. D. Tosteson, E. W. Dong, *et al.*, Maximum androgen blockade in advanced prostate cancer: a meta-analysis of published randomized controlled trials using nonsteroidal antiandrogens. *Urology*, **49** (1997), 71–8.

13. D. J. Samson, J. Seidenfeld, B. Schmitt, *et al.*, Systematic review and meta-analysis of monotherapy compared with combined androgen blockade for patients with advanced prostate carcinoma. *Cancer*, **95** (2002), 361–76.

14. C. J. Tyrrell, A. V. Kaisary, P. Iversen, *et al.*, A randomised comparison of 'Casodex' (bicalutamide) 150 mg monotherapy versus castration in the treatment of metastatic and locally advanced prostate cancer. *Eur Urol*, **33** (1998), 447–56.

15. N. Sharifi, J. L. Gulley, W. L. Dahut, Androgen deprivation therapy for prostate cancer. *JAMA*, **294** (2005), 238–44.

16. K Akakura, N. Bruchovsky, S. L. Goldenberg, *et al.*, Effects of intermittent androgen suppression on androgen-dependent tumors. Apoptosis and serum prostate-specific antigen. *Cancer*, **71** (1993), 2782–90.

17. A. J. Pantuck, A. Zisman, A. S. Belldegrun, Gene therapy for prostate cancer at the University of California, Los Angeles: preliminary results and future direction. *World J Urol*, **18** (2000), 143–7.

18. G. D. Grossfeld, P. R. Carroll, Prostate cancer early detection: a clinical perspective. *Epidemiol Rev*, **23** (2001), 173–80.

19. M. H. Rashid, U. B. Chaudhary, Intermittent androgen deprivation therapy for prostate cancer. *Oncologists*, **9** (2004), 295–301.

20. J. L. Wright, C. S. Higano, D. W. Lin, Intermittent androgen deprivation: clinical experience and practical applications. *Urol Clin North Am*, **33** (2006), 167–79.

21. W. K. Kelly, H. I. Scher, Prostate specific antigen decline after antiandrogen withdrawal: the flutamide withdrawal syndrome. *J Urol*, **149** (1993), 607–9.

22. H. I. Scher, G. J. Kolvenbag, The antiandrogen withdrawal syndrome in relapsed prostate cancer. *Eur Urol*, **31**:Suppl 2 (1997), 3–7; discussion 24–7.

23. H. I. Scher, W. K. Kelly, Flutamide withdrawal syndrome: its impact on clinical trials in hormone-refractory prostatic cancer. *J Clin Oncol*, **11** (1993), 1566–72.

24. H. Miyamoto, M. M. Rahman, C. Chang, Molecular basis for the antiandrogen withdrawal syndrome. *J Cell Biochem*, **91** (2004), 3–12.

25. M. Scholz, M. Jennrich, R. Strum, *et al.*, Long-term outcome for men with androgen independent prostate cancer treated with ketoconazole and hydrocortisone. *J Urol*, **173** (2005), 1947–52.

26. C. R. Pound, A. W. Partin, J. I. Epstein, *et al.*, Prostate-specific antigen after anatomic radical retropubic prostatectomy. Patterns of recurrence and cancer control. *Urol Clin North Am*, **24** (1997), 395–406.

27. M. S. Katz, M. J. Zelefsky, E. S. Venkatraman, *et al.*, Predictors of biochemical outcome with salvage conformal radiotherapy after radical prostatectomy for prostate cancer. *J Clin Oncol*, **21** (2003), 483–9.

28. M. J. Moore, D. Osoba, K. Murphy, *et al.*, Use of palliative end points to evaluate the effects of mitoxantrone and low-dose prednisone in patients with hormonally resistant prostate cancer. *J Clin Oncol*, **12** (1994), 689–94.

29. I. F. Tannock, D. Osoba, M. R. Stockler, *et al.*, Chemotherapy with mitoxantrone plus prednisone or prednisone alone for symptomatic hormone-resistant prostate cancer: a Canadian randomized trial with palliative end points. *J Clin Oncol*, **14** (1996), 1756–64.

30. P. W. Kantoff, S. Halabi, M. Conaway, *et al.*, Hydrocortisone with or without mitoxantrone in men with hormone-refractory prostate cancer: results of the cancer and leukemia group B 9182 study. *J Clin Oncol*, **18** (1999), 2506–13.

31. I. F. Tannock, R. deWit, W. R. Berry, *et al.*, Docetaxel plus prednisone or mitoxantrone plus prednisone for advanced prostate cancer. *New Engl J Med*, **351** (2004), 1502–12.

32. D. P. Petrylak, C. M. Tangen, M. H. Hussain, *et al.*, Docetaxel and estramustine compared with mitoxantrone and prednisone for advanced refractory prostate cancer. *New Engl J Med*, **351** (2004), 1513–20.

33. H. I. Scher, C. L. Sawyers, Biology of progressive, castration-resistant prostate cancer: directed therapies targeting the androgen-receptor signaling axis. *J Clin Oncol*, **23** (2005), 8253–61.

34. M. E. Grossmann, H. Huang, D. J. Tindall, Androgen receptor signaling in androgen-refractory prostate cancer. *J Natl Cancer Inst*, **93** (2001), 1687–97.

35. R. Berger, P. G. Febbo, P. K. Majumder, *et al.*, Androgen-induced differentiation and tumorigenicity of human prostate epithelial cells. *Cancer Res*, **64** (2004), 8867–75.

36. L. Cheng, C. X. Pan, X. J. Yang, *et al.*, Small cell carcinoma of the urinary bladder: a clinicopathologic analysis of 64 patients. *Cancer*, **101** (2004), 957–62.

37. G. Han, G. Buchanan, M. Ittmann, *et al.*, Mutation of the androgen receptor causes oncogenic transformation of the prostate. *Proc Natl Acad Sci USA*, **102** (2005), 1151–60.

38. A. N. Serafini, Therapy of metastatic bone pain. *J Nucl Med*, **42** (2001), 895–906.

39. A. N. Serafini, S. J. Houston, J. Resche, *et al.*, Palliation of pain associated with metastatic bone cancer using samarium-153 lexidronam: a double-blind placebo-controlled clinical trial. *J Clin Oncol*, **16** (1998), 1574–81.

40. R. G. Robinson, D. F. Preton, M. Schiefelbein, *et al.*, Stronium 89 therapy for the palliation of pain due to osseous metastases. *JAMA*; **274** (1995), 420–4.

41. F. Saad, D. M. Gleason, R. Murray, *et al.*, A randomized, placebo-controlled trial of zoledronic acid in patients with hormone-refractory metastatic prostate carcinoma. *J Natl Cancer Inst*, **94** (2002), 1458–68.

7

Transrectal ultrasound imaging of the prostate

Mark L. Pe, Edouard J. Trabulsi, and Ethan J. Halpern

Introduction

Over 186 000 men will be diagnosed with prostate cancer in 2008, accounting for approximately 25% of newly diagnosed cancers in the US male population [1]. In the era of prostate-specific antigen (PSA) screening, prostate cancer has undergone a significant downward stage and risk migration, with an increasing proportion of low-risk, organ-confined disease being diagnosed [2].

Transrectal ultrasound (TRUS) imaging of the prostate has played a fundamental role in the diagnosis, staging, and management of prostate cancer. During the past decade, technological innovations have improved the detection of prostate cancer. Clinical research continues to focus on methods to accurately and efficiently identify clinically significant neoplasms. In this chapter, we describe contemporary techniques for TRUS imaging and detection of prostate cancer.

Sonographic anatomy

Accurate evaluation and assessment of the prostate during TRUS requires a fundamental understanding of the underlying sonographic anatomy and histopathology of the gland. The prostate gland is anatomically divided into zones, originally described by McNeal in 1981 [3]. Zonal architecture of the prostate is defined anatomically with respect to glandular drainage into the prostatic urethra, and consists of a total of four glandular zones – the periurethral zone, the transition zone, the central zone, and the peripheral zone – as well as the anterior fibromuscular stroma. The anterior fibromuscular stroma does not contain any glands, whereas the peripheral zone comprises approximately 70% of the glandular tissue in the normal prostate.

Prostate Cancer, eds. Hedvig Hricak and Peter T. Scardino. Published by Cambridge University Press.
© Cambridge University Press 2009.

Benign prostatic hyperplasia (BPH) commonly originates in the transition zone, while most cancers in the prostate arise from the peripheral zone. The zonal architecture is defined by histopathology, but these various zones are not sonographically distinct. Sonographically, an inner gland consisting of the periurethral and transition zones can usually be distinguished from an outer gland composed of the central and peripheral zones. The outer gland normally appears homogeneously echogenic. The inner gland is less echogenic and is commonly heterogeneous in echotexture, likely reflecting changes in the prostate caused by BPH. The surgical capsule demarcates the inner and outer glands and serves as a plane of enucleation for suprapubic prostatectomy. Calcifications known as corpora amylacea are often deposited along the surgical capsule, causing it to appear sonographically hyperechoic.

The seminal vesicles extend superiorly and posteriorly from the base of the prostate. These paired structures demonstrate a smooth, lobulated, and symmetrical appearance, tapering in diameter as they approach the base of the prostate in the midline. Upon transverse imaging just above the prostate, the ampulla of each vas deferens can be seen superior to the ipsilateral seminal vesicle. An ejaculatory duct is formed on each side of midline by the union of the seminal vesicle with the vas deferens.

Histopathology

The glandular architecture of the prostate changes with age as a result of BPH. Glandular alterations of BPH are most prominent in the inner gland, generally arising from the transition zone, and to a lesser extent from the periurethral zone [4]. The hypertrophied inner gland may have a more heterogeneous and nodular appearance, often distorting and compressing the outer gland tissue. Hypoechoic BPH nodules can often be mistaken for lesions of prostate cancer. In addition, dystrophic calcifications and cystic changes may be interspersed throughout the inner gland. Benign prostatic hyperplasia is associated with increased blood flow to the inner gland of the prostate. The typical radial pattern of blood flow found by Doppler evaluation of the normal prostate may be distorted by the enlarged inner gland of BPH. Focal changes in the Doppler pattern with BPH may mimic the Doppler pattern seen in prostate cancer.

In contrast to BPH, which typically develops within the transition zone of the inner gland, prostate adenocarcinoma is predominantly found in the peripheral zone of the outer gland [5]. Based upon examination of radical prostatectomy specimens the likely location of origin of prostatic adenocarcinoma is the peripheral zone in 68% of cases, the central zone in 8% and the transition zone in 24% of cases [6]. Indeed, 85% of prostate cancer is multifocal in origin, with a growth pattern oriented along the thin fibrous capsule in an oblong shape [7, 8]. Prostate cancer is pathologically defined by a loss of glandular architecture, along with increased cellular and microvessel density. The Gleason grading system for prostate cancer is based upon changes in the normal glandular architecture. These microscopic changes can be targeted through various sonographic techniques to aid in the detection of prostatic malignancy. The loss of glandular architecture, particularly in high-grade cancers, causes a reduction in acoustically reflective interfaces, and results in the hypoechoic mass that is characteristic of prostate cancer. Increased cellular density is associated with increased firmness of prostate tissue and decreased tissue elasticity that can be demonstrated by real-time elastography [9]. Prostate cancer results in increased angiogenesis and increased microvessel density. Color and power Doppler can be used to assess blood flow patterns within larger vessels in the prostate, while contrast-enhanced ultrasound may be used to demonstrate the microvessel architecture perfusing a malignant neoplasm.

Ultrasound imaging of the prostate

Patient preparation and positioning

Administration of antibiotic prophylaxis prior to TRUS biopsy of the prostate is considered standard of care, but there is some debate concerning the duration of the antibiotic course. Studies have shown that single-dose fluoroquinolone has a similar efficacy to a 3-day course [10]. At our institution, we prescribe a 3-day course of an oral fluoroquinolone, and provide the first dose approximately 30–60 min prior to biopsy. If a patient is at risk of developing endocarditis or infection of a prosthesis, we generally pre-medicate with intravenous ampicillin and gentamicin. If the patient has an allergy to penicillin, vancomycin is administered instead of ampicillin. He then finishes a 3-day course of fluoroquinolone post-biopsy.

Approximately 1 h prior to the procedure we have patients take an enema to empty the rectal vault. We feel that this provides a better ultrasound image, while reducing the probability of bacterial infection.

In many centers, patients are positioned in the left-lateral decubitus position. However, because patient positioning alters the blood flow distribution of the prostate, we prefer positioning the patient in the dorsal lithotomy position when Doppler and contrast-enhanced imaging are used to visualize blood flow patterns [11].

A local prostatic block using 2% lidocaine is used to provide analgesia. This is administered using a 22-gauge spinal needle through the biopsy channel of the ultrasound probe. Under TRUS guidance, 5 ml of 2% lidocaine is injected on each side of the midline at the junction of the seminal vesicle with the prostate.

Conventional gray-scale ultrasound

Once the patient is positioned, the ultrasound probe is lubricated and gently inserted. Brightness (gain control) is set such that the peripheral zone is medium gray. Volumetric measurements are calculated based upon transverse, anterior-posterior, and longitudinal diameters from transverse and sagittal images. For the purpose of these calculations, the prostate is approximated by a prolate ellipse and prostate volume is calculated by the following formula: :/6 × (transverse diameter) × (anterior–posterior diameter) × (longitudinal diameter).

Diagnostic imaging of the prostate is performed in both transverse and sagittal planes. Transverse imaging of the prostate allows for a systematic comparison of the right and left sides of the gland and aids in the identification of any asymmetry in contour, echogenicity, tissue elasticity, or blood flow distribution (Figure 7.1). Abnormalities on transverse imaging should be confirmed in the sagittal imaging plane. Any lesion should be documented and sampled by biopsy under ultrasound guidance.

In addition to evaluation for focal abnormality within the prostate, ultrasound should be used for surveillance of the outer borders of the gland and the seminal vesicles. Disruption of the white, hyperechoic periprostatic fat plane suggests extracapsular extension of the tumor. Cancer infiltrating the seminal vesicles may be seen as asymmetry between the two vesicles or as loss of medial tapering. Lastly, one must be gentle when manipulating the ultrasound probe; excessive pressure may compress the gland and lead to false detection of irregular bulges, changes in the Doppler pattern, and more discomfort to the patient.

Prostate cancer is often difficult to detect through conventional gray-scale imaging alone. Prostate cancer is typically described as a hypoechoic lesion on sonography [12]. However, approximately 40% of malignant lesions are isoechoic and an additional 1% may appear hyperechoic [13]. Furthermore, prostate cancer differs from other visceral neoplasms in that it is frequently multifocal in origin [7].

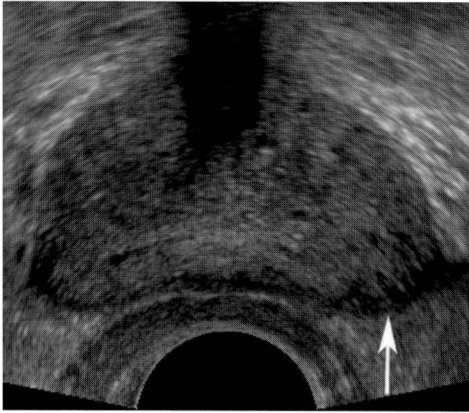

(a)

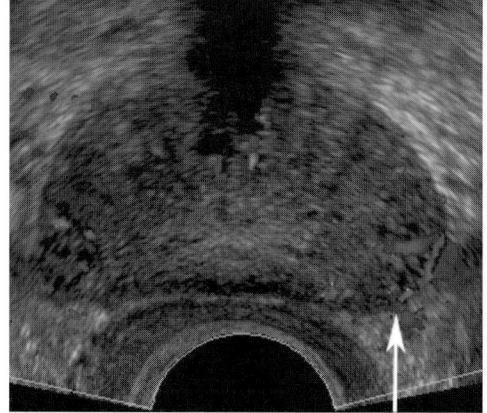

(b)

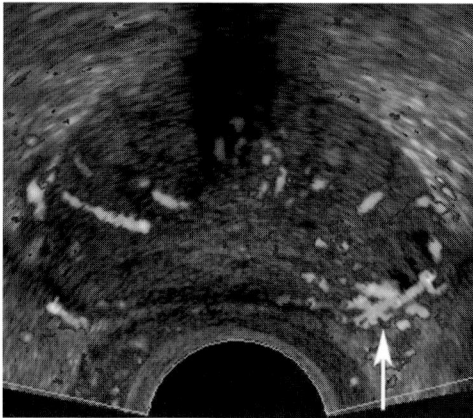

(c)

Figure 7.1. Gleason 6 prostate adenocarcinoma. Transverse images through the midgland of the prostate. (a) Conventional gray-scale demonstrates a slightly hypoechoic peripheral rim along the left midgland (arrow), but no definite focal mass. (b) Color Doppler demonstrates increased flow to this area, corresponding to the area of cancer. (c) Power Doppler shows increased flow to the left midgland area as well, confirming the focus of hypervascularity. See color plate section for full color versions of parts (b) and (c).

Benign processes that occur within the prostate may mimic the gray-scale characteristics of malignancy, further complicating the detection of prostate cancer. Benign prostatic hyperplasia nodules, although classically found in the transition zone of the inner gland, are present in the outer gland in up to 18.5% of prostate specimens [14]. Furthermore, BPH originating in the inner gland can compress and even protrude into the outer gland. Prostatitis is another benign condition that may imitate the gray-scale appearance of prostate cancer. Patients with prostatitis may present with hypoechoic lesions or heterogeneous areas in the outer gland that are often confused for malignancy. Other less common findings that may mimic the sonographic appearance of prostate cancer include infarction and lymphoma [15, 16].

Given the diverse presentation of prostate cancer, its multifocality, and the similarity of its gray-scale appearance to that of other prostatic conditions, conventional gray-scale ultrasound is not adequate to provide accurate detection of cancer. In fact, gray-scale sonography offers little advantage compared to digital rectal examination for discovering cancer [17].

Color and power Doppler ultrasound

Ultrasound Doppler identifies the presence of blood flow within the prostate gland by detecting a frequency/phase shift in the signal reflected from blood traveling through the vasculature. Prostate cancer is associated with increased vascularity and local angiogenesis. Ultrasound imaging of the prostate using color Doppler to detect blood flow patterns has been shown to be a useful adjunct to increase the sensitivity of detecting prostate cancer [18, 19]. In addition, tumor stage and grade as well as risk of recurrence of disease demonstrate a positive correlation with increased color Doppler signal [20].

Power Doppler is a relatively new technique that is often used in conjunction with color Doppler. Power Doppler differs from color Doppler in that it does not show direction of flow. Rather, power Doppler detects the presence of blood flow, and represents the amplitude of the Doppler signal. Power Doppler can enhance the identification of blood flow in areas of relatively diminished or low-velocity perfusion. The addition of power Doppler has been shown to increase sensitivity for cancer detection compared to color Doppler, and is another tool that can be used to augment the identification of cancer [21, 22].

Doppler imaging of the prostate in the transverse plane allows for identification of areas of blood flow asymmetry when comparing both sides of the prostatic parenchyma. Normal prostatic flow is typically characterized as a radial and evenly distributed pattern. Areas of increased perfusion secondary to malignancy will have a more irregular and asymmetric distribution (Figures 7.1, 7.2 and 7.3). Asymmetric changes in the Doppler flow pattern should be used as an adjunct to changes in the gray-scale pattern for the detection of prostate cancer.

Detection of prostate cancer with Doppler imaging is complicated by benign conditions that may alter the normal blood flow pattern of the prostate. For example, BPH nodules demonstrate increased flow patterns. While most lesions of BPH are located in the inner gland, BPH nodules within or protruding into the outer gland will display increased perfusion as well. Benign prostate hyperplasia within the transition zone of the inner gland often compresses and deforms the

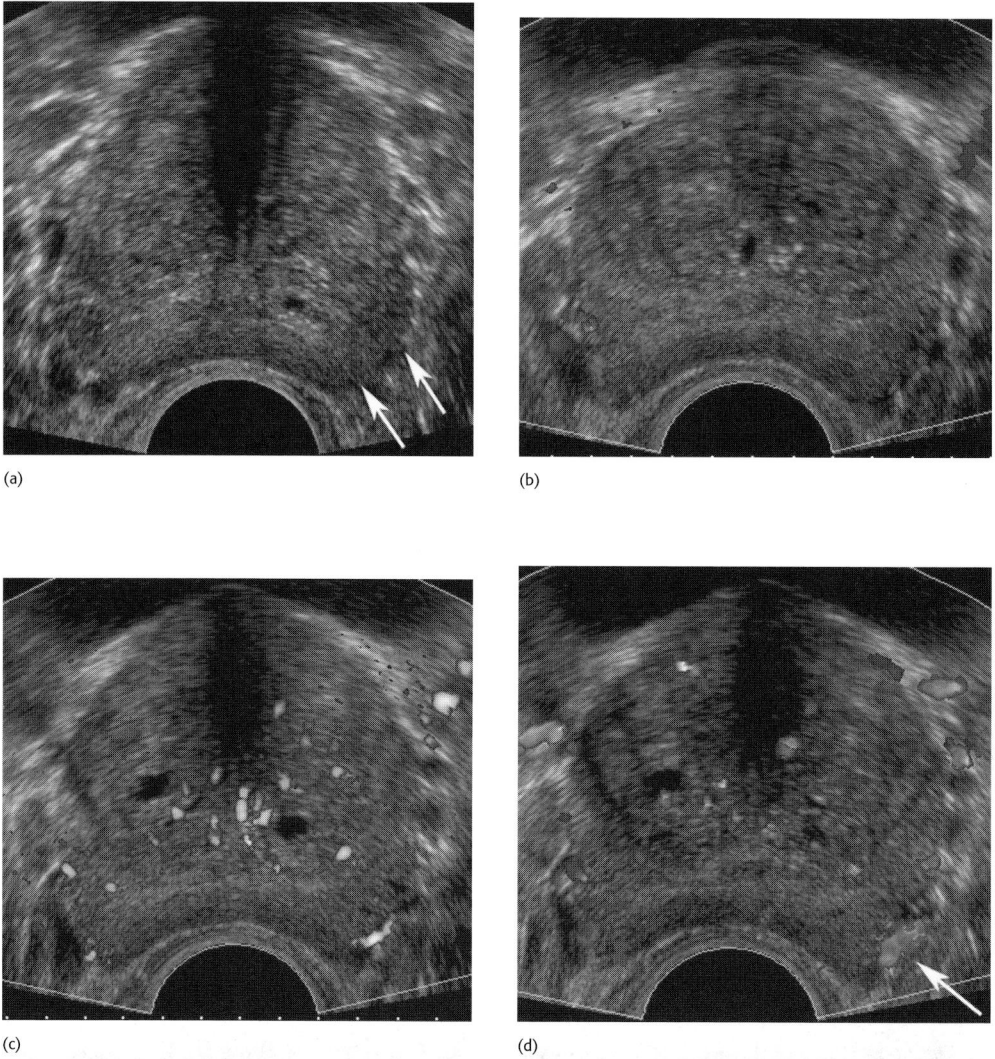

Figure 7.2. Gleason 6 prostate adenocarcinoma. Transverse images through the midgland of the prostate. (a) Conventional gray-scale image demonstrates an enlarged gland, compatible with benign prostatic hyperplasia (BPH), with a subtle hypoechoic appearance along the left outer gland (arrows). Color (b) and power (c) Doppler demonstrate blood flow within the enlarged inner gland and along the neurovascular bundles at the posterolateral aspect of the prostate, but there is no Doppler evidence of malignancy. Contrast-enhanced color (d) and power (e) Doppler show increased blood flow to capsular vessels in the left midgland (arrows). (f) Contrast-enhanced harmonic gray scale with intermittent imaging demonstrates asymmetric parenchymal enhancement of microvessels corresponding to the site of cancer at targeted biopsy (arrows). See color plate section for full color versions of parts (b), (c), (d), (e).

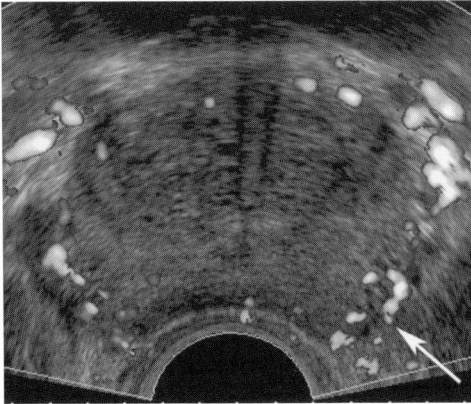

(e)

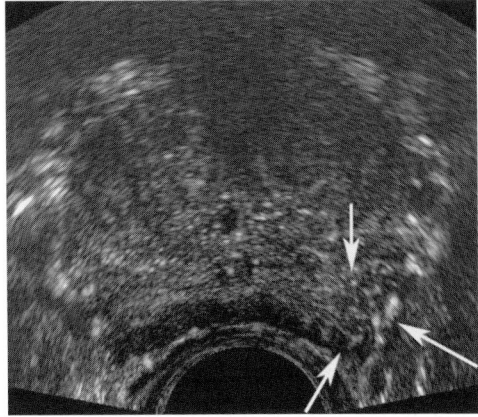

(f)

Figure 7.2. (cont.)

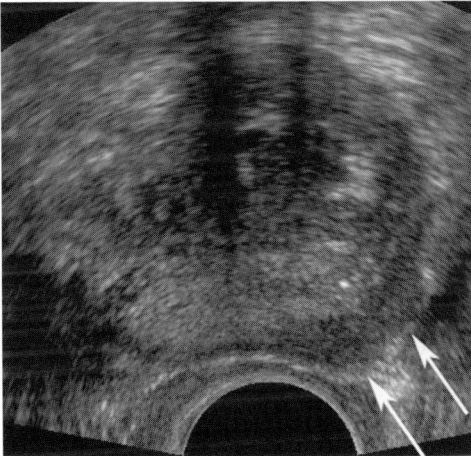

(a)

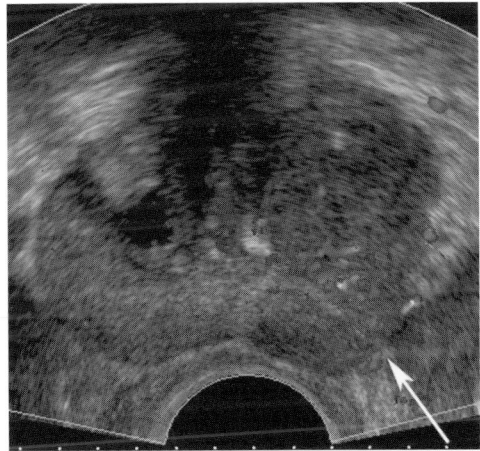

(b)

Figure 7.3. Gleason 8 prostate adenocarcinoma. Transverse images through the midgland of the prostate.
(a) Conventional gray-scale image demonstrates a hypoechoic contour bulge of the left midgland
indicative of prostate cancer (arrows). Color (b) and power (c) Doppler show a subtle asymmetric
increase in blood flow along the lateral aspect of the left midgland (arrows). (d) and (e)
Contrast-enhanced harmonic gray scale with intermittent imaging reveals a larger parenchymal area of
enhancement with visualization of increased neovasculature, providing a better delineation of the
extent of the cancer (arrows). Contrast-enhanced color (f) and power Doppler (g) again demonstrate
augmented asymmetric blood flow on the side of the cancer (arrows), but do not demonstrate details of
the microvascularity. See color plate section for full color versions of parts (b), (c), (f), (g).

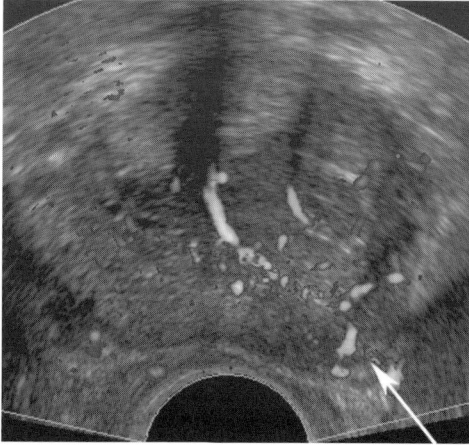

(c)

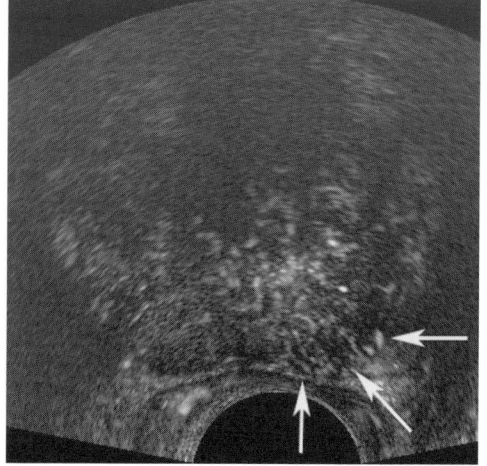

(d)

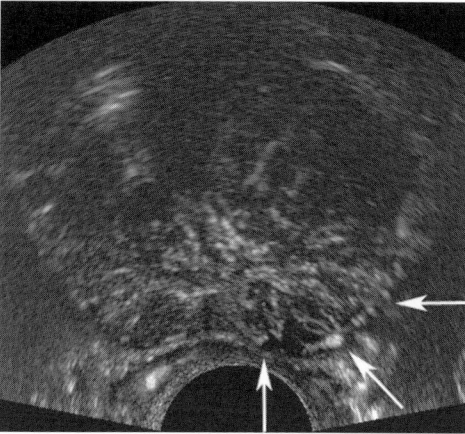

(e)

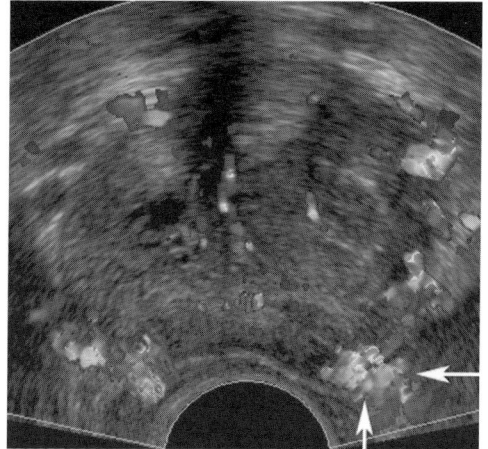

(f)

Figure 7.3. (cont.)

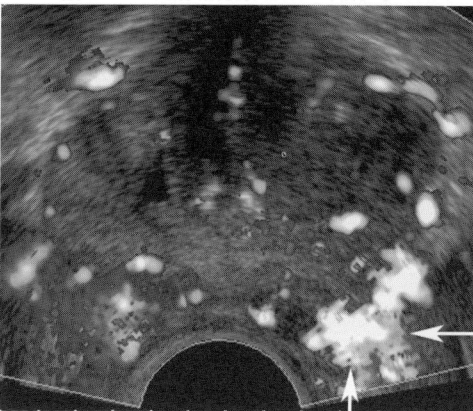

(g)

outer gland, often distorting the typical radial pattern of flow. Furthermore, the augmented blood flow from BPH may be so prominent that it may distract the examiner from noticing asymmetric perfusion patterns in the outer gland. Prostatitis, like BPH, is associated with focal areas of hypervascularity which may mimic prostate cancer [23]. Ejaculation within 24 h prior to evaluation may increase prostatic blood flow as well [24]. As noted earlier, patient positioning alters the blood flow distribution of the prostate. Patients imaged in the lateral decubitus position have been shown to have increased flow in the dependent portion of the prostate. We therefore recommend that all patients are examined in the dorsal lithotomy position for assessment of Doppler flow [11].

Although color and power Doppler are valuable tools that may be used with conventional gray-scale imaging to increase the sensitivity of detection of prostate cancer, they do not improve detection sufficiently to eliminate standard systematic biopsy [25, 26, 27, 28]. Color and power Doppler can identify blood flow in vessels approximately 1 mm in diameter and larger, which represent the larger feeding vessels for cancerous lesions. However, the microvessels infiltrating prostate cancer tumors are approximately 10–50 µm in diameter. New methods, particularly contrast-enhanced ultrasound, have emerged to help visualize and identify the microvessel anatomy associated with prostate cancer.

Contrast-enhanced ultrasound

Increased neovascularity and angiogenesis in prostate cancer is associated with an increase in microvessel density. When compared with normal prostate tissue, malignant lesions contain smaller microvessels with a more uniform distribution [29, 30]. There have been reports showing a correlation between increased micro-vessel density and disease-specific survival [31, 32]. Similarly, an increase in both the microvasculature and tumor angiogenesis is associated with metastases as well as disease stage [33, 34, 35, 36]. Since the microvasculature is too small to be detected by conventional color and power Doppler, another method is needed to recognize the patterns of blood flow through these small vessels.

Microbubble contrast agents are small enough to pass through the microvascu-lature, and can be used to augment the visualization of microvessels in prostate cancer [37, 38]. These agents are between 1 µm 10 µm in diameter and are made of air or gas coated with an outer shell consisting of either albumin or a polymer containing phospholipids. After they pass through the pulmonary circulation, the microbubbles reach various vascular organs. When microbubbles are exposed to acoustic energy by insonation they may rupture or resonate, causing enhancement of the parenchyma and vascular architecture. The agents have intravascular residence times of several minutes; however, parenchymal enhancement of the prostate can be prolonged by slow intravenous infusion during prostate imaging and biopsy.

Doppler and gray-scale harmonic imaging are the two main technologies used to visualize microbubble contrast agents. Doppler signal is significantly increased by microbubble infusion, particularly in areas of increased vascular density such as prostatic neoplasms [39, 40]. Studies have shown improved Doppler detection of prostate cancer through the use of microbubble contrast agents [41, 42]. This results in a more efficient and high-yield detection of prostate cancer through the use of targeted biopsies, diagnosing more cancers with fewer needle cores [43, 44].

Unfortunately, color and power Doppler imaging technology use high energy levels that destroy a large proportion of the microbubbles during imaging. The rupture/destruction of microbubbles produces an intense Doppler signal that results in vascular enhancement. However, Doppler imaging destroys most microbubbles in the larger feeding vessels before they enter the smaller neovessels of malignant tissue. As a result, the enhancement and visibility of the microcirculation are limited with conventional color/power Doppler imaging of microbubble contrast agents.

Gray-scale harmonic imaging uses a lower energy of insonation to evaluate contrast agents and therefore avoids the premature destruction of microbubbles in larger vessels [38, 45, 46]. Most of the reflected ultrasound signal from unenhanced tissue is received at the fundamental frequency of insonation, while resonance of microbubble contrast agents supplies the majority of harmonic signals. Selective gray-scale imaging of reflected harmonic frequencies allows improved visualization of the reflected signal from the vasculature with lower energy levels than those used for insonation with color and power Doppler imaging [47]. The application of low-energy gray-scale harmonic imaging technology allows the microbubbles to persist into the microcirculation and provides harmonic imaging of microbubbles as they perfuse the microvessels within cancerous lesions (Figures 7.2, 7.3) [48, 49]. The parenchyma and microvascular architecture are highlighted, providing an improved enhancement compared to Doppler imaging. Finally, when compared to conventional color and power Doppler imaging, both the spatial and temporal resolution of gray-scale harmonic imaging are superior.

Further improvements in microbubble contrast enhancement have been made through the development of intermittent harmonic imaging. By using a reduced frame rate, this technology lowers the energy of insonation compared to

conventional continuous harmonic imaging. The lower energy of insonation pro-
longs the survival of the microbubble contrast agents and allows for increased
perfusion through the microcirculation. As a result, additional enhancement of
the parenchyma can be noticed [50, 51, 52]. The use of intermittent harmonic
imaging has been shown to improve delineation of the microvascular anatomy of
prostate cancer when compared to continuous harmonic imaging [53].

A more recent advance in harmonic imaging is the development of
flash-replenishment techniques. A high power flash destroys the microbubbles,
while subsequent low-power pulses permit contrast replenishment. Although
only a small number of microbubbles may pass into the microcirculation, harmonic
signals are added from multiple frames in order to track the movement of individual
microbubbles over time. A composite image, constructed from the multiple frames,
shows an outline of the microcirculation based upon tracking of individual microbubbles. Flash-replenishment imaging can provide a better illustration and understanding of the microvasculature that might not be noticeable from a single frame
imaged in real-time.

At the Jefferson Prostate Diagnostic Center of Thomas Jefferson University, we
have conducted a number of clinical trials establishing the efficacy of both
Doppler and contrast-enhanced ultrasound to aid in the detection of prostate
cancer. Between October 1999 and November 2000, 100 subjects in whom prostate cancer was suspected were enrolled in a study comparing contrast-enhanced
harmonic imaging to standard sextant biopsy [54]. Sensitivity for cancer detection
was significantly improved after administration of contrast, from 38% at baseline
to 65% post-contrast infusion. The contrast-enhanced lesions that were biopsied
were also found to be more clinically significant, demonstrating higher Gleason
scores and larger size. Furthermore, in the last 40 patients of this study, a
statistically significant increase in the positive biopsy rate was seen when targeted
biopsies were obtained from areas of intense enhancement with contrast administration [55].

In 2005, we evaluated 301 subjects who were referred for prostate biopsy with
color and power Doppler ultrasound along with harmonic gray-scale ultrasound
[56]. Cancer was found in 363 biopsy cores from 104 of 301 subjects (35%). Of
1133 targeted biopsy cores, 175 (15.5%) detected cancer while 10.4% (188/1806) of
sextant biopsy cores were positive ($p < 0.01$). Targeted cores were twice as likely to
be positive compared to sextant biopsy (odds ratio = 2.0, $p < 0.001$). Unfortunately,
targeted biopsy did not detect 20% (21/104) of cancers. The majority of positive
sites missed by targeted biopsy were found to be at the apex of the prostate. These

findings suggest that systematic biopsy still cannot be eliminated, but that a targeted biopsy strategy with additional systematic biopsies at the apex may provide more efficient detection of prostate cancer.

Increased blood flow with BPH can result in false-positive areas of contrast enhancement in both the inner and outer portions of the prostate gland [57]. As a result, the specificity of targeted biopsy is decreased. 5α-reductase inhibitors, common in the treatment of BPH, have been shown to decrease prostate volume through cellular atrophy and apoptosis [58]. Additionally, their short-term use reduces bleeding in patients undergoing transurethral resection of the prostate due to a decrease in microvessel density [59, 60]. In order to assess pre-treatment with a 5α-reductase inhibitor to suppress blood flow caused by BPH, 11 prostate biopsy patients were evaluated with conventional gray-scale, color, and power Doppler ultrasound at baseline, and then weekly for a total of 3 weeks while taking a 5α-reductase inhibitor [61]. Significant Doppler flow suppression was seen in all patients after 1 week, which was found to be greatest in the peripheral zone ($p < 0.01$). Targeted biopsy cores obtained after treatment with a 5α-reductase inhibitor had improved cancer detection compared to systematic sextant biopsy cores; 20% (8/40) targeted cores were positive while only 7.6% (5/66) of the sextant cores were found to have cancer. We are currently conducting a larger scale clinical trial exploring contrast-enhanced ultrasound detection of prostate cancer in patients pre-treated with a 5α-reductase inhibitor.

Elastography

Prostate cancer is defined by increased cellular proliferation, loss of normal glandular architecture, and focal tissue growth. These pathologic findings are associated with increased tissue firmness that is palpable on digital rectal examination, and reduced tissue elasticity that can be measured by elastography. Elastography is a form of sonographic signal processing that measures tissue stiffness based upon changes in the received radiofrequency (RF) signal [62]. The feasibility of real-time elastography has been demonstrated for the characterization of breast and prostate malignancies [63, 64]. Through slight compression and decompression of the prostate gland with the ultrasound probe, elastograms can be acquired in real-time (Figures 7.4, 7.5). Recent studies have shown significantly improved cancer detection rates among biopsies performed under elastographic guidance [9, 65, 66]. At our institution, we evaluated 137 patients who underwent routine systematic prostate biopsy along with targeted cores under the guidance of

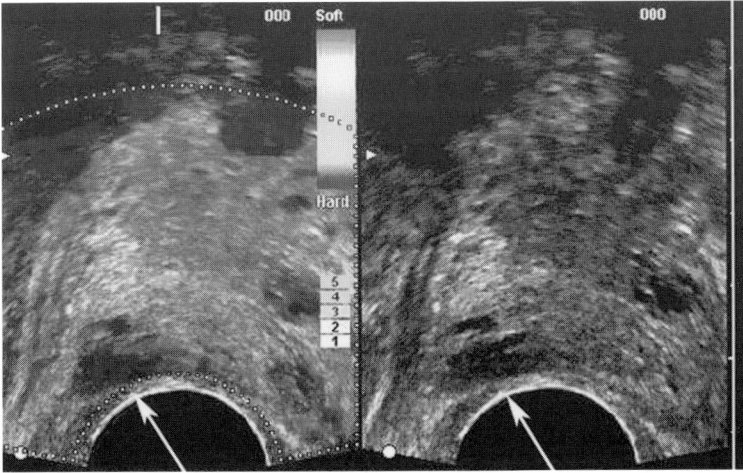

Figure 7.4. Gleason 7 prostate adenocarcinoma. Transverse images through the midgland of the prostate. Gray-scale imaging (right) reveals a hypoechoic lesion in right midgland (arrow), corresponding to an area of increased tissue stiffness on the corresponding elastogram (left). See color plate section for full color version.

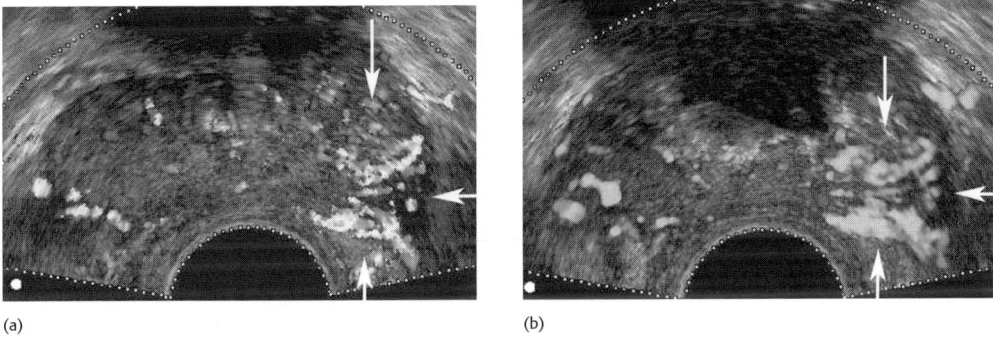

(a)   (b)

Figure 7.5. Gleason 10 prostate adenocarcinoma. Transverse images through the base of the prostate. Color (a) and power (b) Doppler demonstrate an area of increased perfusion in the left base of the prostate (arrows). (c) Elastogram shows increased tissue stiffness in the same area, corresponding to the site of cancer at targeted biopsy. See color plate section for full color version.

gray-scale, color Doppler, and real-time elastography [67]. Positive elastography was found to be predictive of both moderate- and high-grade cancers. In addition, areas of increased elasticity were found to be twice as likely to demonstrate malignancy when compared to systematic biopsy cores. However, similar to other imaging modalities, elastography alone was not sufficient to efficiently diagnose

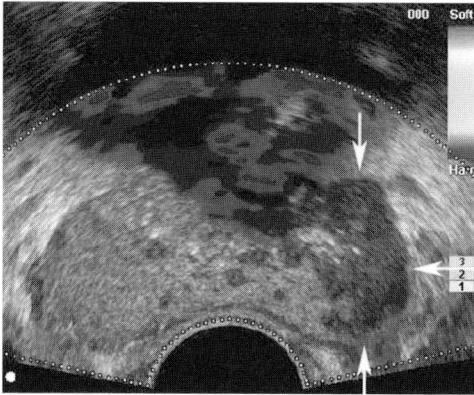

Figure 7.5. (cont.)

(c)

prostate cancer, as 40% of patients with prostate cancer were found to have no sonographic or elastographic abnormality to biopsy.

Conclusion

Transrectal ultrasound imaging of the prostate has played a central role in revolu-tionizing the imaging and diagnosis of prostate cancer. Conventional gray-scale sonography is the established standard for diagnostic prostate evaluation. Over the past two decades, advances in TRUS technology that allow improved identification of malignancy in the prostate have increased cancer detection rates. Color and power Doppler detect abnormal blood flow patterns within the prostate. Contrast-enhanced ultrasound using microbubbles enhances the parenchymal microcirculation of the prostate and highlights the microvascu-lature perfusing malignant lesions. Elastography measures increased tissue stiffness corresponding to areas of suspected cancer. These imaging modalities are useful adjuncts to conventional gray-scale ultrasound for the targeted detection of prostate cancer. The long-term goal of research efforts in advanced TRUS imaging is to provide a non-invasive technique that can detect clinically significant prostate cancer and eliminate the need for prostate biopsy in patients without clinically significant cancer. Transrectal ultrasound is ideally suited to provide an inexpensive, non-invasive technique for character-ization of prostate cancer based upon vascularity and tissue stiffness charac-teristics. Future development of targeted contrast agents may further enhance the ability to discriminate prostate cancer with TRUS.

REFERENCES

1. A. Jemal, R. Siegel, E. Ward, *et al.*, Cancer statistics, 2008. *CA Cancer J Clin* **58** (2008), 71–96.
2. M. R. Cooperberg, J. W. Moul, P. R. Carroll, The changing face of prostate cancer. *J Clin Oncol* **23** (2005), 8146–51.
3. J. E. McNeal, Normal and pathologic anatomy of the prostate. *Urology*, **17**:Suppl (1981), 11–16.
4. J. E. McNeil, Origin and evolution of benign prostatic enlargement. *Investig Urol*, **15** (1978), 340–5.
5. J. E. McNeal, Origin and development of carcinoma in the prostate. *Cancer*, **23** (1969), 24–33.
6. J. E. McNeal, E. A. Redwine, F. S. Freiha, *et al.*, Zonal distribution of prostatic adenocarcinoma: correlation with histologic pattern and direction of spread. *Am J Surg Pathol*, **12** (1988), 897–906.
7. D. P. Byar, F. K. Mostofi, Carcinoma of the prostate: evaluation of certain pathologic features in 208 radical prostatectomies. *Cancer*, **30** (1972), 5–13.
8. J. E. McNeal, E. A. Redwine, F. S. Freiha, *et al.*, Zonal distribution of prostatic adenocarcinoma: correlation with histologic pattern and direction of spread. *Am J Surg Pathol*, **12** (1988), 897–906.
9. K. Konig, U. Scheipers, A. Pesavento, *et al.*, Initial experiences with real-time elastography guided biopsies of the prostate. *J Urol*, **174** (2005), 115–17.
10. R. Sabbagh, M. McCormack, F. Peloquin, *et al.*, A prospective randomized trial of 1-day versus 3-day antibiotic prophylaxis for transrectal ultrasound guided prostate biopsy. *Can J Urol*, **11** (2004), 2216–19.
11. E. J. Halpern, F. Frauscher, F. Forsberg, *et al.*, High frequency Doppler imaging of the prostate: effect of patient position. *Radiology*, **222** (2002), 634–9.
12. M. D. Rifkin, W. Dahnert, A. B. Kurtz, State of the art: endorectal sonography of the prostate gland. *AJR Am J Roentgenol*, **154** (1990), 691–700.
13. K. Shinohara, T. M. Wheeler, P. T. Scardino, The appearance of prostate cancer on transrectal ultrasonography: correlation of imaging and pathological examinations *J Urol*, **142** (1989), 76–82.
14. W. M. Van de Voorde, R. H. Oyen, H. P. Van Poppel, *et al.*, Peripherally localized benign hyperplastic nodules of the prostate. *Mod Pathol*, **8** (1995), 46–50.
15. R. S. Purohit, K. Shonohara, M. V. Meng, *et al.*, Imaging clinically localized prostate cancer. *Urol Clin N Am*, **30** (2003), 279–93.
16. S. L. Varghese, G. D. Grossfeld, The prostatic gland: malignancies other than adenocarcinomas. *Radiol Clin N Am*, **38** (2000), 179–202.
17. R. G. Aarnink, H. P. Beerlage, J. J. De La Rosette, *et al.*, Transrectal ultrasound of the prostate: innovations and future applications. *J Urol*, **159** (1998), 1568–79.
18. M. D. Rifkin, G. S. Sudakoff, A. A. Alexander, Prostate: techniques, results, and potential applications of color Doppler US scanning. *Radiology*, **186** (1993), 509–13.
19. S. Kravchick, S. Cytron, R. Peled, *et al.*, Using gray-scale and two different techniques of color Doppler sonography to detect prostate cancer. *Urology*, **61** (2003), 977–81.
20. M. Ismail, R. O. Petersen, A. A. Alexander, *et al.*, Color Doppler imaging in predicting the biologic behavior of prostate cancer: correlation with disease-free survival. *Urology*, **50** (1997), 906–12.
21. J. Y. Cho, S. H. Kim, S. E. Lee, Diffuse prostatic lesions: role of color Doppler and power Doppler ultrasonography. *J Ultrasound Med*, **17** (1998), 283–7.
22. K. Okihara, M. Kojima, Y. Naya, *et al.*, Ultrasonic power Doppler imaging for prostatic cancer: a preliminary report. *Tohoku J Exp Med*, **82** (1997), 277–81.
23. U. Patel, D. Rickards, The diagnostic value of colour Doppler flow in the peripheral zone of the prostate, with histologic correlation. *BJU Int*, **74** (1994), 590–5.
24. T. S. Keener, T. C. Winter, R. Berger, *et al.*, Prostate vascular flow: the effect of ejaculation as revealed on transrectal power Doppler sonography. *AJR Am J Roentgenol*, **175** (2000), 1169–72.

25. I. M. G. Kelly, W. R. Lees, D. Rickards, Prostate cancer and the role of color Doppler US. *Radiology*, **189** (1993), 153–6.

26. J. S. Newman, R. L. Bree, J. M. Rubin, Prostate cancer: diagnosis with color Doppler sonography with histologic correlation of each biopsy site. *Radiology*, **195** (1995), 86–90.

27. F. Cornud, X. Belin, D. Piron, *et al.*, Color Doppler-guided biopsies in 591 patients with an elevated serum PSA level: impact on Gleason score for non-palpable lesions. *Urology*, **49** (1997), 709–15.

28. E. J. Halpern, F. Frauscher, S. E. Strup, *et al.*, Prostate: high frequency Doppler US imaging for cancer detection. *Radiology*, **225** (2002), 71–7.

29. P. A. Kay, R. A. Robb, D. G. Bostwick, Prostate cancer microvessels: a novel method for three-dimensional reconstruction and analysis. *Prostate*, **37** (1998), 270–7.

30. E. Louvar, P. J. Littrup, A. Goldstein, *et al.*, Correlation of color flow in the prostate with tissue microvascularity. *Cancer*, **83** (1998), 135–40.

31. I. F. Lissbrant, P. Stattin, J. E. Damber, *et al.*, Vascular density is a predictor of cancer-specific survival in prostatic carcinoma. *Prostate*, **33** (1997), 38–45.

32. M. Borre, B. V. Offersen, B. Nerstrom, *et al.*, Microvessel density predicts survival in prostate cancer patients subjected to watchful waiting. *Br J Cancer*, **78** (1998), 940–4.

33. N. Weidner, P. R. Carroll, J. Flax, *et al.*, Tumor angiogenesis correlates with metastasis in invasive prostate carcinoma. *Am J Pathol*, **143** (1993), 401–9.

34. T. A. Fregene, P. S. Khanuja, A. C. Noto, *et al.*, Tumor-associated angiogenesis in prostate cancer. *Anticancer Res*, **13** (1993), 2377–82.

35. M. K. Brawer, R. E. Deering, M. Brown, *et al.*, Predictors of pathologic stage in prostate carcinoma, the role of neovascularity. *Cancer*, **73** (1994), 678–87.

36. D. G. Bostwick, T. M. Wheeler, M. Blute, *et al.*, Optimized microvessel density analysis improves prediction of cancer stage from prostate needle biopsies. *Urology*, **48** (1996), 47–57.

37. B. B. Golberg, J. B. Liu, F. Forsberg, Ultrasound contrast agents: a review. *Ultrasound Med Biol*, **20** (1994), 319–33.

38. B. B. Goldberg, J. S. Raichlen, F. Forsberg, In: *Ultrasound Contrast Agents: Basic Principles and Clinical Applications*, 2nd edn. London: Dunitz, 2001.

39. J. P. Sedelaar, G. J. van Leenders, C. A. Hulsbergen-van de Kaa, *et al.*, Microvessel density: correlation between contrast ultrasonography and histology of prostate cancer. *Eur Urol*, **40** (2001), 285–93.

40. D. Strohmeyer, F. Frauscher, A. Klauser, *et al.*, Contrast-enhanced transrectal color Doppler ultrasonography (TRCDUS) for assessment of angiogenesis in prostate cancer. *Anticancer Res*, **21** (2001), 2907–13.

41. H. A. Bogers, J. P. Sedelaar, H. P. Beerlage, *et al.*, Contrast-enhanced three-dimensional power Doppler angiography of the human prostate: correlation with biopsy outcome. *Urology*, **54** (1999), 97–104.

42. C. Roy, X. Buy, H. Lang, *et al.*, Contrast enhanced color Doppler endorectal-sonography of the prostate: efficiency for detecting peripheral zone tumors and role for biopsy procedure. *J Urol*, **170** (2003), 69–72.

43. F. Frauscher, A. Klauser, E. J. Halpern, *et al.*, Detection of prostate cancer with a microbubble ultrasound contrast agent. *Lancet*, **357** (2001), 1849–50.

44. F. Frauscher, A. Klauser, H. Volgger, *et al.* Comparison of contrast-enhanced color Doppler targeted biopsy to conventional systematic biopsy: impact on prostate cancer detection. *J Urol*, **167** (2002), 1648–52.

45. N. De Jong, R. Cornet, C. T. Lancee, Higher harmonics of vibrating gas-filled microspheres. Part one: simulations. *Ultrasonics*, **32** (1994), 447–53.

46. N. De Jong, R. Cornet, C. T. Lance, Higher harmonics of vibrating gas-filled microspheres. Part two: measurements. *Ultrasonics*, **32** (1994), 455–9.

47. F. Forsberg, B. B. Goldberg, J. B. Liu , *et al.*, On the feasibility of real-time, in vivo harmonic imaging

with proteinaceous microspheres. *Ultrasound Med*, **15** (1996), 853–60.

48. B. A. Schrope, V. L. Newhouse, V. Uhlendorf, Simulated capillary blood flow measurement using a nonlinear ultrasonic contrast agent. *Ultrason Imaging*, **14** (1992), 134–58.

49. B. A. Schrope, V. L. Newhouse, Second harmonic ultrasound blood perfusion measurement. *Ultrasound Med Biol*, **19** (1993), 567–79.

50. T. R. Porter, F. Xie, Transient myocardial contrast after initial exposure to diagnostic ultrasound pressures with minute doses of intravenously injected microbubbles. *Circulation*, **92** (1995), 2391–5.

51. P. J. Colon, D. R. Richards, C. A. Moreno, *et al.*, Benefits of reducing the cardiac cycle-triggering frequency of ultrasound imaging to increase myocardial opacification with FS069 during fundamental and second harmonic imaging. *J Am Soc Echocardiogr*, **10** (1997), 602–7.

52. A. Broillet, J. Puginier, R. Ventrone, *et al.*, Assessment of myocardial perfusion by intermittent harmonic power Doppler using SonoVue, a new ultrasound contrast agent. *Invest Radiol*, **33** (1998), 209.

53. E. J. Halpern, L. Verkh, F. Forsberg, *et al.*, Initial experience with contrast-enhanced sonography of the prostate. *AJR Am J Roentgenol*, **174** (2000), 1575–80.

54. E. J. Halpern, M. Rosenberg, L. G. Gomella, Prostate cancer: contrast-enhanced US for detection. *Radiology*, **219** (2001), 219–25.

55. E. J. Halpern, F. Frauscher, M. Rosenberg, *et al.*, Directed biopsy during contrast enhanced sonography of the prostate. *AJR Am J Roentgenol*, **178** (2001), 915–19.

56. E. J. Halpern, J. R. Ramey, S. E. Strup, *et al.*, Detection of prostate cancer with contrast-enhanced sonography using intermittent harmonic imaging. *Cancer*, **104** (2005), 2373–83.

57. E. J. Halpern, P. A. McCue, A. K. Aksnes, *et al.*, Contrast enhanced sonography of the prostate with Sonazoid: comparison with prostatectomy specimens in twelve patients. *Radiology*, **222** (2002), 361–6.

58. R. S. Rittmaster, R. W. Norman, L. N. Thomas, *et al.*, Evidence for atrophy and apoptosis in the prostates of men given finasteride. *J Clin Endocrinol Metab*, **81** (1996), 814–9.

59. J. F. Donohue, H. Sharma, R. Abraham, *et al.*, Transurethral prostate resection and bleeding: a randomized, placebo controlled trial of role of finasteride for decreasing operative blood loss. *J Urol*, **168** (2002), 2024–6.

60. D. A. Hochberg, J. B. Basillote, N. A. Armenakas, *et al.*, Decreased suburethral prostatic microvessel density in finasteride treated prostates: a possible mechanism for reduced bleeding in benign prostatic hyperplasia. *J Urol*, **167** (2002), 1731–3.

61. E. P. Ives, L. G. Gomella, E. J. Halpern, Effect of dutasteride therapy on Doppler evaluation of the prostate: preliminary results. *Radiology*, **237** (2005), 197–201.

62. L. S. Taylor, B. C. Porter, D. J. Rubens, *et al.*, Three-dimensional sonoelastography: principles and practices. *Phys Med Biol*, **45** (2000), 1477–94.

63. F. Lee, J. P. Bronson, R. M. Lerner, *et al.*, Sonoelasticity imaging: results in vitro tissue specimens. *Radiology*, **181** (1991), 237–9.

64. T. A. Krouskop, T. M. Wheeler, F. Kallel, *et al.*, Elastic moduli of breast and prostatic tissues under compression. *Ultrason Imaging*, **20** (1998), 260–74.

65. J. Ophir, I. Cespedes, H. Ponnekanti, *et al.*, Elastography: a quantitative method for imaging the elasticity of biological tissues. *Ultrason Imaging*, **13** (1991), 111–34.

66. D. L. Cochlin, R. H. Ganatra, D. F. Griffiths, Elastography in the detection of prostatic cancer. *Clin Radiol*, **57** (2002), 1014–20.

67. E. D. Nelson, C. B. Slotoroff, L. G. Gomella, *et al.*, Targeted biopsy of the prostate: the impact of color Doppler and elastography on prostate cancer detection and Gleason score. *Urology*, **70**:6 (2007), 1136–40.

8

Computed tomography imaging in patients with prostate cancer

Jingbo Zhang

Introduction

Prostate cancer has attracted a great deal of resources and effort in the scientific community not only because it is the most common malignancy and the third leading cause of cancer-related mortality in American men [1], but also because of its complex, often baffling nature. It demonstrates a wide clinical spectrum, from indolent disease that the patient will die with, rather than from, to highly aggressive disease that threatens the patient's life. One of the most important questions in managing prostate cancer, therefore, is how to stratify patients by their disease characteristics in order to design appropriate, individualized treatment plans. The use of imaging, which is an integral part of prostate cancer management, should also be guided by the patient's risk category, as determined by the patient's age, prostate-specific antigen (PSA) level, Gleason score, and number of positive biopsy cores [1].

In recent years computed tomography (CT) has undergone substantial technical improvements. With the introduction of high-speed multidetector helical scanners, it is now possible to acquire a CT study with high spatial resolution in a very short time. However, compared to magnetic resonance imaging (MRI), CT has poor soft-tissue resolution in the pelvis and therefore is not the modality of choice for evaluating primary prostate cancer.

It has been shown that in patients with low-risk prostate cancer the likelihood of positive findings on abdominal/pelvic CT is extremely low [2, 3]. Therefore, it has been recommended that CT be reserved for the staging of prostate cancer in high-risk patients. The American College of Radiology has recommended CT in patients with a PSA level higher than 10.0 ng/ml and a Gleason score higher than 6 [4], while the American Urological Association has recommended CT in patients with a PSA level higher than 25.0 ng/ml [5]. However, it appears that such

Prostate Cancer, eds. Hedvig Hricak and Peter T. Scardino. Published by Cambridge University Press.

evidence-based staging guidelines have not been broadly accepted by physicians. Medicare claims data from 1991 and 1996 showed that significant variation was found in the use of diagnostic imaging tests in patients with prostate cancer undergoing different therapeutic modalities, or from different geographic regions within the United States [6]. Another study found that, judging by the recommendations in the literature, urologists were overusing imaging studies for tumor staging in patients with clinically low-risk disease [7].

This chapter will discuss the role of CT imaging in the management of patients with prostate cancer. Potential future developments that may improve the utilization of CT in this setting will also be discussed.

Detection and staging of primary prostate cancer

Diagnostic tests aimed at local staging must differentiate between disease confined to the prostate (stage T1–2) and locally invasive disease extending beyond the prostatic capsule into the periprostatic fat and neurovascular structures (stage T3) or adjacent organs (stage T4) [8]. Most investigators agree that CT has a very limited role in the detection, localization, and staging of primary prostate cancer. This is mainly because the soft-tissue contrast of CT (either contrast-enhanced or unenhanced) is inadequate for differentiating tumor from adjacent normal parenchyma and for delineating the prostatic anatomy. Therefore, a prostate that contains tumor confined within the capsule manifests as a normal-sized or enlarged prostate gland on CT and cannot be differentiated from a benign prostate gland that contains no tumor. Due to the inability of CT to detect cancer and to visualize the prostatic capsule, a smooth outer prostatic margin does not exclude the presence of cancer within the gland, and an apparently irregular margin does not predict accurately the presence of extracapsular extension, unless there is sufficient soft-tissue extending into the periprostatic fat to suggest advanced extracapsular extension (Figure 8.1). Unilateral enlargement of a seminal vesicle with obliteration of the fat plane between the seminal vesicle and prostatic base is suggestive of seminal vesicle invasion (Figure 8.2) [9]. However, this finding needs to be considered with caution, as anatomic distortion from a distended rectum or bladder or tilting of the patient may lead to a false impression of unilateral enlargement of the seminal vesicle on axial CT images [8]. When tumor invasion of adjacent tissues such as bladder, rectum, and levator ani muscles is present, one may see a thickened or irregular posterior bladder wall, irregular thickening of the anterior rectal wall, and/or unilateral enlargement of levator ani muscles on CT (Figure 8.3) [8].

(a)

(b)

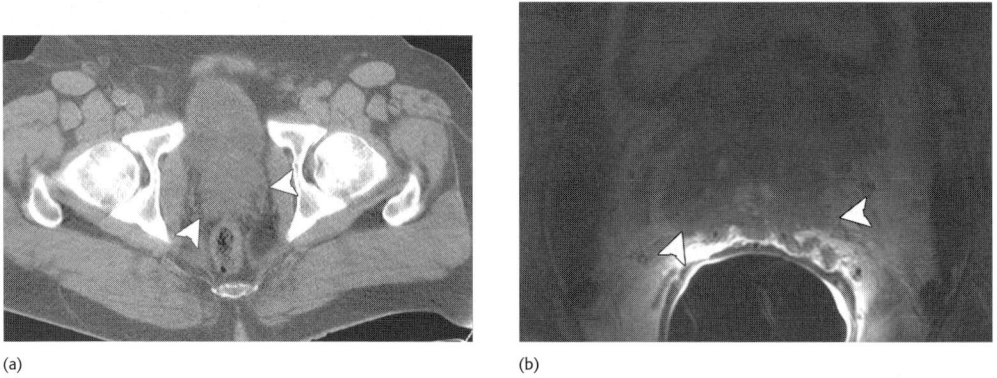

Figure 8.1. A 60-year-old man with prostate cancer. (a) Axial unenhanced CT image of the pelvis demonstrates bulging, angulation, and irregularity of the prostate capsule suggestive of extracapsular extension (arrowheads). (b) Axial T_2-weighted endorectal MRI image of the prostate confirms the presence of gross extracapsular extension (arrowheads).

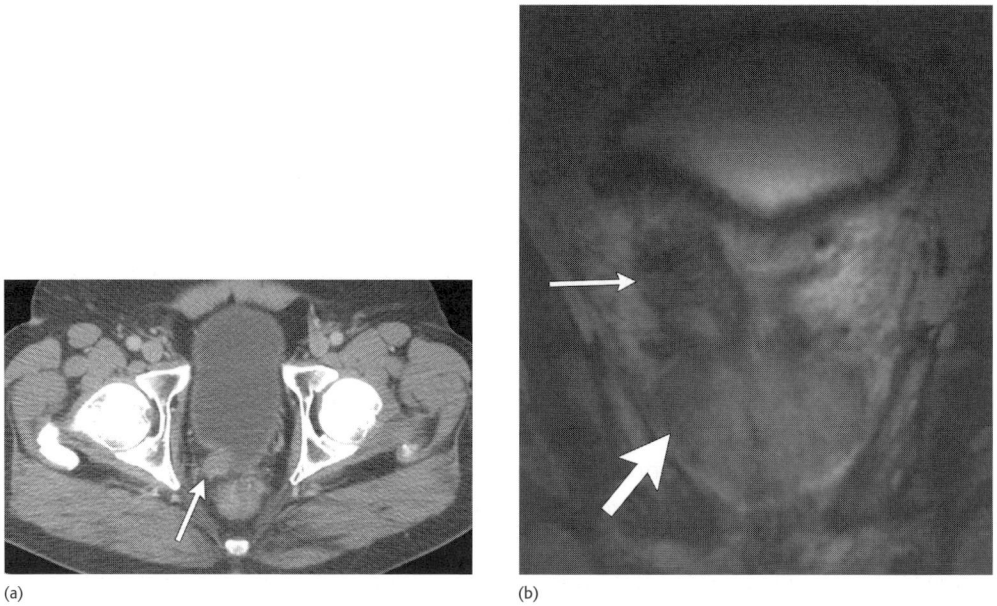

(a)

(b)

Figure 8.2. 64-year-old man with prostate cancer. (a) Axial contrast-enhanced CT image of the pelvis demonstrates asymmetric enlargement of the right seminal vesical (arrow) with enhancement. (b) Coronal T_2-weighted endorectal MRI image of the prostate confirms the presence of a dominant tumor in the right prostate gland (lower arrow) with gross seminal vesical invasion (upper arrow).

(a)

(b)

(c)

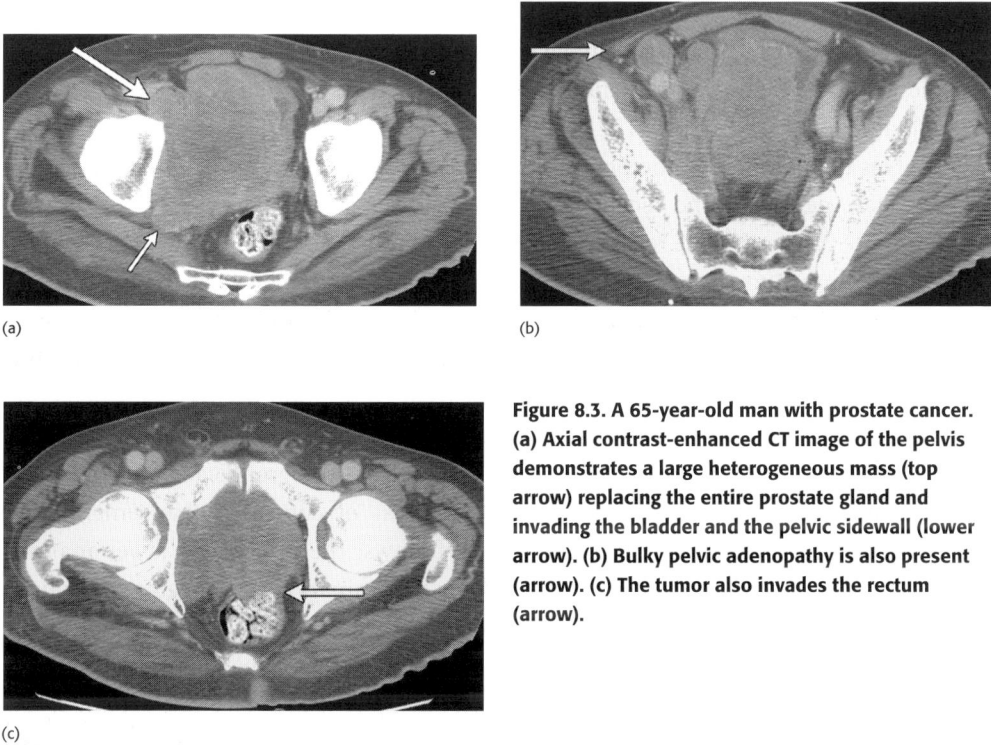

Figure 8.3. A 65-year-old man with prostate cancer. (a) Axial contrast-enhanced CT image of the pelvis demonstrates a large heterogeneous mass (top arrow) replacing the entire prostate gland and invading the bladder and the pelvic sidewall (lower arrow). (b) Bulky pelvic adenopathy is also present (arrow). (c) The tumor also invades the rectum (arrow).

The reported accuracy of CT in the local staging of prostate cancer is low. A study from the early 1990s showed that CT had an accuracy of 24% for extracapsular extension and of 69% for seminal vesicle invasion [10]. Studies in the late 1980s showed an overall accuracy of 65%–67% in staging of prostate cancer with CT, with little difference from the accuracy of clinical staging [11, 12]. Therefore, CT is not recommended for local staging of prostate cancer. Although significant advances have been achieved in the speed and resolution of CT, it is unlikely that the inherent limitation of low soft-tissue contrast can be sufficiently overcome to improve local staging accuracy [8].

One area under active investigation is the role of perfusion or "functional" imaging in the evaluation of prostate cancer [13]. Microvessel density within the prostate is associated with presence of cancer, disease stage, and disease-specific survival [14]. Both dynamic contrast-enhanced (DCE) CT and DCE MRI have been used as imaging methods for evaluating cancer angiogenesis. On DCE CT, unlike DCE MRI, there is a direct linear relationship between changes in iodine concentration and enhancement. However, compared with DCE MRI, DCE CT has had far less validation using accepted surrogate markers for angiogenesis, and the substantial radiation exposure associated with DCE CT remains an important drawback. In addition, the signal-to-noise ratio obtained with DCE CT remains poorer than that obtained with DCE MRI [15].

Ives *et al.* evaluated the potential role of multidetector CT imaging in assessing prostate perfusion and localizing prostate cancer in a series of ten patients with prostate cancer. Visible focal CT enhancement was noted in only one patient with a high-volume tumor and a Gleason score of 10. Correlation between quantitative CT perfusion and tumor location was statistically significant only in subjects with localized high-volume, poorly differentiated prostate cancer [14]. Again, this reflects the fact that CT may lack the soft-tissue resolution necessary for detection of prostate cancer even with administration of contrast. However, another study showed that prostate cancer detected at transrectal, sonographically guided biopsy appears on helical CT as focal or diffuse areas of contrast enhancement [16]. The technique used in this study was as follows: the upper and lower margins of the prostate were demarcated based on preliminary axial images; contiguous 7-mm-thick helical images through the prostate were then obtained during the arterial phase (50 s after the initiation of intravenous injection of contrast material). Patients were given 120 ml of contrast material (300 mg I/ml) at a rate of 3 ml/s. The helical images were then reconstructed at 3.5-mm intervals. Images were viewed at a narrow window width and a low window level [16]. Another more recent study also demonstrated that it is potentially feasible to detect both small and large prostatic lesions using 3D quantitative blood flow mapping of the prostate obtained from DCE multidetector CT, with a spatial resolution as high as 0.1 ml and an average noise level of 3.8 HU [17]. Formal prospective studies are needed to determine the accuracy, sensitivity, and specificity of contrast-enhanced multislice helical CT in the detection and localization of primary prostate cancer.

Staging of systemic disease

The major role of CT is in evaluation of the extent of disease in a patient with prostate cancer, including assessment of the presence of metastases to lymph nodes, distant organs or bones (Figure 8.4). Although all patients with newly diagnosed prostate cancer should be assessed for risk of metastatic disease using clinical parameters, CT is indicated only in selected patients of higher risk categories. Nomograms based on clinical data (PSA level, Gleason score, digital rectal examination findings, etc.) provide risk stratification estimates that guide the ordering of

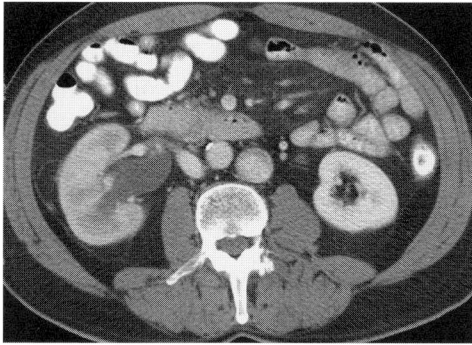

(a)

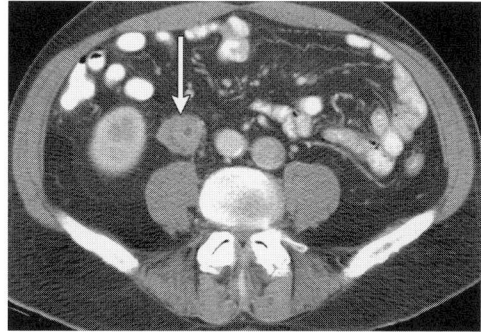

(b)

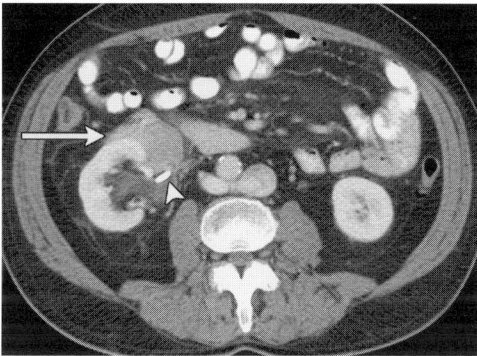

(c)

Figure 8.4. A 61-year-old man with prostate cancer. (a) Axial contrast-enhanced CT image of the abdomen demonstrated right hydronephrosis and delayed right nephrogram. (b) Marked circumferential soft-tissue thickening is seen surrounding a long segment of the right ureter (arrow). The distal right ureteral lumen is obliterated by this abnormal soft tissue (not shown). Subsequent biopsy of the peri-ureteric soft tissue showed metastatic prostate adenocarcinoma. (c) One year later the patient also developed a right perirenal mass (arrow), which proved to be metastatic prostate adenocarcinoma on biopsy (arrowhead, a right ureteral stent).

appropriate imaging tests, including CT [1]. With widespread PSA testing and the resultant stage reduction at diagnosis in prostate cancer, currently the majority of patients with newly diagnosed, localized prostate cancer are at low risk for metastases, and the diagnostic yield of CT is low in these patients. For example, in a cohort of 459 men who had prostate cancer detected through screening, bone or lymph node metastases were present in only 1.7% of cases [18]. Nevertheless, high-risk patients with clinically apparent, grossly advanced local disease, such as gross extraprostatic extension or seminal vesical invasion, and invasion of adjacent structures, will almost always meet the recommended clinical criteria for the appropriate use of CT imaging for staging.

It has been shown that Gleason score, PSA, and clinical stage are independent predictors for a positive CT scan of the abdomen and pelvis in patients with newly diagnosed prostate cancer [19]. In asymptomatic patients with newly diagnosed, untreated prostate cancer and serum PSA levels of less than 20 ng/ml the likelihood of positive findings on abdominal/pelvic CT is extremely low (<1.0%) [20, 21]. Therefore, abdominal/pelvic CT does not appear necessary in this setting. With more than 200 000 cases of prostate cancer being diagnosed each year in the United States, elimination of unnecessary staging abdominal/pelvic CT could reduce medical expenditures by $20–50 million per year [20]. It is generally recommended that CT should be performed only in patients with a PSA level greater than 15–20 ng/ml, a Gleason score greater than 7, and/or clinical tumor stage T3 or higher, or a probability of lymph node involvement of >20% as predicted by clinical nomogram [19, 20, 22, 23, 24] NCCN. One exception is patients with the anaplastic or small-cell variant of prostate cancer [25, 26]. Unlike patients with advanced typical adenocarcinoma of the prostate, patients with the anaplastic or small-cell variant of prostate cancer may have extensive metastatic disease at CT despite relatively low PSA levels.

Bone is the most common site of hematogenous metastases from prostate cancer. Osseous metastases from prostate cancer are typically osteoblastic (80%), and less commonly osteolytic (5%) or mixed osteoblastic-osteolytic (10%–15%). Therefore, osseous metastases from prostate cancer most commonly manifest as sclerotic foci on CT, occasionally lytic or mixed in attenuation (Figure 8.5). However, CT is generally not used as a screening modality for osseous metastases, because radio-nuclide bone scan and MR imaging appear to have a higher sensitivity than CT in detecting osseous metastases. However, compared with bone scan, CT has better spatial resolution that may allow more accurate differentiation between malignant and benign abnormal radioisotope uptake seen on bone scan.

For detection of soft-tissue metastases, a CT study is typically acquired approximately 70 s after injection of intravenous contrast to maximize the detection of metastatic lesions and to differentiate between blood vessels and lymph nodes. Axial images are obtained through the abdomen and pelvis to assess for retroperitoneal and pelvic lymphadenopathy as well as distant metastases to the liver or other organs [8]. Using helical CT technology, thin (5 mm collimation) slices can now be obtained quickly through the entire abdomen and pelvis during one breath-hold with little motion artifact.

In terms of nodal staging of prostate cancer, CT scanning has replaced bipedal lymphography in the detection of pelvic adenopathy at most centers (Figure 8.6). While the reported efficacy of CT is similar to that of MRI, CT has the advantages of better availability in most centers, decreased scan time, and the concomitant ability to perform CT-guided biopsy [27]. The accuracy of CT as a diagnostic tool in detecting nodal metastases is highly correlated with the patient's pre-test

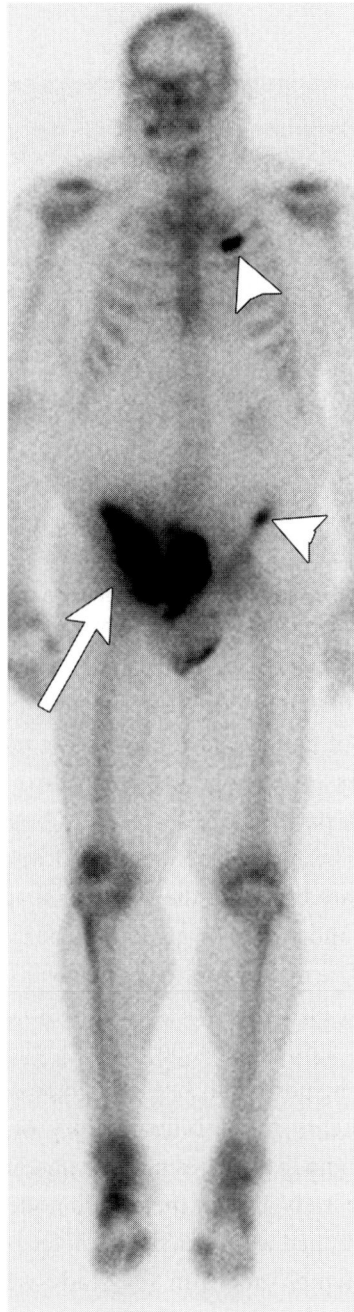

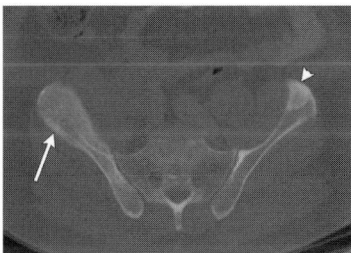

(a)   (b)

Figure 8.5. A 65-year-old man with prostate cancer and osseous metastases. (a) Axial unenhanced CT image of the pelvis viewed with bone window demonstrates a sclerotic lesion in the left iliac bone (arrowhead) and a large sclerotic lesion with periosteal thickening in the right iliac bone (arrow). (b) Whole-body bone scan image demonstrates markedly increased uptake in the right iliac bone (arrow), as well as other foci of increased uptake in the left iliac bone and left third anterior rib (arrowheads).

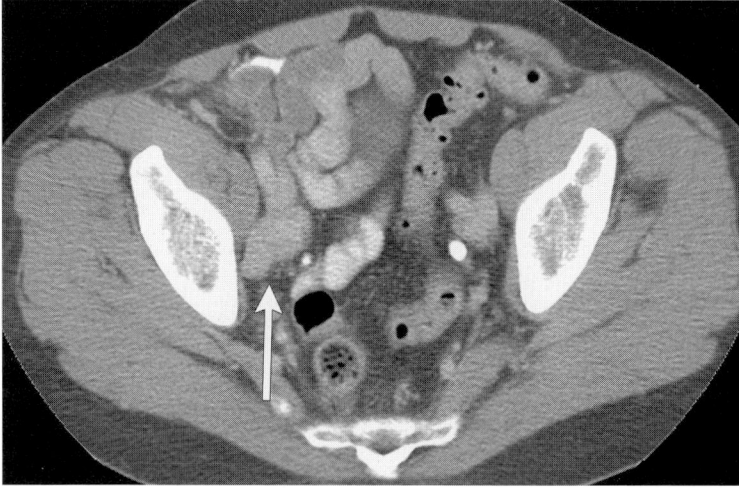

Figure 8.6. A 62-year-old man with prostate cancer and nodal metastases. Axial contrast-enhanced CT image of the pelvis demonstrates an enlarged right obturator lymph node (arrow).

probability. Therefore, it is more cost-effective to perform CT for nodal staging only in a select group of patients at high risk for nodal metastases, as determined by clinical parameters or nomograms based on clinical parameters [21]. However, even in higher risk patients, CT scans are suboptimal in predicting nodal involvement by tumor. The most widely accepted imaging criteria for the diagnosis of nodal metastases are based on the size and shape of the node. Based on the ratio between the short and long axes, a node will be classified as round (ratio of 0.8–1) or oval (ratio <0.8). The malignancy of a node will be determined by the minimal axial diameter (>10 mm for oval nodes and >8 mm for round nodes). However, these criteria are neither sensitive nor specific, as a lymph node harboring a small amount of metastasis may be normal in size and shape, whereas a benign lymph node may be enlarged secondary to an inflammatory or hyperplastic process. One study showed that lymph node size does not correlate with the presence of prostate cancer metastasis. In this study 74% of metastatic nodes had a short axis diameter of less than 1 cm and 26% had a short axis diameter of less than 5 mm. In addition, the dissected benign lymph nodes in the study were overall larger in size than the metastatic lymph nodes [28]. The reported sensitivity of CT for the detection of nodal metastases varies, but it is typically less than 40% [29].

The accuracy of CT as a diagnostic tool in diagnosing nodal metastases obviously is related to the size criteria being used. Some investigators in the past have adopted different imaging criteria and found them more accurate. For instance, Oyen *et al.*

considered any pelvic lymph node that was 6 mm or greater and asymmetric when compared to the contralateral side as pathologic [30]. Thus they were able to achieve a sensitivity of 78% and a specificity of 97% in diagnosing nodal metastases. However, their criteria are not widely adopted. It should also be noted that the reported frequency of positive lymph nodes in this study was 15.8%, much higher than the 2%–5% frequency expected in the modern screened patient population.

It is believed that nodal disease in prostate cancer often progresses in a step-wise fashion [31]. Therefore, if metastatic lymph nodes are present outside the pelvis, they are frequently accompanied by pelvic lymphadenopathy. Thus CT staging studies of newly diagnosed prostatic cancer do not need to include the abdominal retroperitoneum if there is no lymphadenopathy at or below the aortic bifurcation [32].

Treatment planning

Computed tomography has an established role in treatment planning, especially planning for radiotherapy or brachytherapy of the prostate gland.

It has been shown that in patients treated with either external radiotherapy or interstitial brachytherapy, conventional treatment planning may result in an under-estimation of tumor volume. Because the prostate gland moves in relation to the bones, CT is useful for radiation planning and has been shown to be a better guide than conventional bony structure for prostate localization [33]; therefore, CT is a reliable method for determining the adequacy of portals for external beam radiation and calculating prostatic size and volume for correct dosimetry of iodine-125 seeds. Treatment plan modifications prompted by CT scan findings are most frequent in patients with locally advanced disease [34]. Pilepich *et al.* showed that up to 53% of patients with involvement of the seminal vesicles required an enlargement of treatment fields to adequately encompass the target volume [35]. Mens *et al.* showed that the introduction of CT-based information resulted in a significant increase of field sizes, leading to an almost doubling of the treated volume, with some increase in late rectal toxicity, but also in local control [36]. In addition, the degree of pubic arch interference is highly variable from one patient to the next and the prostatic volume measured on transrectal ultrasound is not a reliable indicator of which patients do or do not need pelvic CT to detect potential arch interference [37]. Therefore, in general, CT simulations are used for establishing the treatment volume for radiation therapy in modern practice [34]. Magnetic resonance imaging may be more accurate than CT or urethrography in localizing the prostatic apex for radiation planning [38], but it is costly and limited in availability. Pre-operative CT is also beneficial in planning the target volume for patients who need adjuvant radiation therapy after radical prostatectomy [39].

Patients with prostate cancer localized to the pelvis without nodal or distant metastases can be treated with radiation therapy. Three-dimensional conformal radiation therapy has been developed to improve safe, targeted delivery of radiation dose to the prostate while minimizing radiation exposure to surrounding tissues [40]. CT, MRI and transrectal ultrasound have all been used for 3D treatment planning in this setting. There appears to be a tendency to overestimate the prostate volume by CT compared to MRI or transrectal ultrasound [40, 41, 42]. This could be related to uncertainty in defining the apex of the prostate and thereby the length of the prostate [43, 44]. In addition, the administration of intravenous contrast on CT makes a difference in how the prostate and seminal vesicles are outlined by the observer, and can lead to an increase in estimated target volume [45]. Therefore, when defining a target for radiotherapy, it is important to be aware of the effects that the imaging technique used may have on volume estimation [46].

Brachytherapy is one of the oldest techniques in radiation therapy of prostate cancer. It has evolved over time, with clinical outcomes improving consistently [47]. It is a form of less-invasive, low-morbidity radiation therapy in which iodine-125 or other radioactive seeds are implanted directly into the prostate, typically via a transperineal approach. This treatment modality is desirable due to its ability to deliver a high dose of radiation to a confined volume with relative sparing of adjacent normal tissue. Brachytherapy can deliver more radiation to the prostate with less dose to the surrounding normal organs than conventional external beam radiation therapy [8]. Pre-implant CT allows precise radiation planning by determining prostate volume and contour. Gore and Moss showed that the prostate gland volumes measured by pre-implant CT were on average 25%–30% greater than clinical estimates [48].

For tumor-targeted radiation therapy, dose escalation to intra-prostatic tumor deposits can be performed by brachytherapy. Because treatment planning for prostate brachytherapy is based on ultrasound or CT images, a technique has been developed for mapping areas suspected of harboring tumor on MR or MR spectroscopy onto the ultrasound or CT image used for guiding tumor-targeted dose escalation in brachytherapy [49].

In terms of surgical planning, it has been shown that while a larger prostatic volume is predictive of a greater operative duration, pelvimetric measurements on

CT fail to predict either operative duration or the perioperative blood transfusion requirement. However, a narrower transverse pelvic diameter on CT predicted a higher likelihood of a positive margin due to capsular breech [50].

Treatment follow-up

Computed tomography may detect local recurrence of prostate cancer at the surgical bed, although the reported sensitivity is relatively low (Figures 8.7 and 8.8). Kramer *et al.* showed that even in retrospect CT could only definitively identify recurrent tumor that manifested as a soft-tissue mass of 2 cm or larger [51]. The role of CT in prostate cancer treatment follow-up is focused on the assessment of metastatic disease in the lymph nodes, bone, and visceral organs (Figure 8.9). However, in post-treatment patients, PSA is a reliable follow-up tool. A study showed that the post-treatment detection of progressive disease by imaging was always preceded by an abnormal PSA [52]. Therefore, the National Comprehensive Cancer Network (NCCN) recommends that, in patients whose PSA levels fail to fall to an undetect-able level or remain detectable and rising on at least two subsequent measurements after radical prostatectomy, CT, among other imaging modalities, can be consid-ered for detection of remaining disease and for selection of patients for salvage

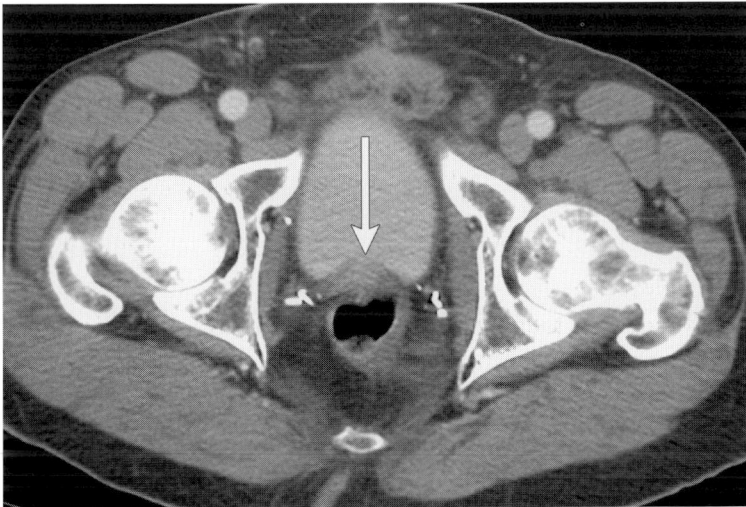

Figure 8.7. A 66-year-old patient with rising PSA, status post-radical prostatectomy for prostate cancer. Axial contrast-enhanced CT image of the pelvis demonstrates an enhancing mass at the prostatectomy bed (arrow). Subsequent biopsy confirmed the presence of recurrent prostate adenocarcinoma.

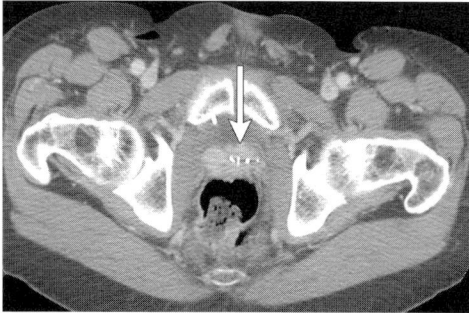

(a)

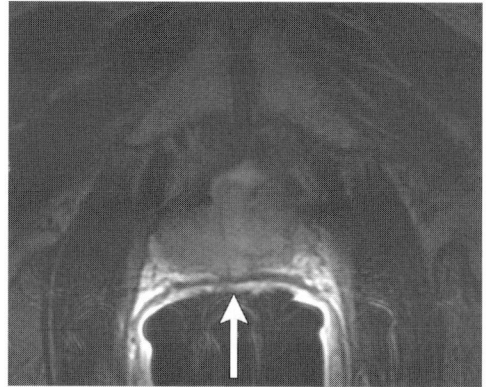

(b)

Figure 8.8. A 63-year-old patient with rising PSA, status post-radical prostatectomy for prostate cancer. (a) Axial contrast-enhanced CT image of the pelvis demonstrates an enhancing mass at the prostatectomy bed (arrow). (b) Axial T_2-weighted endorectal MR image of the pelvis also confirms the presence of a mass (arrow) at the vesicourethral anastomotic site. Subsequent biopsy confirmed the presence of recurrent prostate adenocarcinoma.

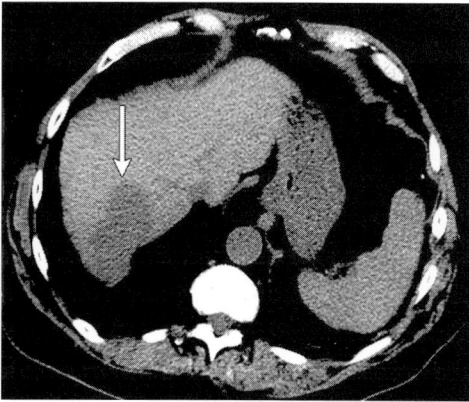

(a)

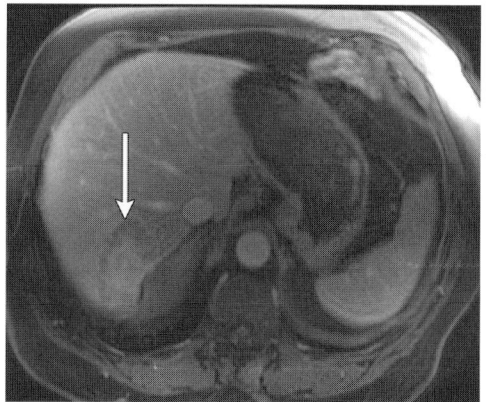

(b)

Figure 8.9. A 77-year-old man with a history of prostate and colon cancer, status post-radical prostatectomy and right hemi-colectomy, presenting with rising PSA and carcinoembryonic antigen (CEA). (a) Axial unenhanced CT image of the abdomen demonstrates a large hypoattenuating mass (arrow) in the right hepatic lobe. (b) Axial T_1-weighted fat-saturated MR image of the abdomen confirms the presence of a heterogeneously enhancing mass (arrow) in the right hepatic lobe. (c) Fluorodeoxyglucose positron emission tomography (FDG-PET) shows high uptake in the right hepatic lesion (arrow). Subsequent biopsy of the liver lesion showed poorly differentiated metastatic prostate adenocarcinoma.

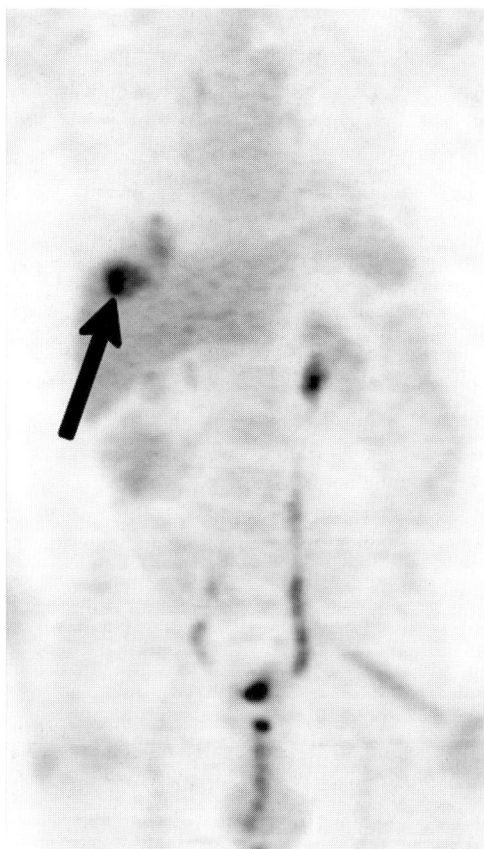

Figure 8.9. (cont.)

(c)

therapy. The NCCN also recommends that CT is considered for patients who have a rising PSA or positive digital rectal examination after radiation therapy who are still considered candidates for local salvage therapy.

Computed tomography is not the modality of choice for screening osseous metastases. However, individual bone lesions can be better visualized on CT than on a bone scan. Therefore, CT is often used to monitor therapeutic responses. Caution should be exercised though, when the size of a bone lesion is interpreted as a therapeutic marker, as a bone metastasis that is responding to systemic therapy may have a relatively high level of osteoblastic activity and may demonstrate as an enlarging sclerotic lesion on CT [53]. Interpreting an enlarging osseous lesion that is responding to therapy as a progressing metastatic lesion may lead to misguided clinical management decisions.

Computed tomography scanning has supplanted bipedal lymphography in the detection of enlarged pelvic and retroperitoneal lymph nodes in patients with prostate cancer after radical prostatectomy or radiation therapy in most centers. Although the nodal disease in prostate cancer prior to treatment often progresses in a stepwise fashion, in patients with disease recurrence following radical prostatectomy, the usual pattern of vertical nodal spread beginning in the pelvis may be absent. These patients may demonstrate predominant retroperitoneal disease or even a "pseudolymphoma" pattern of massive retroperitoneal disease with contiguous invasion of the perirenal space and adrenal glands in advanced cases [54]. Therefore Spencer and Golding suggested that whilst staging examinations with cross-sectional imaging at initial diagnosis of clinically localized prostate cancer may be confined to the pelvis, evaluation of suspected recurrent disease requires examination of the abdomen and pelvis (Figure 8.10) [54].

In patients undergoing brachytherapy, post-implant CT can be used to evaluate seed distribution, tumor response, and periprostatic tumor spread (Figure 8.11) [48, 55]. Post-implant CT could demonstrate errors in implantation, including inhomogeneous distribution and extraprostatic seeds. Serial post-implantation

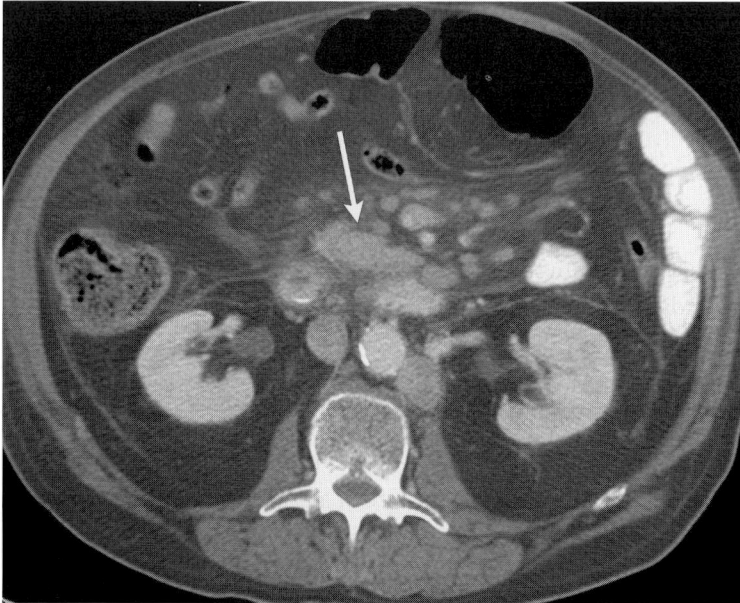

Figure 8.10. A 66-year-old man status post-radical prostatectomy for prostate cancer with subsequent nodal metastases. Axial contrast-enhanced CT image of the abdomen demonstrates bulky retroperitoneal and mesenteric (arrow) adenopathy.

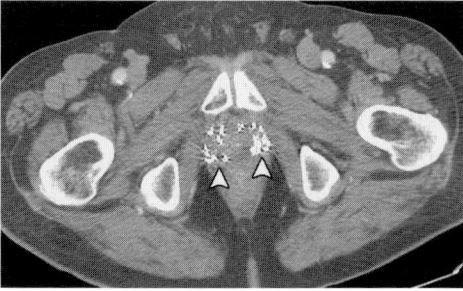

(a)

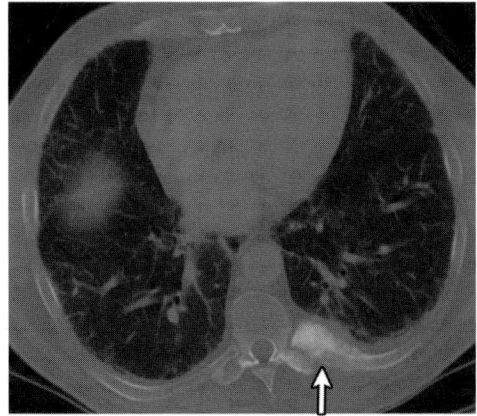

(b)

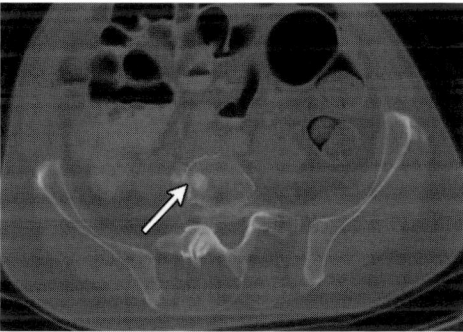

(c)

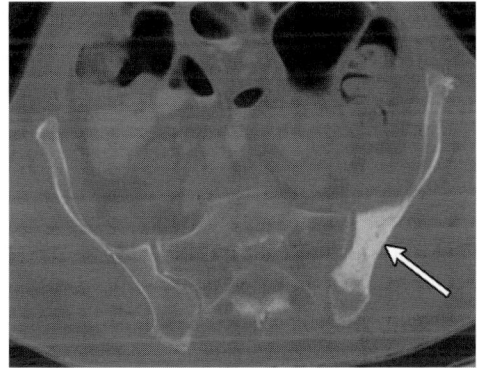

(d)

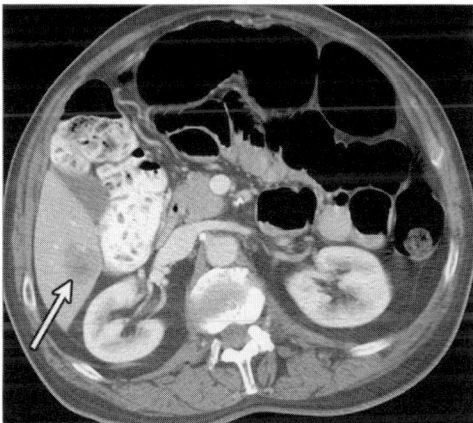

(e)

Figure 8.11. A 72-year-old man status post-brachytherapy for prostate cancer with subsequent widespread metastases. (a) Axial contrast-enhanced CT image of the pelvis demonstrates numerous brachytherapy seeds (arrowheads) in the prostate gland. (b) Axial contrast-enhanced CT image of the chest viewed at bone window demonstrates a sclerotic metastasis in a left rib (arrow). (c) Axial contrast-enhanced CT image of the abdomen viewed at bone window demonstrates a sclerotic metastasis in the spine (arrow). (d) Axial contrast-enhanced CT image of the pelvis viewed at bone window demonstrates a large sclerotic metastasis in the left iliac bone (arrow). (e) Axial contrast-enhanced CT image of the abdomen demonstrates a liver metastasis (arrow).

scans can be used to monitor change in prostate volume, which correlates with clinical assessment of response to therapy. Computed tomography may also identify clinically unsuspected tumor spread in post-implantation patients [48]. Although CT is the modality of choice for visualizing seed distribution, soft-tissue anatomy cannot be well delineated on CT. However, MRI delineates soft-tissue anatomy well but seed visualization on MRI can be inferior to that on CT. Therefore, overlaying of CT and MR images has been used to exploit the advantages of both of these modalities when assessing the quality of a prostate seed implant [56]. Depending on clinical and imaging findings, adjunctive external beam radiation may be directed to areas that are not treated adequately by the seed implants [8].

Functional CT, with its capability to measure perfusion and permeability, has also been investigated in terms of its role in evaluating patients following radiation therapy. It has been shown that an acute hyperemic response occurs following radiation therapy to the prostate gland and remains for 6–12 weeks [57, 58, 59]. Dynamic CT may have the potential to measure pathophysiologic indices in response to therapy but further studies are needed.

Conclusion

Computed tomography has a limited role in detection, localization, and staging of primary prostate cancer due to the inadequate soft-tissue contrast. The potential role of multidetector functional CT in assessing prostate perfusion and localizing prostate cancer needs to be further validated. The major role of CT is in evaluation of the extent of disease, including assessment of the presence of metastases to lymph nodes, distant organs or bones, in selected prostate cancer patients of higher risk categories. Computed tomography has an established role in treatment planning, especially for radiotherapy or brachytherapy of the prostate gland. The role of CT in prostate cancer treatment follow-up is focused on the assessment of recurrent or metastatic disease in patients with rising PSA levels after therapy.

REFERENCES

1. H. Hricak, P. L. Choyke, S. C. Eberhardt, *et al.*, Imaging prostate cancer: a multidisciplinary perspective. *Radiology*, **243** (2007), 28–53.

2. M. Huncharek, J. Muscat, Serum prostate-specific antigen as a predictor of radiographic staging studies in newly diagnosed prostate cancer. *Cancer Invest*, **13** (1995), 31–5.

3. S. Abuzallouf, I. Dayes, H. Lukka, Baseline staging of newly diagnosed prostate cancer: a summary of the literature. *J Urol*, **171** (2004), 2122–7.

4. E. S. Amis, Jr., L. R. Bigongiari, E. I. Bluth, *et al.*, Pretreatment staging of clinically localized prostate cancer. American College of Radiology. ACR Appropriateness Criteria. *Radiology* **215**:Suppl (2000), 703–8.

5. P. Carroll, C. Coley, D. McLeod, *et al.*, Prostate-specific antigen best practice policy – part II: prostate cancer staging and post-treatment follow-up. *Urology*, **57** (2001), 225–9.

6. C. S. Saigal, C. L. Pashos, J. M. Henning, *et al.*, Variations in use of imaging in a national sample of men with early-stage prostate cancer. *Urology*, **59** (2002), 400–4.

7. A. V. Kindrick, G. D. Grossfeld, D. M. Stier, *et al.*, Use of imaging tests for staging newly diagnosed prostate cancer: trends from the CaPSURE database. *J Urol*, **160** (1998), 2102–6.

8. K. K. Yu, H. Hricak, Imaging prostate cancer. *Radiol Clin North Am*, **38** (2000), 59–85, viii.

9. O. Akin, H. Hricak, Imaging of prostate cancer. *Radiol Clin North Am*, **45** (2007), 207–22.

10. C. E. Engeler, N. F. Wasserman, G. Zhang, Preoperative assessment of prostatic carcinoma by computerized tomography. Weaknesses and new perspectives. *Urology*, **40** (1992), 346–50.

11. J. F. Platt, R. L. Bree, R. E. Schwab, The accuracy of CT in the staging of carcinoma of the prostate. *AJR Am J Roentgenol*, **149** (1987), 315–18.

12. H. Hricak, G. C. Dooms, R. B. Jeffrey, *et al.*, Prostatic carcinoma: staging by clinical assessment, CT, and MR imaging. *Radiology*, **162** (1987), 331–6.

13. E. Henderson, M. F. Milosevic, M. A. Haider, *et al.*, Functional CT imaging of prostate cancer. *Phys Med Biol*, **48** (2003), 3085–100.

14. E. P. Ives, M. A. Burke, P. R. Edmonds, *et al.*, Quantitative computed tomography perfusion of prostate cancer: correlation with whole-mount pathology. *Clin Prostate Cancer*, **4** (2005), 109–12.

15. A. R. Padhani, C. J. Harvey, D. O. Cosgrove, Angiogenesis imaging in the management of prostate cancer. *Nat Clin Pract Urol*, **2** (2005), 596–607.

16. A. Prando, S. Wallace, Helical CT of prostate cancer: early clinical experience. *AJR Am J Roentgenol*, **175** (2000), 343–6.

17. C. R. Jeukens, C. A. van den Berg, R. Donker, *et al.*, Feasibility and measurement precision of 3D quantitative blood flow mapping of the prostate using dynamic contrast-enhanced multi-slice CT. *Phys Med Biol*, **51** (2006), 4329–43.

18. J. B. Rietbergen, R. F. Hoedemaeker, A. E. Kruger, *et al.*, The changing pattern of prostate cancer at the time of diagnosis: characteristics of screen detected prostate cancer in a population based screening study. *J Urol*, **161** (1999), 1192–8.

19. N. Lee, J. H. Newhouse, C. A. Olsson, *et al.*, Which patients with newly diagnosed prostate cancer need a computed tomography scan of the abdomen and pelvis? An analysis based on 588 patients. *Urology*, **54** (1999), 490–4.

20. M. Huncharek, J. Muscat, Serum prostate-specific antigen as a predictor of staging abdominal/pelvic computed tomography in newly diagnosed prostate cancer. *Abdom Imaging*, **21** (1996), 364–7.

21. J. A. Spencer, W. J. Chng, E. Hudson, *et al.*, Prostate specific antigen level and Gleason score in predicting the stage of newly diagnosed prostate cancer. *Br J Radiol*, **71** (1998), 1130–5.

22. G. J. O'Dowd, R. W. Veltri, R. Orozco, *et al.*, Update on the appropriate staging evaluation for newly diagnosed prostate cancer. *J Urol*, **158** (1997), 687–98.

23. Z. Levran, J. A. Gonzalez, A. C. Diokno, *et al.*, Are pelvic computed tomography, bone scan and pelvic lymphadenectomy necessary in the staging of prostatic cancer? *Br J Urol*, **75** (1995), 778–81.

24. R. C. Flanigan, T. C. McKay, M. Olson, *et al.*, Limited efficacy of preoperative computed tomographic scanning for the evaluation of lymph node metastasis in patients before radical prostatectomy. *Urology*, **48** (1996), 428–32.

25. L. H. Schwartz, L. R. LaTrenta, E. Bonaccio, *et al.*, Small cell and anaplastic prostate cancer: correlation between CT findings and prostate-specific antigen level. *Radiology*, **208** (1998), 735–8.

26. J. W. Moul, C. J. Kane, S. B. Malkowicz, The role of imaging studies and molecular markers for selecting candidates for radical prostatectomy. *Urol Clin North Am*, **28** (2001), 459–72.

27. H. Hricak, H. Schoder, D. Pucar, *et al.*, Advances in imaging in the postoperative patient with a rising prostate-specific antigen level. *Semin Oncol*, **30** (2003), 616–34.

28. R. Tiguert, E. L. Gheiler, M. V. Tefilli, *et al.*, Lymph node size does not correlate with the presence of prostate cancer metastasis. *Urology*, **53** (1999), 367–71.

29. J. S. Wolf, Jr., M. Cher, M. Dall'era , *et al.*, The use and accuracy of cross-sectional imaging and fine needle aspiration cytology for detection of pelvic lymph node metastases before radical prostatectomy. *J Urol*, **153** (1995), 993–9.

30. R. H. Oyen, H. P. van Poppel, F. E. Ameye, *et al.*, Lymph node staging of localized prostatic carcinoma with CT and CT-guided fine-needle aspiration biopsy: prospective study of 285 patients. *Radiology*, **190** (1994), 315–22.

31. R. H. Flocks, D. Culp, R. Porto, Lymphatic spread from prostatic cancer. *J Urol*, **81** (1959), 194–6.

32. J. Spencer, S. Golding, CT evaluation of lymph node status at presentation of prostatic carcinoma. *Br J Radiol*, **65** (1992), 199–201.

33. A. Y. Fung, S. Y. Grimm, J. R. Wong, *et al.*, Computed tomography localization of radiation treatment delivery versus conventional localization with bony landmarks. *J Appl Clin Med Phys*, **4** (2003), 112–19.

34. D. J. Lee, S. Leibel, R. Shiels, *et al.*, The value of ultrasonic imaging and CT scanning in planning the radiotherapy for prostatic carcinoma. *Cancer*, **45** (1980), 724–7.

35. M. V. Pilepich, S. C. Prasad, C. A. Perez, Computed tomography in definitive radiotherapy of prostatic carcinoma, part 2: definition of target volume. *Int J Radiat Oncol Biol Phys*, **8** (1982), 235–9.

36. J. W. Mens, B. J. Slotman, O. W. Meijer, *et al.*, Effect of CT-based treatment planning on portal field size and outcome in radiation treatment of localized prostate cancer. *Radiother Oncol*, **55** (2000), 27–30.

37. J. Bellon, K. Wallner, W. Ellis, *et al.*, Use of pelvic CT scanning to evaluate pubic arch interference of transperineal prostate brachytherapy. *Int J Radiat Oncol Biol Phys*, **43** (1999), 579–81.

38. M. Milosevic, S. Voruganti, R. Blend, *et al.*, Magnetic resonance imaging (MRI) for localization of the prostatic apex: comparison to computed tomography (CT) and urethrography. *Radiother Oncol*, **47** (1998), 277–84.

39. S. Hocht, T. Wiegel, D. Bottke, *et al.*, Computed tomogram prior to prostatectomy. Advantage in defining planning target volumes for postoperative adjuvant radiotherapy in patients with stage C prostate cancer? *Strahlenther Onkol*, **178** (2002), 134–8.

40. M. Roach, 3rd, P. Faillace-Akazawa, C. Malfatti, *et al.*, Prostate volumes defined by magnetic resonance imaging and computerized tomographic scans for three-dimensional conformal radiotherapy. *Int J Radiat Oncol Biol Phys*, **35** (1996), 1011–18.

41. S. C. Hoffelt, L. M. Marshall, M. Garzotto, *et al.*, A comparison of CT scan to transrectal ultrasound-measured prostate volume in untreated prostate cancer. *Int J Radiat Oncol Biol Phys*, **57** (2003), 29–32.

42. G. L. Sannazzari, R. Ragona, M. G. Ruo Redda, *et al.*, CT-MRI image fusion for delineation of volumes in three-dimensional conformal radiation therapy in the treatment of localized prostate cancer. *Br J Radiol*, **75** (2002), 603–7.

43. S. Wachter, N. Wachter-Gerstner, T. Bock, *et al.*, Interobserver comparison of CT and MRI-based prostate apex definition. Clinical relevance for conformal radiotherapy treatment planning. *Strahlenther Onkol*, **178** (2002), 263–8.

44. E. Berthelet, M. C. Liu, A. Agranovich, *et al.*, Computed tomography determination of prostate volume and maximum dimensions: a study of interobserver variability. *Radiother Oncol*, **63** (2002), 37–40.

45. S. M. Zhou, G. C. Bentel, C. G. Lee, *et al.*, Differences in gross target volumes on contrast vs. noncontrast CT scans utilized for conformal radiation therapy treatment planning for prostate carcinoma. *Int J Radiat Oncol Biol Phys*, **42** (1998), 73–8.

46. K. M. Kalkner, G. Kubicek, J. Nilsson, *et al.*, Prostate volume determination: differential

volume measurements comparing CT and TRUS. *Radiother Oncol*, **81** (2006), 179–83.

47. A. T. Porter, J. C. Blasko, P. D. Grimm, *et al.*, Brachytherapy for prostate cancer. *CA Cancer J Clin*, **45** (1995), 165–78.

48. R. M. Gore, A. A. Moss, Value of computed tomography in interstitial ^{125}I brachytherapy of prostatic carcinoma. *Radiology*, **146** (1983), 453–8.

49. T. Mizowaki, G. N. Cohen, A. Y. Fung, *et al.*, Towards integrating functional imaging in the treatment of prostate cancer with radiation: the registration of the MR spectroscopy imaging to ultrasound/CT images and its implementation in treatment planning. *Int J Radiat Oncol Biol Phys*, **54** (2002), 1558–64.

50. M. G. Neill, G. A. Lockwood, S. A. McCluskey, *et al.*, Preoperative evaluation of the "hostile pelvis" in radical prostatectomy with computed tomographic pelvimetry. *BJU Int*, **99** (2007), 534–8.

51. S. Kramer, J. Gorich, H. W. Gottfried, *et al.*, Sensitivity of computed tomography in detecting local recurrence of prostatic carcinoma following radical prostatectomy. *Br J Radiol*, **70** (1997), 995–9.

52. W. L. Strohmaier, T. Keller, K. H. Bichler, Follow-up in prostate cancer patients: which parameters are necessary? *Eur Urol*, **35** (1999), 21–5.

53. K. K. Yu, R. A. Hawkins, The prostate: diagnostic evaluation of metastatic disease. *Radiol Clin North Am*, **38** (2000), 139–57, ix.

54. J. A. Spencer, S. J. Golding, Patterns of lymphatic metastases at recurrence of prostate cancer: CT findings. *Clin Radiol*, **49** (1994), 404–7.

55. N. Glajchen, R. D. Shapiro, R. G. Stock, *et al.*, CT findings after laparoscopic pelvic lymph node dissection and transperineal radioactive seed implantation for prostatic carcinoma. *AJR Am J Roentgenol*, **166** (1996), 1165–8.

56. R. J. Amdur, D. Gladstone, K. A. Leopold, *et al.*, Prostate seed implant quality assessment using MR and CT image fusion. *Int J Radiat Oncol Biol Phys*, **43** (1999), 67–72.

57. C. J. Harvey, M. J. Blomley, P. Dawson, *et al.*, Functional CT imaging of the acute hyperemic response to radiation therapy of the prostate gland: early experience. *J Comput Assist Tomogr*, **25** (2001), 43–9.

58. C. Harvey, J. Morgan, M. Blomley, *et al.*, Tumor responses to radiation therapy: use of dynamic contrast material-enhanced CT to monitor functional and anatomical indices. *Acad Radiol*, **9**: Suppl 1 (2002), S215–219.

59. C. Harvey, A. Dooher, J. Morgan, *et al.*, Imaging of tumour therapy responses by dynamic CT. *Eur J Radiol*, **30** (1999), 221–6.

9

Magnetic resonance imaging of prostate cancer

Oguz Akin

Introduction

Magnetic resonance imaging (MRI) is one of the most useful imaging methods for the non-invasive evaluation of prostate cancer. The prostate and periprostatic structures can be depicted with excellent soft-tissue resolution with MRI, allowing assessment of the local extent of disease. Currently, the role of MRI in prostate cancer is evolving to improve disease detection and staging, to determine the aggressiveness of disease, and to optimize individualized treatment planning and follow-up.

This article reviews the role of MRI in the diagnosis and management of prostate cancer, from diagnosis to post-treatment follow-up. Specific imaging features of prostate cancer as seen on MR imaging are described, and the advantages, limitations, and clinically relevant uses of various MRI techniques are discussed.

Magnetic resonance imaging techniques

A magnetic field strength of at least 1.5 Tesla (T) is required for a high-quality MRI study of the prostate. A magnetic field strength of 3 T provides a greater signal-to-noise ratio that allows higher resolution imaging. The advantages of higher resolution imaging are the detection of small tumors and more accurate local staging.

The use of an endorectal coil with a pelvic phased-array coil markedly improves image quality and is recommended. Magnetic resonance imaging parameters applied in prostate imaging depend on the type of MRI system used and the field strength. In general, T_1-weighted transverse images of the entire pelvis are obtained for the assessment of post-biopsy hemorrhage in the prostate, pelvic lymph nodes, and bones. High-resolution T_2-weighted images with a small field of view (~14 cm) and thin sections (3 mm) acquired with fast spin-echo sequences in the transverse, sagittal, and coronal planes are essential in prostate cancer detection, localization, and staging.

Prostate Cancer, eds. Hedvig Hricak and Peter T. Scardino. Published by Cambridge University Press.
© Cambridge University Press 2009.

Post-biopsy hemorrhage may cause under- or over-estimation of the tumor presence and local extent. Therefore, MRI must be delayed for at least 4–8 weeks after prostate biopsy.

Dynamic contrast-enhanced magnetic resonance imaging

Dynamic contrast-enhanced MRI may improve the accuracy of prostate cancer detection by MR imaging alone. It is believed that in dynamic contrast-enhanced imaging, tumor angiogenesis results in different contrast enhancement in cancerous tissues than in normal tissues. Numerous contrast-enhancement parameters can be used to differentiate cancerous from benign tissue, including onset time, time to peak enhancement, peak enhancement, relative peak enhancement, and washout time.

Although a standard MRI protocol for dynamic contrast-enhanced MRI has not been established, a fast imaging sequence with minimal artifacts is obtained after rapid bolus administration of intravenous contrast. Typically, serial acquisitions through the prostate are obtained every 2–5 s after contrast injection.

The main challenge in dynamic contrast-enhanced MRI is to establish an optimized balance between temporal and spatial resolution. More studies are necessary to refine the dynamic imaging protocols and standardize parameters that could be of clinical value.

Diffusion-weighted magnetic resonance imaging

Diffusion-weighted MRI is used to depict variations in water diffusion in different tissues. The cellular structure and organization of cancerous cells are different from those of normal cells, therefore water diffusion is different in cancerous tissues than in normal tissues.

The advantages of diffusion-weighted imaging are its short acquisition time and high contrast resolution between cancerous and normal tissues. However, its poor spatial resolution is one of the major limitations of this technique. Further studies are necessary to establish the incremental value of diffusion-weighted imaging to other MRI techniques in assessment of prostate cancer.

Magnetic resonance spectroscopy

Magnetic resonance spectroscopy provides metabolic information about prostatic tissue by displaying the relative concentrations of citrate, creatine, choline, and polyamines. Normal prostate tissue contains high levels of citrate. In the presence of prostate cancer, the citrate level is diminished or not detectable and the choline is elevated due to the high phospholipid cell membrane turnover in the proliferating malignant tissue. Therefore, regions containing prostate cancer depict an increased choline-to-citrate ratio. Because the creatine peak is very close to the choline peak in the spectral trace, the two may be inseparable; therefore, for practical purposes, the [choline+creatine]/citrate ratio is used in practice. With the latest spectroscopic sequences, polyamine peaks can be resolved as well. The polyamine peak decreases in the presence of prostate cancer.

Commonly used MR spectroscopic imaging techniques include chemical shift imaging with point resolved spectroscopy (PRESS) voxel excitation and band-selective inversion with gradient dephasing (BASING) for water and lipid suppression. Nowadays, three-dimensional (3D) proton MR spectroscopic mapping of the entire prostate is possible.

Addition of MR spectroscopy as a supplement to T_2-weighted MRI can improve overall tumor detection and increase readers' confidence in their assessment. Limitations of MR spectroscopy include its long acquisition time and the dependency of MR spectral quality on post-processing or shimming.

The role of MR spectroscopy in the assessment of prostate cancer is further discussed in detail in Chapter 10.

Magnetic resonance imaging appearance of normal prostate

Among all imaging modalities, MRI offers the most exquisite depiction of the zonal anatomy of the prostate due to its high spatial resolution and superior contrast resolution.

The zonal anatomy of the prostate gland is best seen on high-resolution T_2-weighted images [1] (Figure 9.1). The prostate gland is composed of peripheral, central, and transition zones and a fibromuscular stroma. The fibromuscular stroma is located anteriorly and has low signal intensity on T_2-weighted images. The peripheral zone, the major glandular constituent, forms the posterior, lateral, and apical portions of the prostate. Normal peripheral zone demonstrates high signal intensity. The low-signal-intensity central zone is located posteriorly and superiorly between the peripheral zone and the proximal prostatic urethra. The heterogeneous-signal-intensity transition zone is located anteriorly and laterally to the prostatic urethra. A hair-thin rim with low signal intensity around the peripheral zone represents the anatomic capsule of the prostate. The boundary

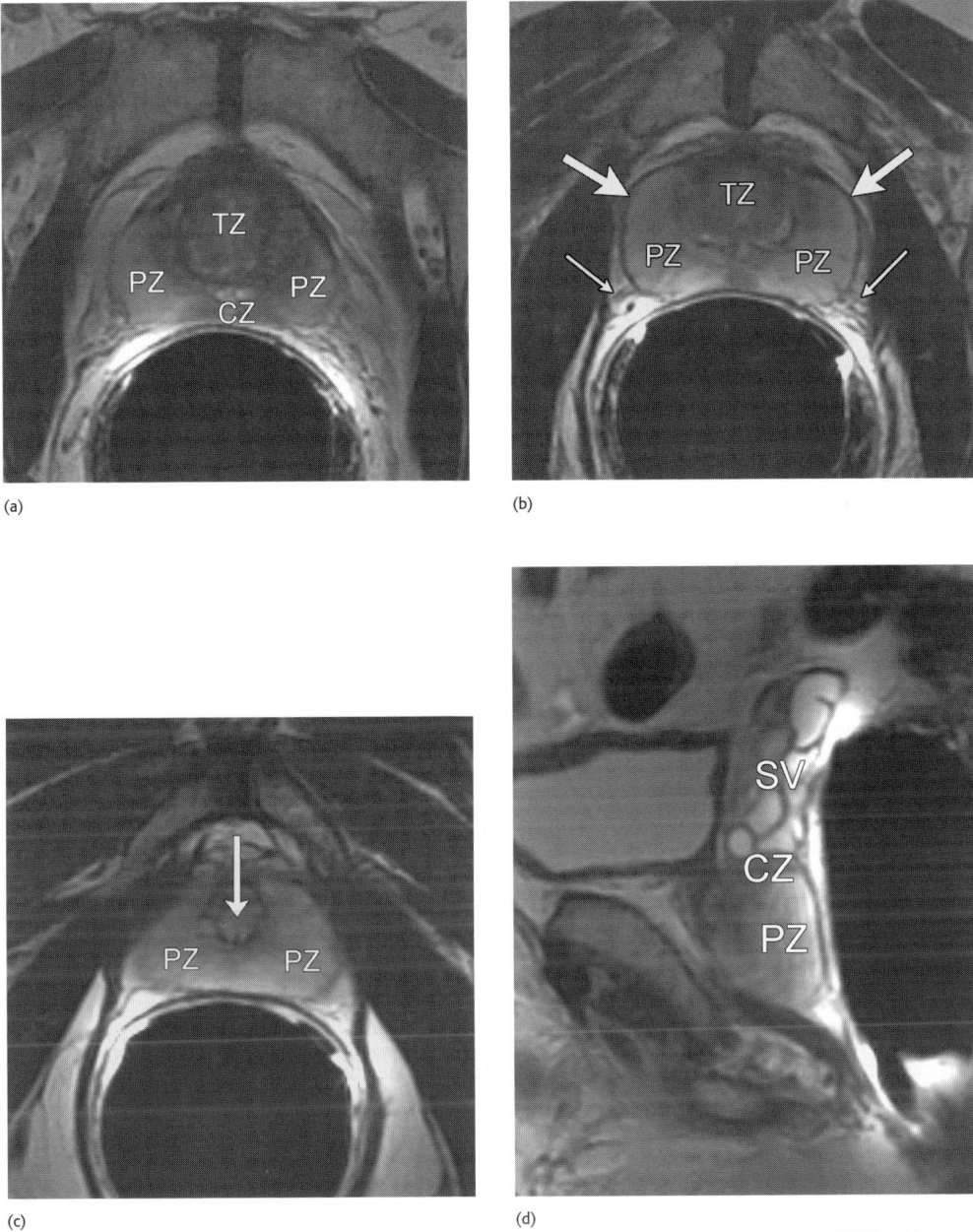

Figure 9.1. Normal zonal anatomy of the prostate in a 62-year-old man seen on transverse T$_2$-weighted MR images obtained at the level of the base of the prostate (a), the midgland (b), and the apex (c); parasagittal (d), midsagittal (e), and coronal (f) MR images are also shown. PZ, peripheral zone; TZ, transition zone; CZ, central zone; SV, seminal vesicles. The large arrows on (b) indicate the prostatic capsule; the small arrows on (b) indicate neurovascular bundles. The arrows on (c) and (f) indicate the urethra. The arrows on (e) indicate anterior fibromuscular stroma.

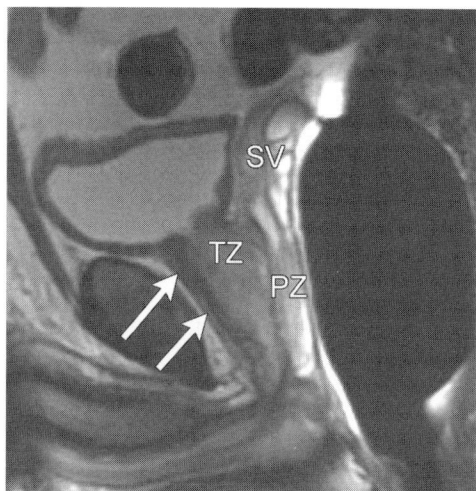
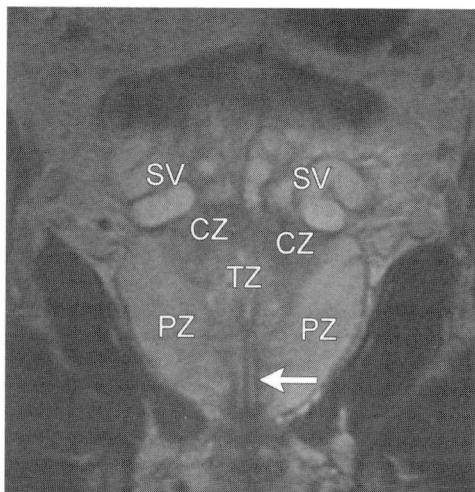

(e)

(f)

Figure 9.1. (cont.)

between the transition and peripheral zones can be seen as a thin line, which represents the pseudocapsule or surgical capsule of the prostate. The neurovascular bundles are seen posterolaterally to the prostate capsule on both sides. The seminal vesicles and the vasa deferentia are located just above the base of the prostate and behind the urinary bladder and both demonstrate high signal intensity. The ducts of the seminal vesicles join the vasa deferentia to form the ejaculatory ducts, which open into the prostatic urethra at the level of the verumontanum. The proximal prostatic urethra is less distinct on T_2-weighted images but the distal prostatic urethra is seen as a well-defined low-signal-intensity structure in the lower prostate.

Magnetic resonance imaging appearance of prostate cancer

On MRI, foci of prostate cancer are best seen on T_2-weighted images (Figure 9.2). Most commonly prostate cancer occurs in the peripheral zone of the prostate. In the peripheral zone, prostate cancer appears as focal low-signal-intensity lesions on the background of a high-signal-intensity peripheral zone. However, low signal intensity can also be caused by several other conditions such as biopsy-related changes, prostatitis, atrophy, or changes due to prior radiation or hormonal treatment [1]. Although less commonly than the peripheral zone, the transition zone of the prostate may also harbor cancer. Evaluation of transition zone cancers on MRI

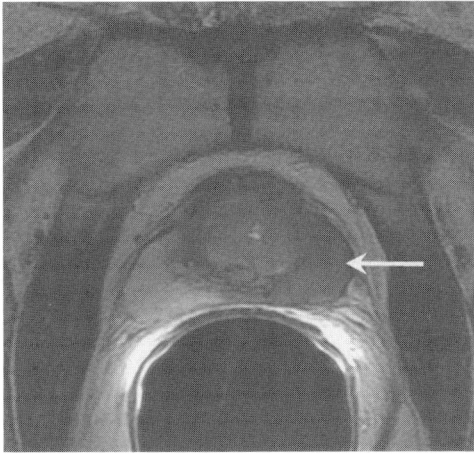

(a)

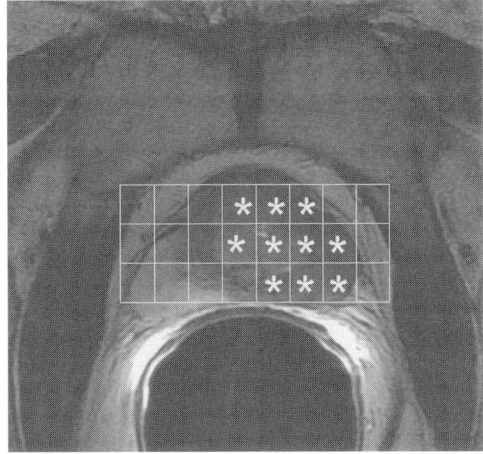

(b)

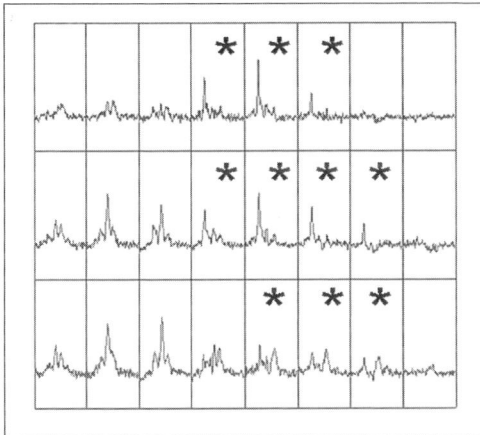

(c)

Figure 9.2. MR imaging appearance with corresponding MR spectroscopy of prostate cancer in a 65-year-old man (a–c). Transverse T_2-weighted MR image (a) shows a focal low-signal-intensity lesion (arrow) representing tumor involving the peripheral and transition zones of the prostate on the left. A multi-voxel MR spectroscopy grid superimposed on a T_2-weighted image (b) and corresponding spectra (c) show voxels (asterisks), with elevated choline and reduced citrate, which are consistent with tumor.

is complicated by the fact that the transition zone is commonly affected by benign prostatic hyperplasia and, thus, demonstrates heterogeneous signal intensity on T_2-weighted images. It is especially difficult to distinguish transition zone cancers from fibromuscular (stromal) benign prostatic hyperplasia nodules, because both conditions can demonstrate low T_2 signal intensity on MR images. However, transition zone cancers have certain distinguishing MRI features such as homogeneous low T_2 signal intensity, ill-defined margins without a well-defined capsule, lenticular shape, and invasion of the anterior fibromuscular stroma [2, 3].

In order to overcome the limitations of T_2-weighted MRI and to improve the diagnostic performance of MRI in the detection of prostate cancer, other MRI techniques have been proposed [4]. These newer techniques such as dynamic contrast-enhanced MRI, diffusion-weighted MRI and MR spectroscopic imaging offer "physiologic" and "metabolic" information that are generally used to supplement the "morphologic" information provided by T_2-weighted MRI [5, 6].

Data obtained by dynamic contrast-enhanced MRI can be quantitatively analyzed for several contrast-enhancement parameters mentioned above. In general, prostate cancer enhances more rapidly and intensely and shows early washout compared with normal prostate tissue [7, 8, 9, 10]. This pattern of enhancement is predictive of, but is not pathognomonic for, prostate cancer. Some prostate cancers, especially those that are mildly or moderately hypervascular, are not detectable with this method [11].

On diffusion-weighted MRI, prostate cancer appears as foci with restricted diffusion and with a reduction in apparent diffusion coefficient (ADC) values compared to the normal prostate tissue [12, 13, 14, 15, 16]. However, there are variations in the diffusion properties of the cancerous and normal tissues, and overlap in ADC values limits the diagnostic accuracy of this technique [4].

On MR spectroscopic imaging, metabolic data in spectral form can be directly overlaid on the corresponding morphologic T_2-weighted images (Figure 9.2). A voxel is classified as normal, suspicious for cancer, or very suspicious for cancer. Voxels are considered suspicious for cancer if [Cho+Cr]/Cit is at least two standard deviations above the average ratio for the normal peripheral zone, and voxels are considered very suspicious for cancer if [Cho+Cr]/Cit is more than three standard deviations above the average ratio [17, 18]. Although currently the spatial resolution of MR spectroscopy is lower than that of MRI, the combined use of MR spectroscopy and T_2-weighted imaging improves prostate cancer detection [19].

Role of magnetic resonance imaging in assessment of prostate cancer

Magnetic-resonance-imaging-guided prostate biopsy

Biopsy, typically guided by transrectal ultrasound (TRUS), remains the gold standard for the detection and diagnosis of prostate cancer and is safe and cost-effective. Although MRI is not used as an initial imaging modality to detect prostate cancer, it can be useful for targeted biopsy planning especially in patients with clinically suspected prostate cancer and previous negative TRUS-guided biopsy results [20, 21, 22, 23]. Magnetic-resonance-imaging-guided transrectal prostate biopsy is technically possible. However, the use of MRI for biopsy guidance is limited by difficulties in patient access and positioning and by the higher cost of this technique. An alternative approach is to fuse MR images with real-time TRUS to guide biopsy. In this technique, T_2-weighted images are overlaid on corresponding TRUS images using several landmarks within the prostate. Once the MR images and TRUS are fused, suspicious areas on T_2-weighted images can be targeted using TRUS [24].

Tumor detection and localization

A study on prostate cancer detection and tumor localization found that MRI had 61% and 77% sensitivity, and 46% and 81% specificity, with moderate inter-reader agreement. In the same study, MR spectroscopy for the detection of cancer had significantly higher specificity (75%, $p < 0.05$) but lower sensitivity (63%, $p < 0.05$). The investigators reported high specificity (91%) when combined MRI and MR spectroscopy indicated a positive result, and high sensitivity (95%) when either test alone did so [19]. A later study comparing digital rectal examination, TRUS-guided biopsy, and MRI in the detection and localization of prostate cancer showed that MRI significantly increased the accuracy of prostate cancer localization compared with either digital rectal examination or TRUS-guided biopsy ($p < 0.0001$ for each). The area under the receiver operating characteristic (ROC) curve for tumor localization was greater for MRI than for digital rectal examination at the prostatic apex (0.72 vs. 0.66), midgland (0.80 vs. 0.69), and base (0.83 vs. 0.69); it was also higher for MRI than for TRUS-guided biopsy in the midgland (0.75 vs. 0.68) and base (0.81 vs. 0.61) but not in the apex (0.67 vs. 0.70) [25].

Most MR studies focus on tumor detection in the peripheral zone of the prostate, where most cancers originate. Magnetic resonance imaging can also be useful in detecting transition zone prostate cancers. In a recent study on the detection and localization of transition zone cancer by MRI, the areas under the ROC curves of two readers were 0.75 and 0.73 [2].

As noted earlier, combining different MRI techniques can increase accuracy in prostate cancer detection. A recent study reported that, for prostate cancer localization, the areas under the ROC curve for T_2-weighted MRI, dynamic contrast-enhanced MRI, and MR spectroscopy were 0.68, 0.91, and 0.80, respectively [26]. The accuracy in tumor localization with dynamic contrast-enhanced imaging was significantly better than that with MR spectroscopic imaging ($p < 0.01$); and the accuracy in tumor localization with both dynamic contrast-enhanced MRI and MR spectroscopy was significantly better than that with T_2-weighted MRI ($p < 0.01$) [26]. Another recent study showed that the sensitivity, specificity, accuracy, and the area under the ROC curve for the detection of prostate cancer were 73%, 54%, 64%, and 0.71, respectively, with T_2-weighted MRI alone; 84%, 85%, 84%, and 0.90, respectively, with combined T_2-weighted MRI and diffusion-weighted MRI; and 95%, 74%, 86%, and 0.96, respectively, with combined T_2-weighted MRI, diffusion-weighted MRI and dynamic contrast-enhanced MRI [27]. The sensitivity, specificity, and accuracy differed significantly among these three approaches ($p < 0.01$) [27].

Tumor staging

Magnetic resonance imaging plays an important role in local staging of prostate cancer. Local spread of tumor – most importantly extraprostatic extension and seminal vesicle invasion – can be assessed on MRI (Figure 9.3).

Magnetic resonance imaging criteria for extracapsular extension of prostate cancer include a tumor causing contour deformity with a step-off or angulated margin; an irregular capsular bulge or retraction; a breach of the capsule with evidence of direct tumor extension; obliteration of the recto-prostatic angle; and asymmetric thickening or retraction of the neurovascular bundles [1, 5].

Magnetic resonance imaging criteria for seminal vesicle invasion include contiguous low-signal-intensity tumor extension from the base of the gland into the seminal vesicles; tumor extension along the ejaculatory ducts (non-visualization of the ejaculatory ducts); asymmetric decrease in the signal intensity of the seminal vesicles; and decreased conspicuity of the seminal vesicle walls [1, 5, 28].

Previous studies reported varying accuracies (from 50% to 92%) for the local staging of prostate cancer with MRI [29]: MRI has been reported to have 13%–95% sensitivity and 49%–97% specificity for the detection of extracapsular extension and 23%–80% sensitivity and 81%–99% specificity for the detection of seminal vesicle invasion [30, 31, 32, 33, 34, 35, 36, 37, 38]. A recent study showed that for two readers, the areas under the ROC curves were 0.93 and 0.81 for the detection of seminal vesicle invasion at MRI [28].

Although MR spectroscopy alone is not used for the detection of extracapsular extension of prostate cancer, combined use of MRI and MR spectroscopy improves tumor detection and consequently the detection of extracapsular extension.

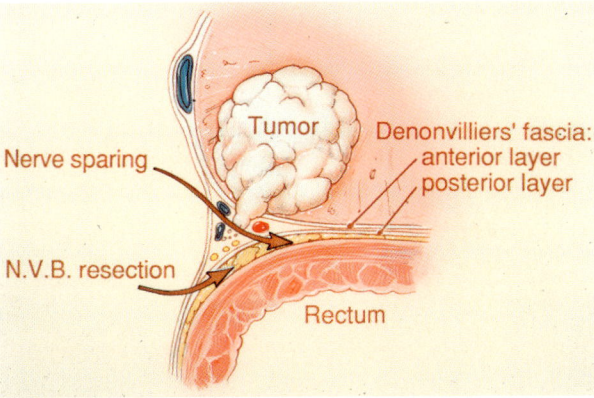

4.2

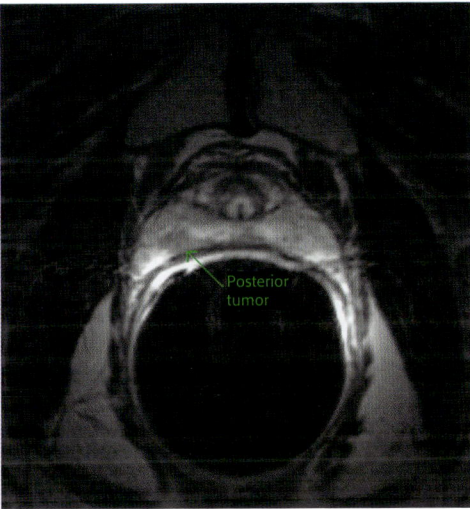

4.3

Posterior
tumor

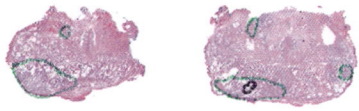

(a)   (b)   (c)

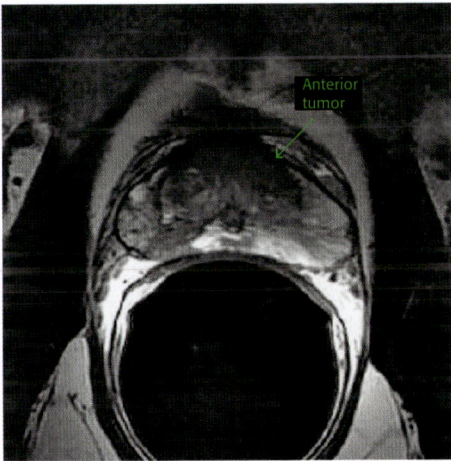

4.4

Anterior
tumor

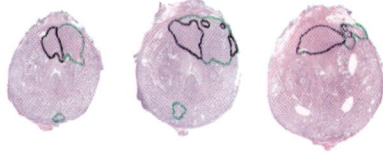

(a)   (b)   (c)   (d)

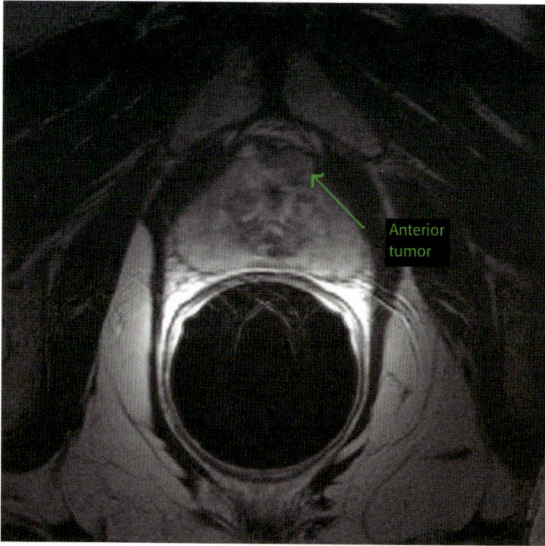

(a)

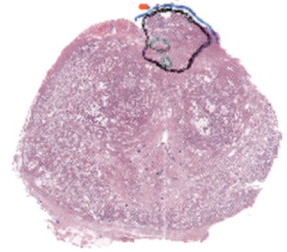

(b)

3D conformal

IMRT

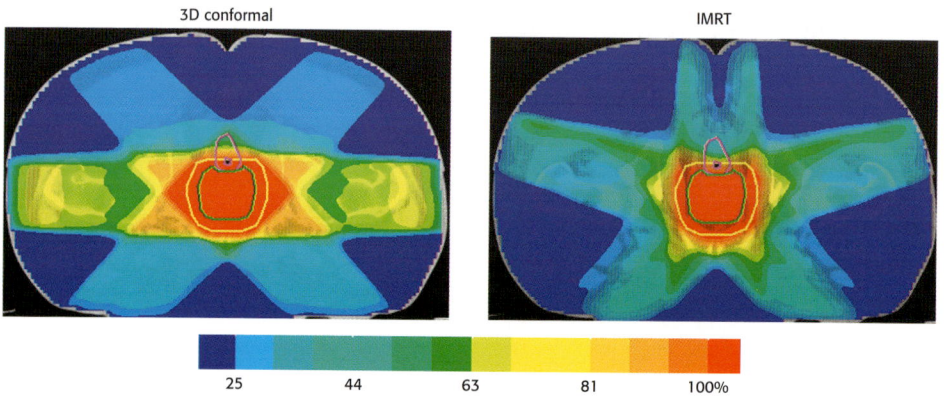

25   44   63   81   100%

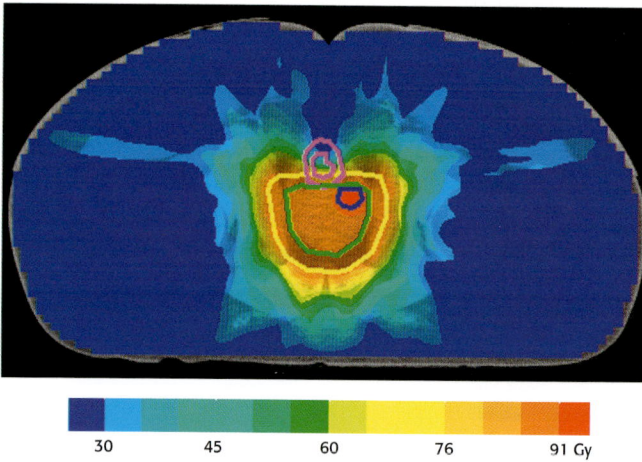

30   45   60   76   91 Gy

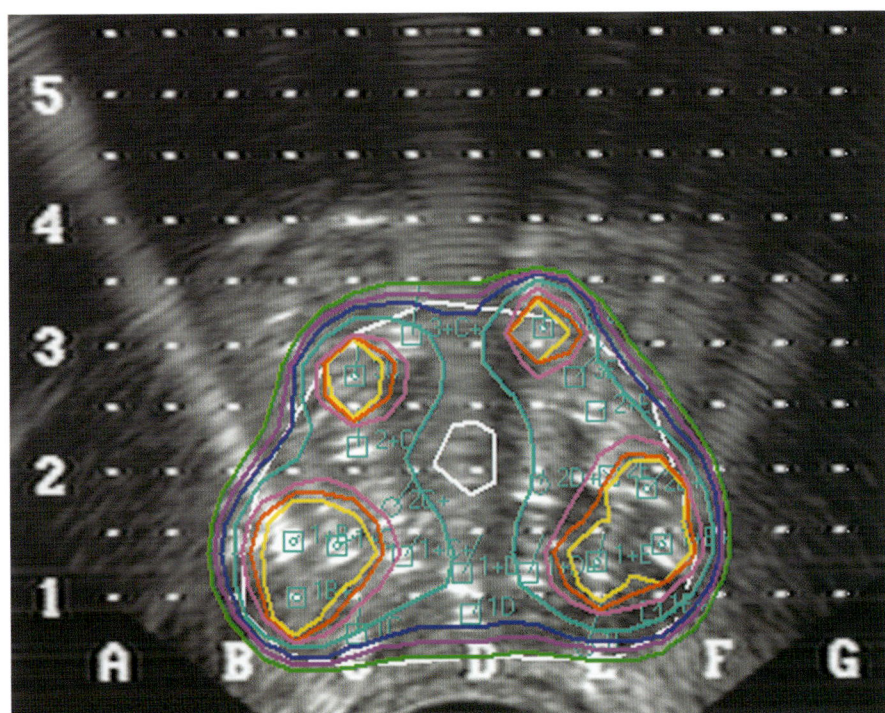

5.6

5.7

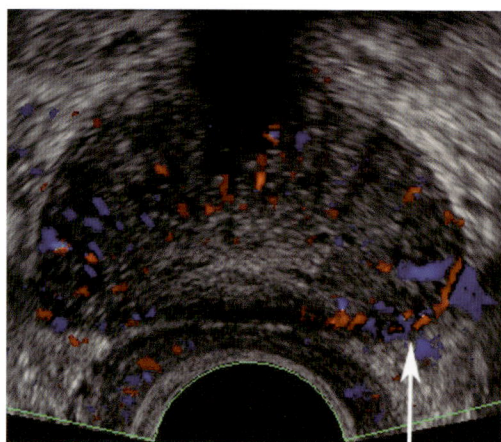

7.1b

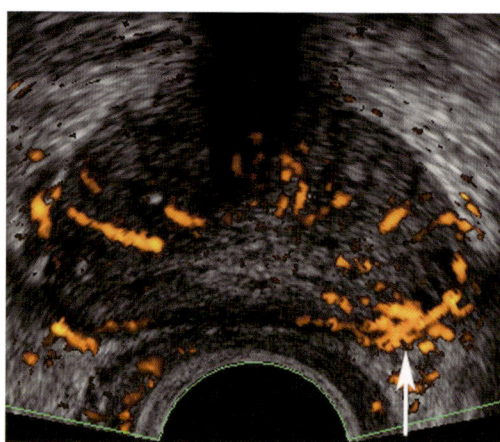

7.1c

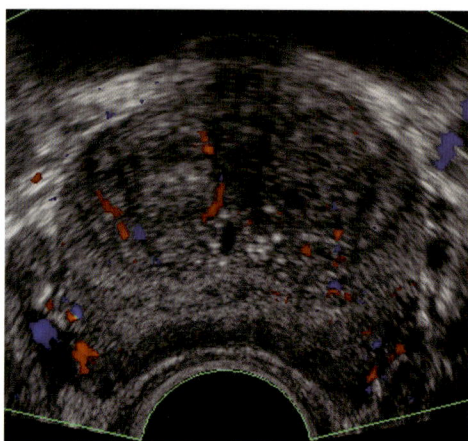

7.2b

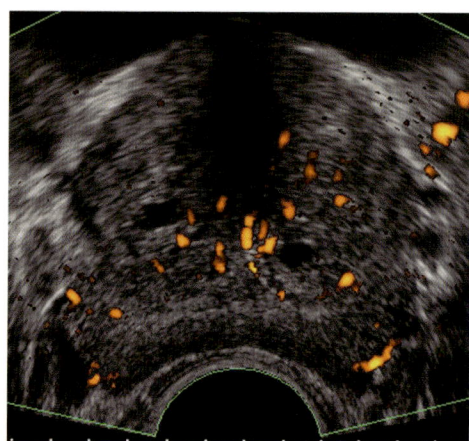

7.2c

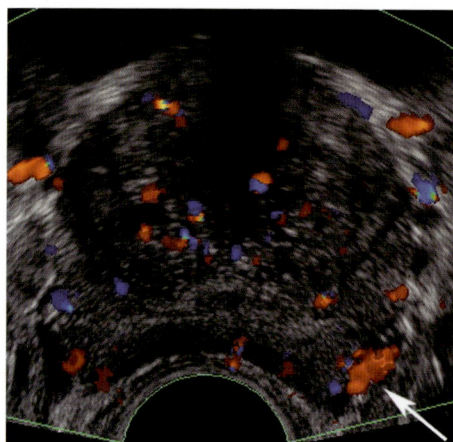

7.2d

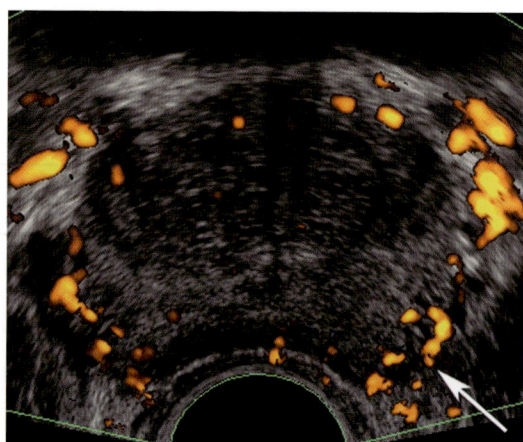

7.2e

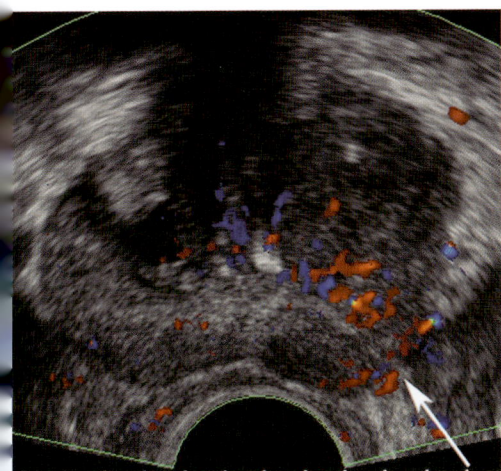

7.3b

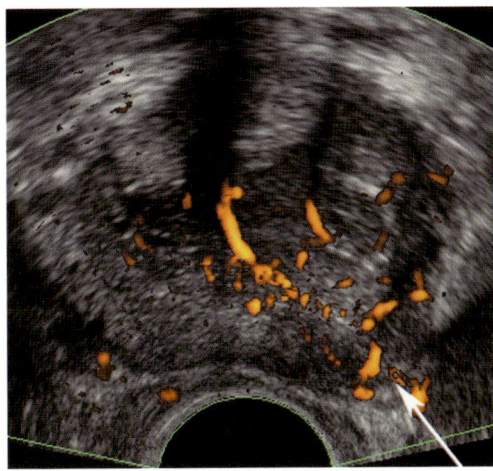

7.3c

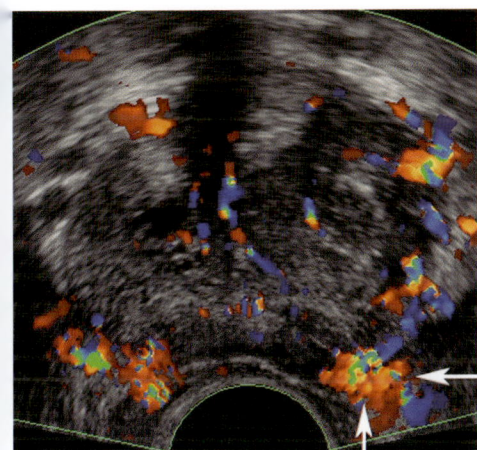

7.3f

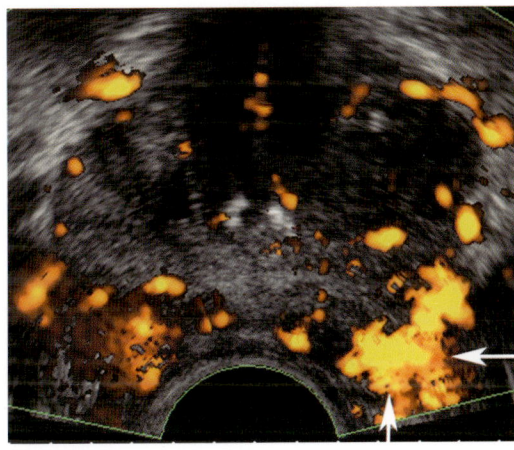

7.3g

7.4

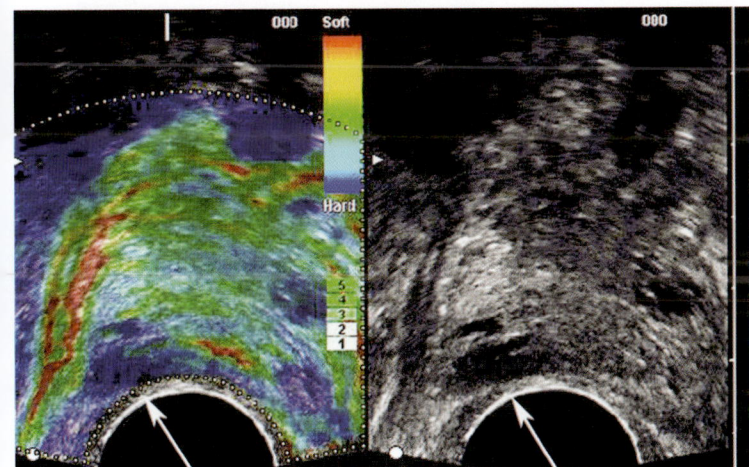

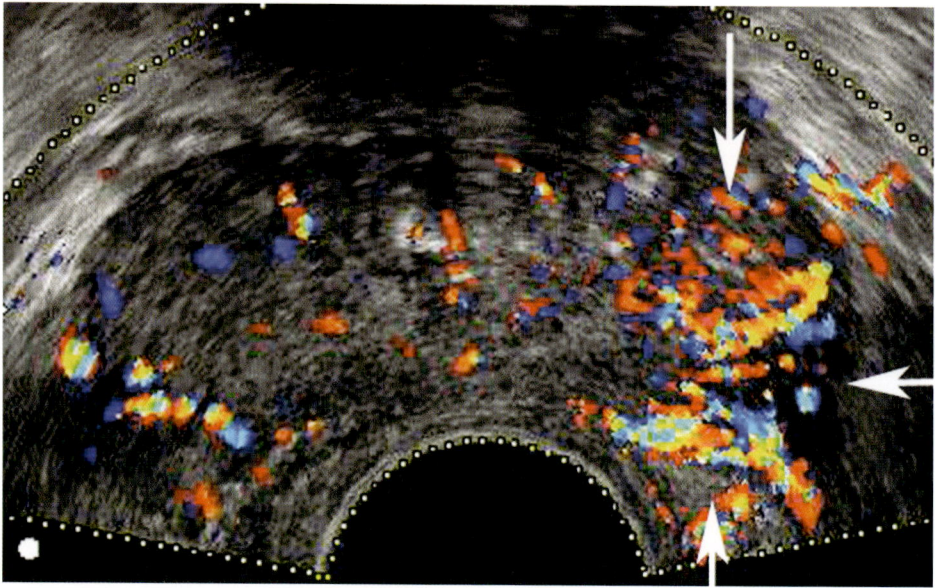

7.5a

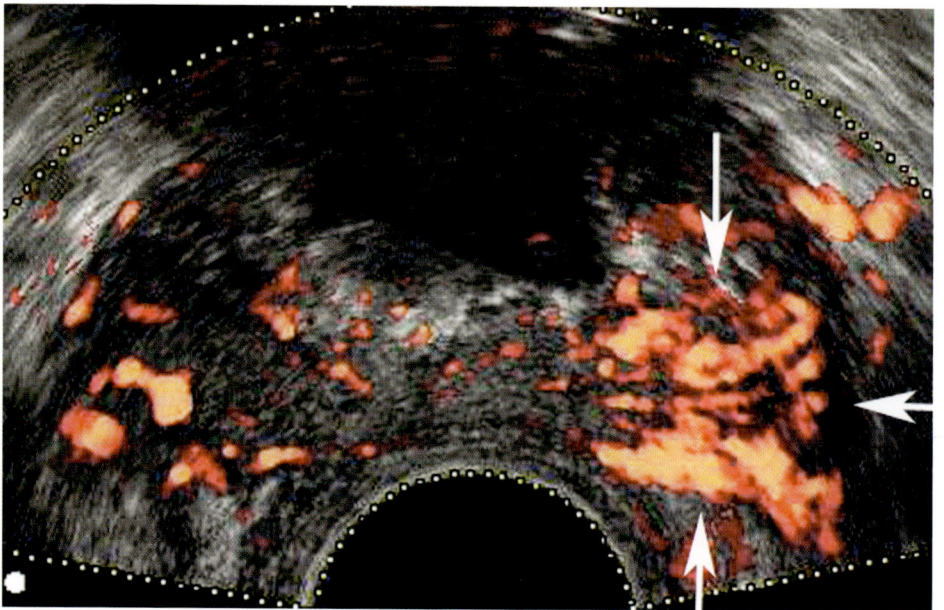

7.5b

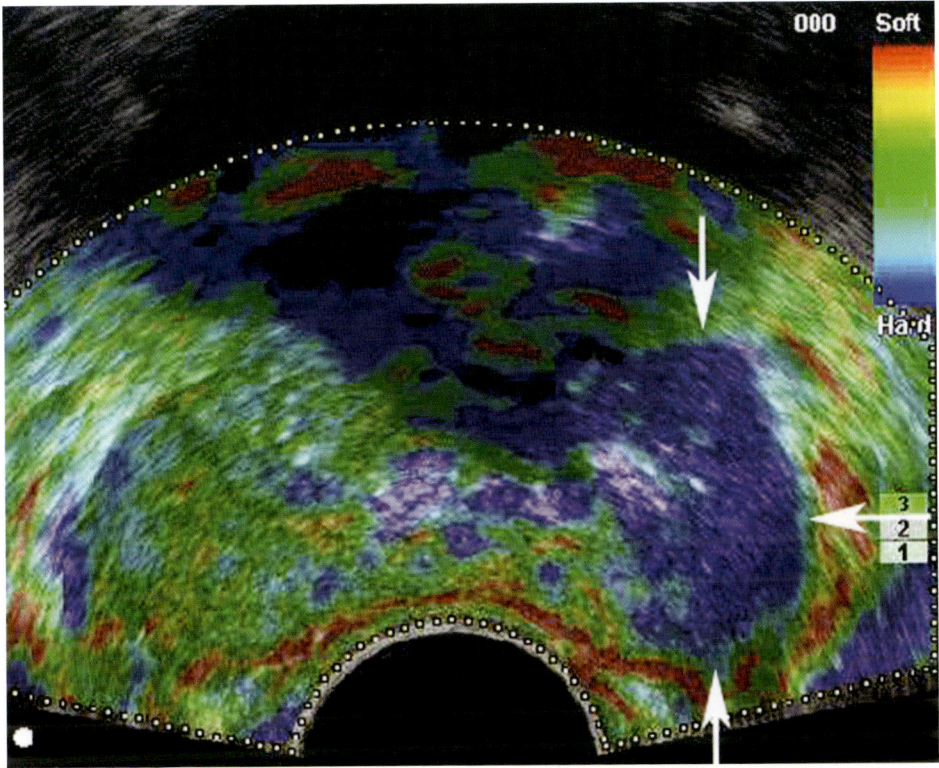

7.5c

10.5b

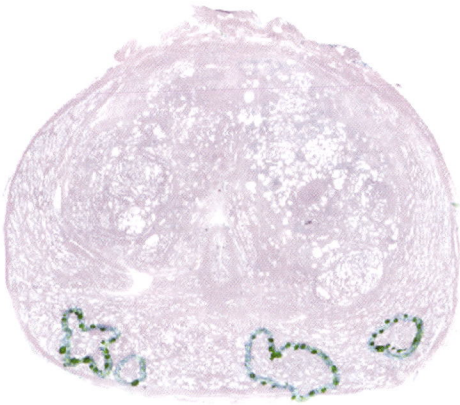

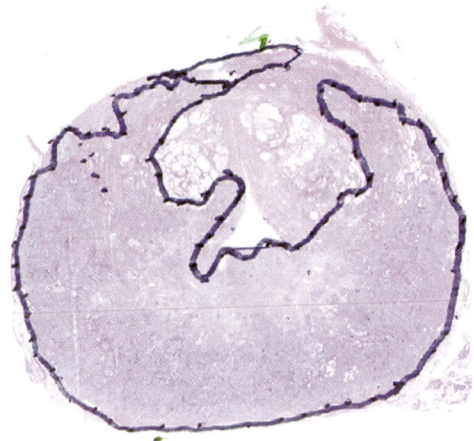

10.5d

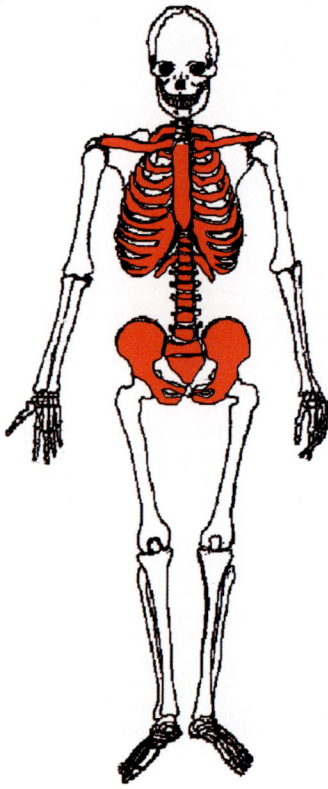
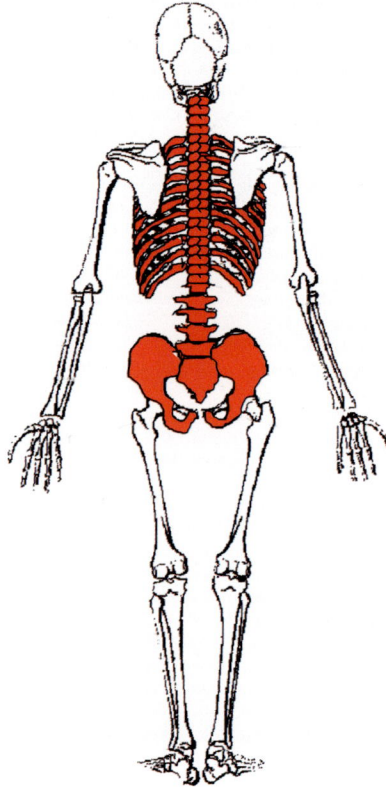

11.2b

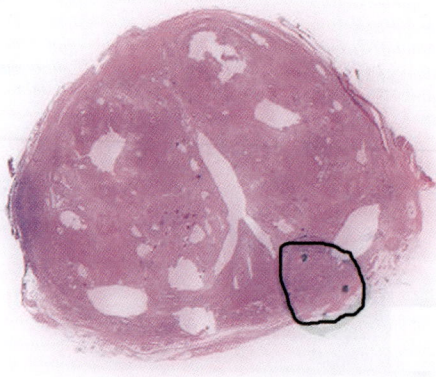

12.4c

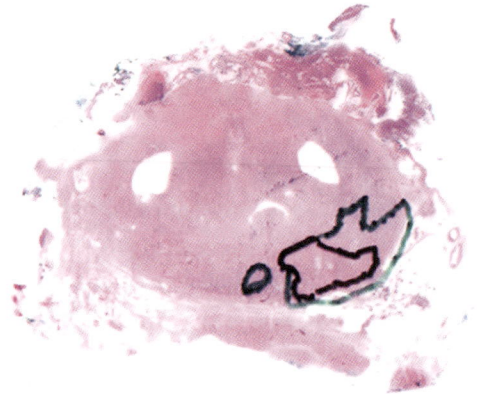

12.5b

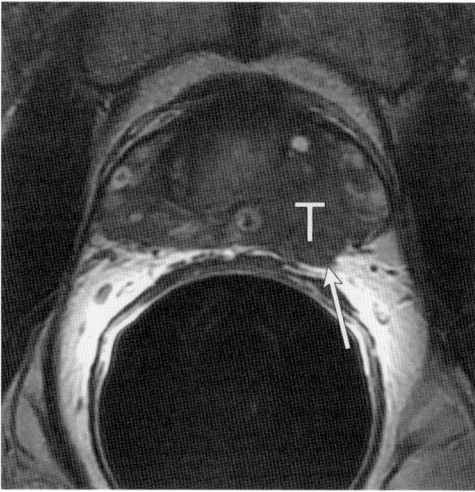

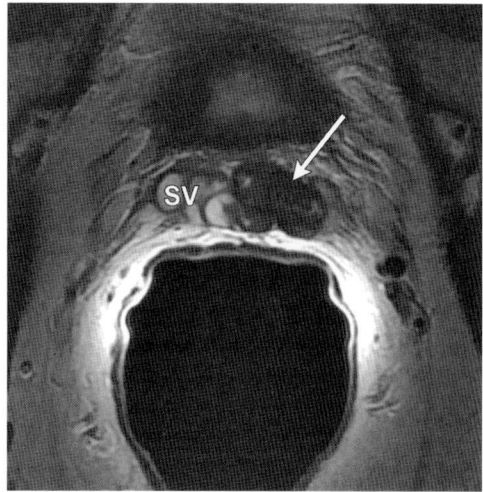

(a)

(b)

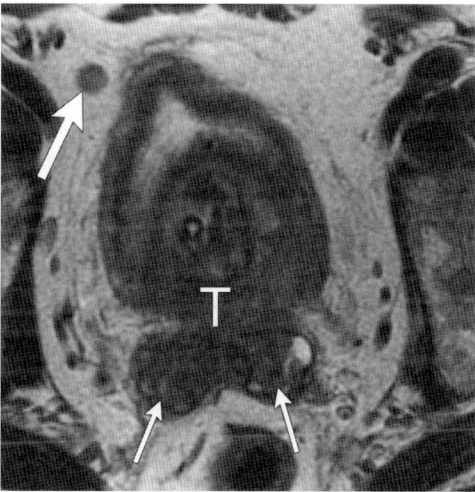

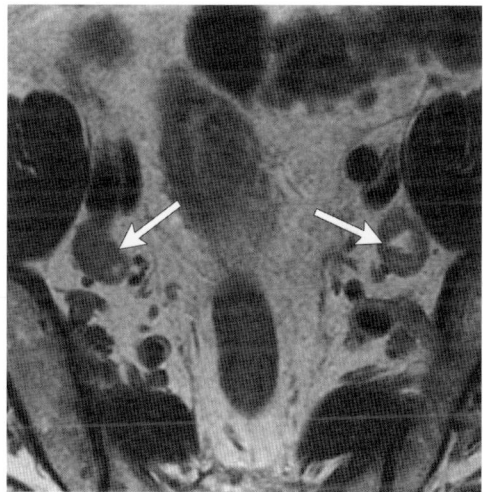

(c)

(d)

Figure 9.3. Local staging of prostate cancer on MR imaging. Transverse T$_2$-weighted MR images in a 55-year-old man show extracapsular extension (arrow) of the tumor (T) on the left side posterolaterally (a); and seminal vesicle (SV) invasion (arrow) (b). Transverse T$_2$-weighted MR images in a 68-year-old man show a large tumor (T) with bilateral seminal vesicle invasion (small arrows) (c); and bilateral pelvic lymphadenopathy (arrows) (c, d). Note that the small round lymph node (c) is considered involved because its signal intensity is similar to that of tumor.

In a study on the detection of extracapsular extension by two readers with different levels of experience, the addition of MR spectroscopy to MRI reduced inter-observer variability and significantly improved accuracy for the less experienced reader (whose area under the ROC curve increased from 0.62 to 0.75, $p < 0.05$); for the more experienced reader, the addition of MR spectroscopy also improved accuracy, but not significantly (the area under the ROC curve increased from 0.78 to 0.86) [39].

Lymph node staging

The accuracy of MRI, like that of other cross-sectional imaging techniques such as CT, is limited in the assessment of lymph node metastasis. On MRI, enlargement of lymph nodes at the usual lymphatic drainage pathways of prostate cancer is suggestive of metastasis. However, lymph nodes that are normal in size may still contain metastatic foci.

The use of MRI with newly developed ultrasmall superparamagnetic iron oxide (USPIO) particles is a promising technique for the detection of lymph node metastases, because it may allow the detection of metastases in normal-sized lymph nodes. The small iron oxide particles are sequestered by the reticuloendothelial system and cause signal loss on T_2^*-weighted images in normal lymph nodes. However, foci of tumor in metastatic lymph nodes do not show signal loss and can therefore be identified on MRI.

A study showed that MRI with these superparamagnetic particles had a significantly higher sensitivity than conventional MRI in the detection of metastasis on a node-by-node basis (90.5% vs. 35.4%, $p < 0.001$); the new technique also had a sensitivity of 100% and a specificity of 95.7% in detecting nodal metastasis on a per-patient basis [40]. Although these are promising results, routine use of these particles is not warranted, as the incidence of lymph node metastasis is low among patients with prostate cancer.

Added value of magnetic resonance imaging to clinical assessment

Determining the local extent of prostate cancer is crucial for selecting and planning an optimal treatment strategy. Findings from MRI can provide invaluable information for this process.

A study has shown that in predicting extracapsular extension of prostate cancer, MRI findings contribute significant added value to clinical variables (areas under the ROC curves for detection of extracapsular extension with and without endo-rectal MRI findings were 0.838 and 0.772, respectively, $p = 0.022$) [41]. However, experience in prostate MRI is an important factor in interpretation. A subsequent study that analyzed the same data [41] demonstrated that the incremental value of MRI in predicting extracapsular extension was only significant when interpretation was performed by genitourinary radiologists with experience in endorectal MRI rather than general body MRI radiologists [42].

Another recent study showed that MRI contributed significant added value ($p \le 0.02$) to staging nomograms in predicting organ-confined prostate cancer; the contribution of MRI findings was significant in all risk groups but was greatest in the intermediate- and high-risk groups ($p < 0.01$ for both) [43]. Accuracy in the prediction of organ-confined prostate cancer of MRI improved when MR spectro-scopy was added, but the difference was not statistically significant [43].

A recent study reported that MRI contributed significant added value to the clinical nomogram for predicting seminal vesicle invasion by prostate cancer [44]. In this study, MRI (0.76) had a larger area under the ROC curve than any other clinical variable (0.62–0.73) in predicting seminal vesicle invasion, and MRI plus the clinical nomogram (0.87) had a significantly larger ($p < 0.05$) area under the ROC curve than either MRI alone (0.76) or the nomogram alone (0.80) [44].

Role of magnetic resonance imaging in treatment planning

The therapeutic options for patients with prostate cancer are numerous and include watchful waiting, androgen ablation (chemical or surgical castration), hormone therapy, radical surgery, and various forms of radiation therapy (brachytherapy, external beam irradiation). In treatment planning, the goal is to improve cancer control while minimizing the risk of complications. This kind of treatment planning requires accurate information about the location and extent of prostate cancer. Clinical decisions are based on tumor stage, Gleason grade and PSA level. In addition, factors such as the patient's age, general medical condition, and personal preference have an effect on the treatment strategy.

In patients who undergo surgery, MRI findings can guide surgical planning by providing a road map to preserve periprostatic tissues (important for recovery of urinary and sexual function) while reducing the risk of positive surgical margins. A study showed that the use of MRI before radical prostatectomy significantly improved the surgeon's decision regarding whether to spare or to resect the neurovascular bundles [45].

Magnetic resonance imaging can also be very helpful in radiation treatment planning by showing tumor location and extent. During treatment planning for intensity-modulated radiation therapy an anatomic map of the prostate and surrounding tissues is created to improve radiation delivery to the target areas while minimizing the radiation dose to the adjacent organs. This mapping is usually done with CT. However, MRI is more accurate than CT in defining contours and the volume of the prostate, the tumor location, and the location of adjacent structures such as rectum, urethra, and penile bulb. A study showed that the radiation dose delivered to the rectal wall and bulb of the penis was significantly reduced when treatment planning was based on MRI-delineated prostate anatomy rather than CT-delineated prostate anatomy [46]. Another area of research is the potential role of MRI in guiding brachytherapy seed placement. Although MRI may improve seed localization and therefore provide better dose distribution to the tumor, the high cost and the technical difficulties associated with MRI interventions limit the use of this method [23].

Role of magnetic resonance imaging in assessment of recurrent disease

After any kind of treatment, patients with prostate cancer are followed with periodic clinical examination and measurement of PSA level. Magnetic resonance imaging is not routinely used for follow-up, but it can be useful when clinical findings suggest recurrence.

Due to its excellent soft-tissue resolution, MRI is superior to the other imaging modalities such as TRUS and CT in the assessment of locally recurrent disease after radical prostatectomy. Recurrent tumor after surgery is best depicted on T_2-weighted MR images and appears as nodular or infiltrative soft-tissue-intensity lesions (Figure 9.4).

Two studies reported that MRI had 95%–100% sensitivity and 100% specificity for detecting local recurrence after surgery [47, 48]. In one of these studies, local recurrences seen on MRI were perianastomotic in 29% of patients and retrovesical in 40%, within retained seminal vesicles in 22%, and at anterior or lateral surgical margins in 9%; the mean diameter of tumors was 1.4 cm (range, 0.8–4.5 cm), and PSA levels ranged from undetectable to 10 ng/ml (mean, 2.18 ng/ml) [47].

Assessment of recurrent prostate cancer after radiation treatment on MRI can be difficult due to the tissue changes related to radiation therapy. Recurrent tumor after radiation treatment appears as low-signal-intensity lesions on T_2-weighted MR images (Figure 9.5). However, tumor conspicuity could be diminished within

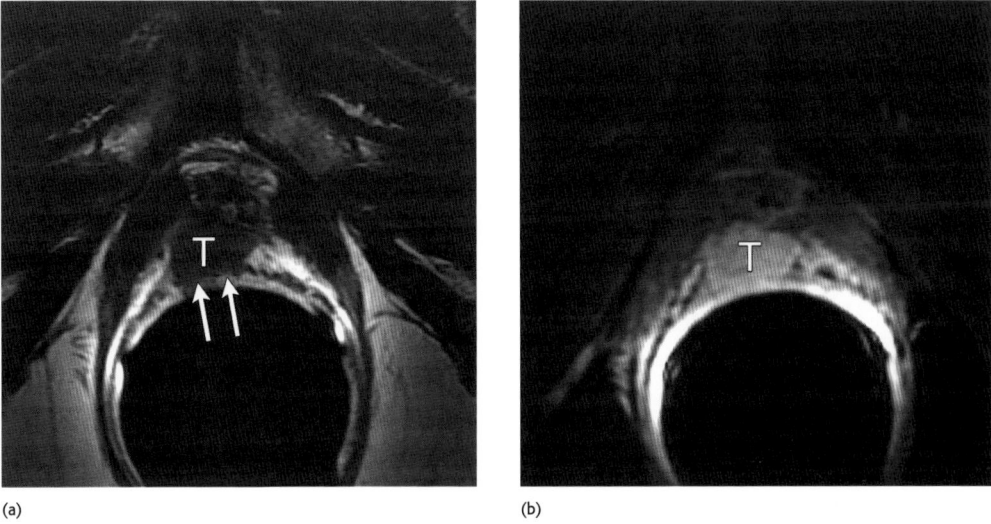

(a)   (b)

Figure 9.4. Recurrent tumor after surgery. Transverse T$_2$-weighted (a) and post-contrast T$_1$-weighted (b) MR images in a 66-year-old man show a nodular recurrent tumor (T) on the right side in the surgical bed just posterior to the urethra. Note that the recurrent tumor (T) invades the anterior rectal wall (arrows) (a).

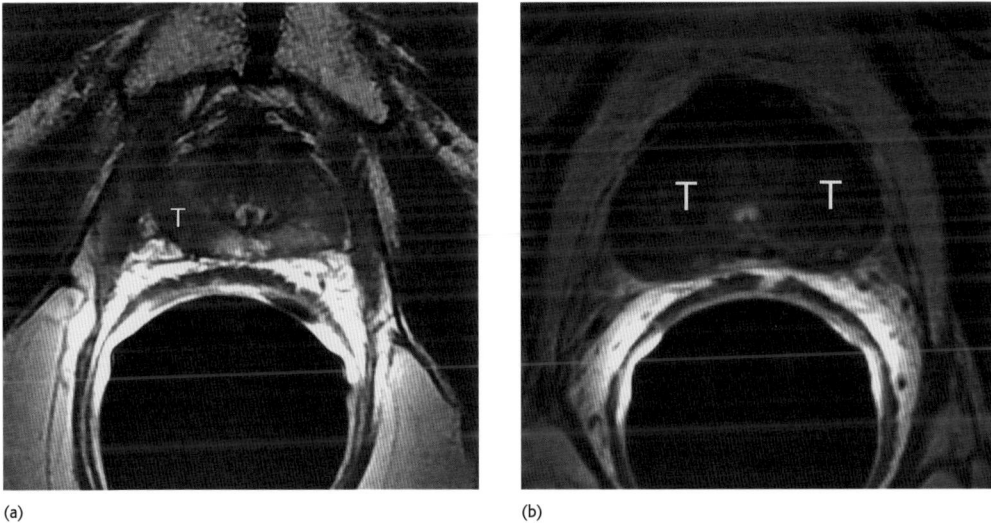

(a)   (b)

Figure 9.5. Recurrent tumor after radiation treatment. Transverse T$_2$-weighted MR image in a 62-year-old man shows a low-signal-intensity focus indicating recurrent tumor (T) in the peripheral zone of the prostate on the right (a). Transverse T$_2$-weighted MR image in a 72-year-old man shows bilateral low-signal-intensity foci indicating recurrent tumor (T) in the transition zone of the prostate (b). Note that in both cases post-radiation changes in the prostate limit conspicuity of the recurrent tumors (a, b) but in both patients MRI findings of recurrent tumor were confirmed with biopsy results.

the background of low signal intensity of the remainder of the prostate due to post-radiation changes.

A study reported that MRI and MR spectroscopy could be more sensitive than sextant biopsy and digital rectal examination for localization of prostate cancer recurrence after external beam radiation therapy [49]. In this study, MRI and MR spectroscopy had sensitivities of 68% and 77%, respectively, whereas the sensitivities of biopsy and digital rectal examination were 48% and 16%, respectively [49]. Magnetic resonance spectroscopy had lower specificity (78%) than the other three tests, each of which had a specificity greater than 90% [49]. A more recent study showed that, in patients who underwent salvage prostatectomy after failed radiation therapy, MRI could help identify tumor sites and depict local extent of disease [50]. In this recent study, areas under the ROC curves for two readers were 0.61 and 0.75 for tumor detection; 0.76 and 0.87 for prediction of extracapsular extension; and 0.70 and 0.76 for prediction of seminal vesicle invasion [50].

Summary

Magnetic resonance imaging is the most extensively studied imaging technique for the assessment of prostate cancer. Research is ongoing in the use of higher magnetic field strengths and new MRI sequences. The use of stronger magnetic fields produces images of higher resolution and could therefore improve tumor detection and staging. The introduction of several new MRI techniques has given rise to the idea of "multiparametric" MRI, in which morphologic information obtained with T_2-weighted imaging for tumor detection and staging is improved by the addition of metabolic and physiologic information obtained with MR spectroscopy, dynamic contrast-enhanced MRI and diffusion-weighted MRI. Each of these techniques has unique advantages and disadvantages. Therefore, current research efforts focus on establishing the optimal use of various MRI techniques in different clinical situations.

As technology continues to advance, so do the understanding of imaging criteria and experience in image interpretation. In addition, there is growing interest in further individualization of treatment plans, which requires the accurate characterization of the location and extent of cancer. This necessitates optimal use of MRI techniques and accurate image interpretation. Future directions for MRI of prostate cancer include more precise patient stratification for different management options and more accurate methods for guidance and assessment of emerging local prostate cancer therapies.

REFERENCES

1. F. G. Claus, H. Hricak, R. R. Hattery, Pretreatment evaluation of prostate cancer: role of MR imaging and 1H MR spectroscopy. *Radiographics*, **24** (2004), S167–180.

2. O. Akin, E. Sala, C. S. Moskowitz, *et al.*, Transition zone prostate cancers: features, detection, localization, and staging at endorectal MR imaging. *Radiology*, **239** (2006), 784–92.

3. H. Li, K. Sugimura, Y. Kaji, *et al.*, Conventional MRI capabilities in the diagnosis of prostate cancer in the transition zone. *AJR Am J Roentgenol*, **186** (2006), 729–42.

4. Y. J. Choi, J. K. Kim, N. Kim, *et al.*, Functional MR imaging of prostate cancer. *Radiographics*, **27** (2007), 63–75.

5. O. Akin, H. Hricak, Imaging of prostate cancer. *Radiol Clin North Am*, **45** (2007), 207–22.

6. S. Katz, M. Rosen, MR imaging and MR spectroscopy in prostate cancer management. *Radiol Clin North Am*, **44** (2006), 723–34.

7. J. K. Kim, S. S. Hong, Y. J. Choi, *et al.*, Wash-in rate on the basis of dynamic contrast-enhanced MRI: usefulness for prostate cancer detection and localization. *J Magn Reson Imaging*, **22** (2005), 639–46.

8. D. L. Buckley, C. Roberts, G. J. Parker, *et al.*, Prostate cancer: evaluation of vascular characteristics with dynamic contrast-enhanced T1-weighted MR imaging – initial experience. *Radiology*, **233** (2004), 709–15.

9. O. Rouviere, A. Raudrant, R. Ecochard, *et al.*, Characterization of time-enhancement curves of benign and malignant prostate tissue at dynamic MRI. *Eur Radiol*, **13** (2003), 931–42.

10. M. R. Engelbrecht, H. J. Huisman, R. J. Laheij, *et al.*, Discrimination of prostate cancer from normal peripheral zone and central gland tissue by using dynamic contrast-enhanced MR imaging. *Radiology*, **229** (2003), 248–54.

11. H. Hricak, P. L. Choyke, S. C. Eberhardt, *et al.*, Imaging prostate cancer: a multidisciplinary perspective. *Radiology*, **243** (2007), 28–53.

12. P. Gibbs, D. J. Tozer, G. P. Liney, *et al.*, Comparison of quantitative T2 mapping and diffusion-weighted imaging in the normal and pathologic prostate. *Magn Reson Med*, **46** (2001), 1054–8.

13. K. Hosseinzadeh, S. D. Schwarz, Endorectal diffusion-weighted imaging in prostate cancer to differentiate malignant and benign peripheral zone tissue. *J Magn Reson Imaging*, **20** (2004), 654–61.

14. C. Sato, S. Naganawa, T. Nakamura, *et al.*, Differentiation of noncancerous tissue and cancer lesions by apparent diffusion coefficient values in transition and peripheral zones of the prostate. *J Magn Reson Imaging*, **21** (2005), 258–62.

15. R. Shimofusa, H. Fujimoto, H. Akamata, *et al.*, Diffusion-weighted imaging of prostate cancer. *J Comput Assist Tomogr*, **29** (2005), 149–53.

16. C. K. Kim, B. K. Park, J. J. Han, *et al.*, Diffusion-weighted imaging of the prostate at 3 T for differentiation of malignant and benign tissue in transition and peripheral zones: preliminary results. *J Comput Assist Tomogr*, **31** (2007), 449–54.

17. J. Kurhanewicz, D. B. Vigneron, H. Hricak, *et al.*, Three-dimensional 1H spectroscopic imaging of the in situ human prostate with high spatial (0.24 to 0.7 cm^3) spatial resolution. *Radiology*, **198** (1996), 795–805.

18. R. Males, D. B. Vigneron, J. Star-Lack, *et al.*, Clinical application of BASING and spectral/spatial water and lipid suppression pulses for prostate cancer staging and localization by in vivo 3D 1H magnetic resonance spectroscopic imaging. *Magn Reson Med*, **43** (2000), 17–22.

19. J. Scheidler, H. Hricak, D. B. Vigneron, *et al.*, Prostate cancer: localization with three-dimensional proton MR spectroscopic imaging – clinicopathologic study. *Radiology*, **213** (1999), 473–80.

20. D. Beyersdorff, M. Taupitz, B. Winkelmann, *et al.*, Patients with a history of elevated prostate-specific antigen levels and negative transrectal US-guided quadrant or sextant biopsy results: value of MR imaging. *Radiology*, **224** (2002), 701–6.

21. D. Beyersdorff, A. Winkel, B. Hamm, *et al.*, MR imaging-guided prostate biopsy with a closed MR unit at 1.5 T: initial results. *Radiology*, **234** (2005), 576–81.

22. R. C. Susil, C. Menard, A. Krieger, *et al.*, Transrectal prostate biopsy and fiducial marker placement in a standard 1.5T magnetic resonance imaging scanner. *J Urol*, **175** (2006), 113–20.

23. E. Atalar, C. Menard, MR-guided interventions for prostate cancer. *Magn Reson Imaging Clin N Am*, **13** (2005), 491–504.

24. I. Kaplan, N. E. Oldenburg, P. Meskell, *et al.*, Real time MRI-ultrasound image guided stereotactic prostate biopsy. *Magn Reson Imaging*, **20** (2002), 295–9.

25. M. Mullerad, H. Hricak, K. Kuroiwa, *et al.*, Comparison of endorectal magnetic resonance imaging, guided prostate biopsy and digital rectal examination in the preoperative anatomical localization of prostate cancer. *J Urol*, **174** (2005), 2158–63.

26. J. J. Futterer, S. W. Heijmink, T. W. Scheenen, *et al.*, Prostate cancer localization with dynamic contrast-enhanced MR imaging and proton MR spectroscopic imaging. *Radiology*, **241** (2006), 449–58.

27. A. Tanimoto, J. Nakashima, H. Kohno, *et al.*, Prostate cancer screening: the clinical value of diffusion-weighted imaging and dynamic MR imaging in combination with T2-weighted imaging. *J Magn Reson Imaging*, **25** (2007), 146–52.

28. E. Sala, O. Akin, C. S. Moskowitz, *et al.*, Endorectal MR imaging in the evaluation of seminal vesicle invasion: diagnostic accuracy and multivariate feature analysis. *Radiology*, **238** (2006), 929–37.

29. M. R. Engelbrecht, G. J. Jager, R. J. Laheij, *et al.*, Local staging of prostate cancer using magnetic resonance imaging: a meta-analysis. *Eur Radiol*, **12** (2002), 2294–302.

30. C. Bartolozzi, I. Menchi, R. Lencioni, *et al.*, Local staging of prostate carcinoma with endorectal coil MRI: correlation with whole-mount radical prostatectomy specimens. *Eur Radiol*, **6** (1996), 339–45.

31. F. Cornud, T. Flam, L. Chauveinc, *et al.*, Extraprostatic spread of clinically localized prostate cancer: factors predictive of pT3 tumor and of positive endorectal MR imaging examination results. *Radiology*, **224** (2002), 203–10.

32. S. Ikonen, P. Karkkainen, L. Kivisaari, *et al.*, Magnetic resonance imaging of clinically localized prostatic cancer. *J Urol*, **159** (1998), 915–19.

33. S. Ikonen, P. Karkkainen, L. Kivisaari, *et al.*, Endorectal magnetic resonance imaging of prostatic cancer: comparison between fat-suppressed T2-weighted fast spin echo and three-dimensional dual-echo, steady-state sequences. *Eur Radiol*, **11** (2001), 236–41.

34. F. May, T. Treumann, P. Dettmar, *et al.*, Limited value of endorectal magnetic resonance imaging and transrectal ultrasonography in the staging of clinically localized prostate cancer. *BJU Int*, **87** (2001), 66–9.

35. M. Perrotti, R. P. Kaufman, Jr., T. A. Jennings, *et al.*, Endo-rectal coil magnetic resonance imaging in clinically localized prostate cancer: is it accurate? *J Urol*, **156** (1996), 106–9.

36. J. C. Presti, H. Hricak, P. A. Narayan, *et al.*, Local staging of prostatic carcinoma: comparison of transrectal sonography and endorectal MR imaging. *AJR Am J Roentgenol*, **166** (1996), 103–8.

37. J. Rorvik, O. J. Halvorsen, G. Albrektsen, *et al.*, MRI with an endorectal coil for staging of clinically localised prostate cancer prior to radical prostatectomy. *Eur Radiol*, **9** (1999), 29–34.

38. K. K. Yu, H. Hricak, R. Alagappan, *et al.*, Detection of extracapsular extension of prostate carcinoma with endorectal and phased-array coil MR imaging: multivariate feature analysis. *Radiology*, **202** (1997), 697–702.

39. K. K. Yu, J. Scheidler, H. Hricak, *et al.*, Prostate cancer: prediction of extracapsular extension with endorectal MR imaging and three-dimensional proton MR spectroscopic imaging. *Radiology*, **213** (1999), 481–8.

40. M. G. Harisinghani, J. Barentsz, P. F. Hahn, *et al.*, Noninvasive detection of clinically occult

lymph-node metastases in prostate cancer. *N Engl J Med*, **348** (2003), 2491–9.

41. L. Wang, M. Mullerad, H. N. Chen, *et al.*, Prostate cancer: incremental value of endorectal MR imaging findings for prediction of extracapsular extension. *Radiology*, **232** (2004), 133–9.

42. M. Mullerad, H. Hricak, L. Wang, *et al.*, Prostate cancer: detection of extracapsular extension by genitourinary and general body radiologists at MR imaging. *Radiology*, **232** (2004), 140–6.

43. L. Wang, H. Hricak, M. W. Kattan, *et al.*, Prediction of organ-confined prostate cancer: incremental value of MR imaging and MR spectroscopic imaging to staging nomograms. *Radiology*, **238** (2006), 597–603.

44. L. Wang, H. Hricak, M. W. Kattan, *et al.*, Prediction of seminal vesicle invasion in prostate cancer: incremental value of adding endorectal MR imaging to the Kattan nomogram. *Radiology*, **242** (2007), 182–8.

45. H. Hricak, L. Wang, D. C. Wei, *et al.*, The role of preoperative endorectal magnetic resonance imaging in the decision regarding whether to preserve or resect neurovascular bundles during radical

retropubic prostatectomy. *Cancer*, **100** (2004), 2655–63.

46. R. J. Steenbakkers, K. E. Deurloo, P. J. Nowak, *et al.*, Reduction of dose delivered to the rectum and bulb of the penis using MRI delineation for radiotherapy of the prostate. *Int J Radiat Oncol Biol Phys*, **57** (2003), 1269–79.

47. T. Sella, L. H. Schwartz, P. W. Swindle, *et al.*, Suspected local recurrence after radical prostatectomy: endorectal coil MR imaging. *Radiology*, **23** (2004), 379–85.

48. J. M. Silverman, T. L. Krebs, MR imaging evaluation with a transrectal surface coil of local recurrence of prostatic cancer in men who have undergone radical prostatectomy. *AJR Am J Roentgenol*, **168** (1997), 379–85.

49. D. Pucar, A. Shukla-Dave, H. Hricak, *et al.*, Prostate cancer: correlation of MR imaging and MR spectroscopy with pathologic findings after radiation therapy – initial experience. *Radiology* **236** (2005), 545–53.

50. E. Sala, S. C. Eberhardt, O. Akin, *et al.*, Endorectal MR imaging before salvage prostatectomy: tumor localization and staging. *Radiology*, **238** (2006), 176–83.

10

Magnetic resonance spectroscopic imaging and other emerging magnetic resonance techniques in prostate cancer

Amita Shukla-Dave and Kristen L. Zakian

Introduction

Combined magnetic resonance imaging (MRI) and magnetic resonance spectroscopic imaging (MRSI) have been applied to the investigation of the prostate gland for more than a decade. In that time much has been learned about the metabolic characteristics of the *in situ* prostate gland. This chapter reviews technical developments and clinical findings arising from combined MRI/MRSI of the prostate gland as well as the challenges in applying this technique. As Chapter 9 is on MRI of the prostate gland, we will focus here on the development and application of MRSI. We will also touch briefly on other emerging MR techniques such as diffusion-weighted imaging (DWI) and dynamic contrast-enhanced MRI (DCE MRI).

Biologic basis of prostate spectral patterns

Proton MR spectroscopy permits the non-invasive assessment of metabolites in the prostate gland. The technology used to acquire proton spectra includes hardware identical to that used for MR imaging and a specific pulse sequence program which captures both spatial location and chemical shift information from hydrogen-containing (proton) metabolites. The proton metabolites that are most commonly detectable *in vivo* are choline-containing compounds (Cho), polyamines (spermine, spermidine, putrescine), creatine + phosphocreatine, and citrate. A proton spectrum acquired on a 1.5-T clinical scanner from the healthy prostate peripheral zone is shown in Figure 10.1. The *in vivo* spectrum reflects what had been demonstrated in early *ex vivo* studies of prostate tissue extracts: high levels of citrate and relatively low levels of choline-containing compounds in the healthy

Prostate Cancer, eds. Hedvig Hricak and Peter T. Scardino. Published by Cambridge University Press.
© Cambridge University Press 2009.

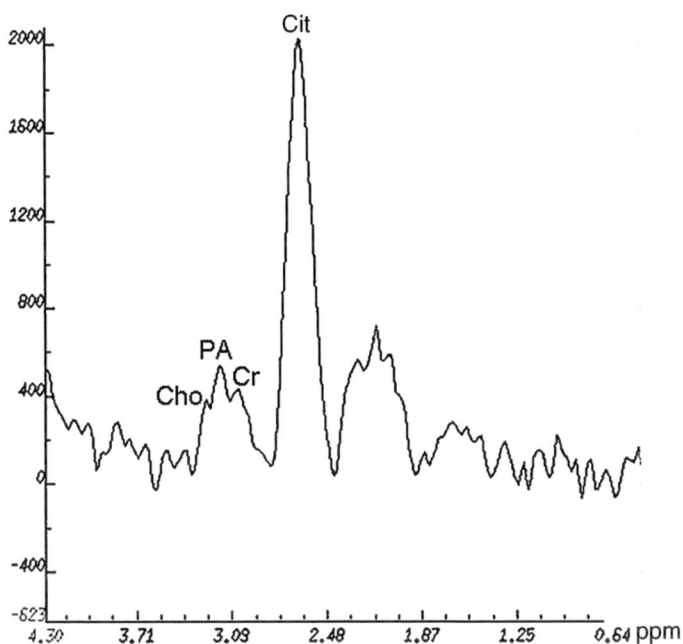

Figure 10.1. Single-voxel ^{1}H MR spectrum extracted from a 3D-MRSI data set. The spectrum corresponds to healthy prostate peripheral zone. Acquisition parameters: body coil transmit/endorectal coil receive, point resolved spectroscopy (PRESS) volume excitation with spectral/spatial water and lipid suppression, 16×8×8 chemical shift imaging, voxel size=0.33 cm³, time to repetition (TR)=1 s, time to echo (TE)=130 ms, 1 average (17-min scan time). Abbreviations: Cho, choline-containing compounds; PA, polyamines; Cr, creatine/phosphocreatine; Cit, citrate; PRESS, point resolved spectroscopy; TE, time to echo; TR, time to repetition.

gland, with the converse being true in prostate cancer [1, 2, 3]. In addition, higher levels of polyamines have been associated with benign prostate tissue [3, 4, 5, 6].

Proton MRS of tumor and benign tissue extracts and *ex vivo* magic angle spinning MRS of prostate samples have identified at high resolution the constituents of the peaks observed *in vivo* and suggested reasons for the differences between healthy and malignant tissue. Glycerophosphocholine (GPC), phosphocholine (PC), and free choline (fCho) have been identified as the metabolites making up the *in vivo* choline (Cho) signal [7, 8]. Numerous investigators have found elevated levels of Cho-containing compounds in tumors [9, 10, 11, 12, 13, 14, 15]. Since these compounds are anabolites (cho, PC) and catabolites (GPC) of phosphatidylcholine, a major membrane phospholipid, it has been suggested that the elevated Cho peak reflects an elevated cell proliferation rate, and there are some data to support this hypothesis [16]. However, it has also been reported that cells in culture with similar proliferation rates have different Cho profiles; specifically, PC/GPC and total choline increased as cells progressed from benign to malignant phenotypes [17]. It was suggested that up-regulation of enzymes in the phosphatidylcholine pathway in more malignant tumors could explain the increased total choline levels. The creatine levels were not significantly different between the benign and tumor tissues [18]. Benign prostate epithelial cells produce high levels of citrate, probably due to the suppression of aconitase, which catalyzes the oxidation of citrate in the Krebs cycle [18]. Large amounts of citrate are secreted into the glands, resulting in the peak shown in Figure 10.1. In prostate cancer, dedifferentiation of prostate epithelial cells may alter cell metabolism and reduce the amount of citrate produced. In addition, displacement of glandular tissue by tumor would result in a reduction of citrate in a spectroscopic volume. These effects may produce the reduced citrate observed in prostate tumor spectra *in vivo*. As mentioned above, *in vitro* MR spectroscopy of tumor tissue identified polyamines (mainly spermine) as markers of healthy prostate tissue [3, 4, 5, 6]. Increased intracellular spermine has been associated with well-differentiated, non-proliferative cells. Furthermore, because spermine is also a secretory product in the prostate, its level would be expected to decrease if ductal volume were reduced (i.e., if tissue morphology changed because of tumor) [6].

Technical developments in prostate MR spectroscopy

Following the first demonstration of *in vivo* magnetic resonance spectroscopy (MRS) of the human prostate [19], single-voxel MRS studies were performed using the stimulated echo acquisition (STEAM) technique [20] and the double spin-echo or point resolved spectroscopy (PRESS) technique [21] using either an external coil or an endorectal probe [22, 23]. The 1995 study demonstrated significant differences in the ratios of citrate to Cho + Cr between cancer and benign tissue [22]. However, using a single-voxel technique to sample multiple areas of the gland is inefficient and also requires prospective targeting of tissue thought to be malignant. Subsequently, chemical shift imaging [24] or MRSI using two- or three-dimensional phase encoding was employed, which mapped the distribution of metabolites over the entire prostate gland [18, 25]. This technique, rendered at a spatial resolution of 6–8 mm, requires the use of an endorectal radiofrequency (RF) receive coil to achieve sufficient sensitivity in a reasonable scan time (less than 20 min) on a 1.5-T magnet. While generating some patient discomfort and also deforming the gland, the endorectal probe is essential to provide the sensitivity needed to acquire a spatial array of spectra that reflect the zonal anatomy of the small prostate gland (approximately 4–7 cm in the right–left dimension) and permits detection of cancers with diameters as small as approximately 5 mm.

Some of the other technical issues that must be addressed for *in vivo* MRSI studies are the need for adequate shimming, exclusion of signal from periprostatic fats, and good water suppression. Good shimming results in higher amplitude and narrower metabolite peaks that are easier to differentiate from nearby peaks and quantifiable with greater accuracy. In addition, good shimming results in a narrower water line, which is more efficiently suppressed and is less likely to contaminate the regions of the spectrum where the metabolites of interest reside.

The issues of water and fat suppression have resulted in a series of developments that have paralleled improved scanner hardware capabilities for delivering complicated RF and gradient waveforms. Initial MRSI studies [18] used chemical-shift-selective (CHESS) water suppression and short-time inversion recovery (STIR) lipid suppression [26, 27]. However, these techniques are dependent on local water and lipid T_1 values and ideally should be optimized on a case-to-case basis. Band-selective inversion and dephasing (BASING) was developed to simultaneously suppress the water (4.77 ppm) and lipid (1.3–0.9 ppm) regions of the spectrum [28]. The addition of two BASING pulse pairs with crusher gradients into the standard PRESS sequence resulted in highly effective, T_1-independent lipid and water suppression. The replacement of standard spatially selective PRESS pulses with spectrally and spatially selective pulses was a further advancement, which used a composite RF pulse combined with oscillating gradient waveforms to select the excitation volume and to select the metabolites of interest while suppressing water and lipids [28, 29, 30]. This combination of complex RF and gradient pulses makes use of the sophisticated MR hardware available today. A specific advantage of the spectral-spatial pulses is their large spectral band width, which minimizes the chemical-shift misregistration effect that occurs for metabolites resonating at different frequencies. While BASING or spectral-spatial pulses theoretically should eliminate lipid signals at their expected resonance frequencies, contamination from the periprostatic lipids outside the voxel of interest may still occur, with signals appearing at frequencies in the passband of these pulses. One solution to this is the use of very selective saturation pulses that have a very sharp slice profile [31]. These sharp saturation bands may be placed along the edges and diagonally across the corners of the rectangular excitation volume in order to tailor the shape of the excited volume to the shape of the prostate gland and exclude periprostatic fat signals more effectively [31]. It has also been recognized that more efficient sampling of k-space can increase signal-to-noise ratio and/or reduce scan time in these three-dimensional data sets which require hundreds of phase encode steps [32]. The current state of the art on 1.5-T scanners results in MRSI data sets with a voxel resolution of 6–8 mm, acquired in 12–17 min.

One of the major limitations of proton MRSI at 1.5 T is the low sensitivity of the metabolites at millimolar concentrations, which results in somewhat limited spatial resolution. Because of the expected increase in signal-to-noise ratio at higher field strength, there is great interest in performing prostate MRSI on 3–T (or higher field) MR systems. Within the past 5 years, 3-T MR spectrometers have been installed at many major research centers. At 3 T, spectral dispersion increases, and, theoretically, the signal-to-noise ratio for MR spectroscopy could double, permitting better resolution of peaks that resonate in close proximity as well as a reduction in voxel size and/or scan time. However, a new series of technical challenges has also arisen. With regard to imaging, T_1 values are longer and T_2 values are shorter, and care must be taken in the selection of appropriate time to repetition (TR) and time to echo (TE) values to obtain the optimal contrast and signal-to-noise ratio in a given scan time. In addition, artifacts induced by magnetic susceptibility differences between tissue, endorectal probe, and air scale with the square of the field and are quite severe at 3 T. Images are affected and spectral quality is highly degraded. This has been addressed satisfactorily by filling the central volume of the inflatable endorectal probe with a fluid such as a perfluorocarbon, thus reducing the magnetic susceptibility differences.

Intense effort has been put forth to develop 3 T pulse sequence programs to address issues of chemical shift artifact, citrate modulation, and increasing spatial resolution while maintaining an acceptable scan time. Chemical shift artifact arises when the PRESS excitation volume for one resonance is offset with respect to another resonance in proportion to their chemical shift difference. At 3 T, this issue is more severe than at 1.5 T because of the doubling in chemical shift difference (in Hz). The implementation of high-bandwidth spectral-spatial pulses is effective at minimizing this problem [29]. The modulation of the strongly coupled methyl protons of citrate with respect to TE has more impact at 3 T. Chen *et al.* have incorporated dual-band spectral-spatial pulses as well as a train of non-selective 180 degrees pulses utilizing Malcolm Levitt's (MLEV) phase-cycling to generate an upright citrate resonance at TE = 85 ms [33]. In order to cover the entire prostate gland with smaller voxel sizes, more phase encodes are needed, lengthening the scan time. Optimized k-space sampling can be applied to this problem. Another way to address this issue is the implementation of a flyback k-space trajectory, which accelerates coverage of k-space and reduces scan time [34]. A three-dimensional MRSI data set with spatial resolution of 5.4 mm (0.157 cm^3 voxel volume) has been obtained in 8.5 min, and the improvement in spatial resolution as well as in spectral resolution as demonstrated by the separation of Cho, polyamine, and Cr is apparent [34].

Criteria for magnetic resonance spectroscopic imaging data interpretation

Multiple studies have assessed the metabolic profile of the prostate gland and proposed criteria for evaluation of the gland on a voxel-by-voxel basis [18, 29, 35, 36]. The criteria for characterizing voxels as benign or malignant are more clear-cut in the peripheral zone than in the transition zone due to the metabolic homogeneity of the benign peripheral zone. The first report on the spectral interpretation of the peripheral zone voxels was given by Kurhanewicz *et al.* using the ratio of (Cho + Cr) to Cit to differentiate between benign and malignant tissue, from a three-dimensional proton MRSI data set of 85 patients [18]. (Cho + Cr)/Cit values in the normal peripheral zone (mean 0.54 ± 0.11) showed no overlap with prostate cancer values (mean 2.10 ± 1.30) ($p = 0.0001$), while central zone, periurethral tissue, and benign prostatic hyperplasia (BPH) metabolite ratios had some overlap with ratios in cancer [18].

Males *et al.* showed that PRESS using either BASING or spectral-spatial pulses resulted in differentiation between healthy peripheral zone (PZ) and cancer: using BASING water and lipid suppression, the mean (Cho + Cr)/Cit value equalled 0.22 ± 0.13 for healthy tissue and 1.6 ± 2.1 for cancer in the PZ, while spectral-spatial suppression resulted in (Cho + Cr)/Cit $= 0.31 \pm 0.17$ for healthy tissue and 3.4 ± 8.7 for cancer in data from 17 patients [29]. For both techniques, the ratio was significant when healthy PZ tissue was compared to cancerous tissue ($p < 0.05$) [29]. In the transition zone (TZ), clear differentiation between cancerous and benign tissue is more difficult because of the heterogeneous metabolic pattern of the benign tissue [37, 38]. Benign prostatic hyperplasia, which arises in the TZ, may consist of glandular or stromal tissue or a combination of both, leading to different spectral patterns. A retrospective study by Zakian *et al.* showed a trend toward elevation of choline and a reduction in or lack of citrate in TZ tumors when they were compared to BPH; however, the broad range of metabolite ratios observed precluded the use of a single ratio to differentiate TZ cancer from benign TZ tissue [38].

Futterer *et al.* recently reported a scoring system which incorporated (Cho + Cr)/ Cit and Cho/Cr to assess regions of interest defined as abnormal on T_2-weighted MRI [39]. This system resulted in a sensitivity of 85%–92% and a specificity of 85%–87% for MRSI detection of cancer in the central gland (central zone + transition zone) [39].

Recently, *in vivo* MRSI data analysis criteria have begun to incorporate the polyamine peak, which resides between the choline and creatine peaks and is not completely resolved. Jung *et al.* were the first to incorporate polyamines into a metabolic assessment that uses a scale of 1 (benign) to 5 (malignant) for data interpretation [35]. They assessed the accuracy of the system for MRSI of the prostate using step-section pathology as the "gold standard." The initial score was assigned based on (Cho + Cr)/Cit and could subsequently be adjusted based on the appearance of the polyamine peak. This system had an accuracy of 74.2% to 85.0% in the differentiation between benign and malignant tissue voxels, with an area under the receiver operator characteristic (ROC) curve of 0.89 for reader 1 and 0.87 for reader 2. When voxel scores of 4 or 5 were used to indicate cancer, specificity values of 84.6% or 89.3% were achieved, respectively, as compared to a previous reported specificity of 75%, achieved in a study that did not incorporate polyamine information [35]. They used in-house software for MRSI acquisition and processing and used only high-quality data with a good signal-to-noise ratio and no artifacts for analysis [35].

With the release of commercial MRSI software such as PROSE (Prostate Spectroscopy Examination, General Electric (GE), Waukeshau, WI, USA), more hospitals worldwide have access to prostate MRSI technology. We have recently performed a retrospective study on 50 consecutive patients who underwent combined MRI/MRSI with PROSE and had whole-mount step-section pathology maps available for comparison with MRI/MRSI [36]. The goal of the study was to generate criteria for classifying voxels as benign or malignant based on both the level of polyamines and (Cho + Cr)/Cit [36]. Specifically, a statistical model was generated using the classification and regression tree (CART) analysis method [40] to optimize the use of (Cho + Cr)/Cit and polyamine information in the voxel characterization process. The PROSE software permits the detection of the polyamine (PA) resonance. The height of the PA signal was judged qualitatively and scored on a scale of 0–2 as follows: 0 = PA undetectable; 1 = PA signal lower than Cho signal; and 2 = PA signal same height as or higher than Cho signal [36] (Figure 10.2). Figure 10.3 shows an example of patient data including the spectral grid superimposed on the corresponding T_2-weighted MRI section, and an

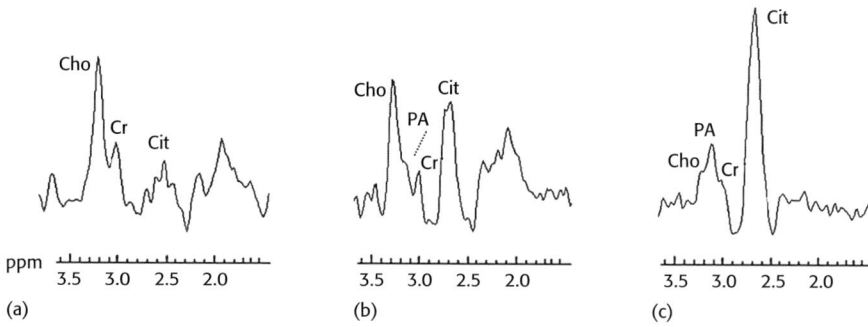

Figure 10.2. Representative prostate ^{1}H MR spectra for (a) polyamine (PA) score=0 (PA undetectable); (b) PA score=1 (PA<Cho), and (c) PA score=2 (PA≥Cho). Adapted with permission from Shukla-Dave *et al.* [36].

extracted voxel indicative of cancer. The (Cho + Cr)/Cit value is >1.11 and the PA score is 0 (undetectable PA). In this study the mean (Cho + Cr)/Cit ratio for benign tissue was 0.59 ± 0.03, and for cancerous tissue it was 1.1 ± 0.2. In the decision tree for classifying voxels as benign or malignant [36] (Figure 10.4), the first tree branching is according to the PA score and the second branching is based on (Cho + Cr)/Cit. When applied to the training data set the tree yielded a sensitivity of 54% and a specificity of 91%, and for the test data set it yielded a sensitivity of 42% and a specificity of 85%. The percentage of cancer in the voxel correlated positively with the sensitivity of the CART rule ($p<0.001$). In voxels with $\geq 90\%$ tumor content, the sensitivity for cancer detection using the rule was 75%. This study demonstrated that polyamines are as important as (Cho+Cr)/Cit in the voxel-characterization process and that MRSI is particularly valuable for identifying benign voxels [36].

Role of magnetic resonance spectroscopic imaging in untreated gland

As has been covered eloquently in the literature [41, 42, 43, 44, 45], MRI/MRSI enables the non-invasive evaluation of anatomic and metabolic features of the prostate gland and, thus, may play an important role in the detection, localization, and assessment of aggressiveness of cancer as well as treatment selection and planning. The first systematic study of the correlation between *in vivo* ^{1}H MRSI parameters and Gleason score was reported by Vigneron *et al.* [46]. In 26 patients who underwent MRI/MRSI, cancer location was based on histopathologic step-sections, correlated with T_2-weighted ^{1}H MRI, and, finally, the MRSI data

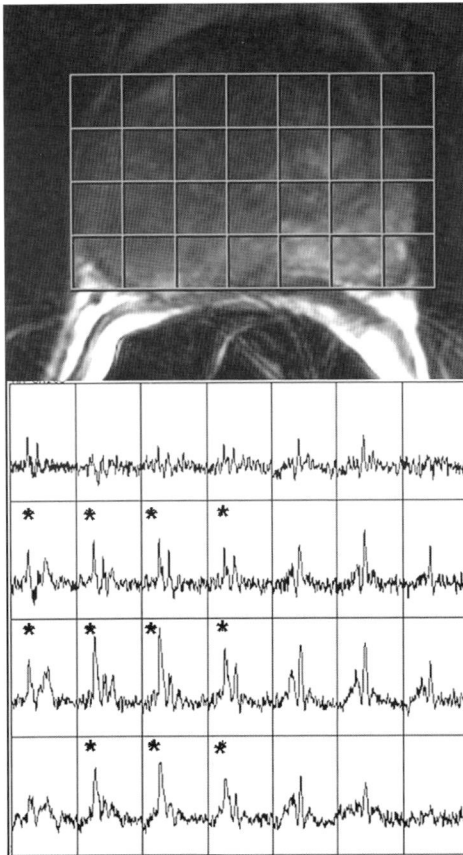

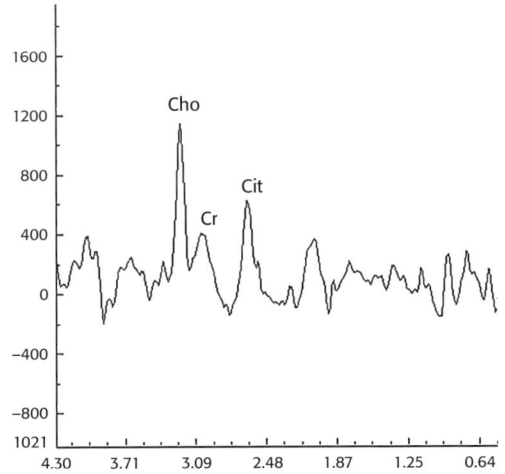

(a)

(b)

Figure 10.3. MRI/MRSI data from a patient with prostate cancer (biopsy Gleason score 7): (a) MRSI grid superimposed on transverse T_2-weighted ^{1}H MR image; MR imaging parameters were as follows: TR/TE, 4000/102; echo-train length, 12; field of view, 14 cm; acquisition matrix, 256×192; section thickness, 3 mm; no section gap; number of acquisitions, 4. MRSI imaging parameters were as follows: volume excitation with water and lipid suppression by spectral-spatial pulses; TR/TE, 1000/130; chemical shift imaging matrix, $16 \times 8 \times 8$; field of view, 110 mm $\times$ 55 mm $\times$ 55 mm; spatial resolution, 6.9 mm; number of acquisitions, 1; imaging time, 17 min. (b) Extracted single voxel suggestive of cancer with (Cho+Cr)/Cit=>1.11 and PA score=0 (undetectable polyamines).

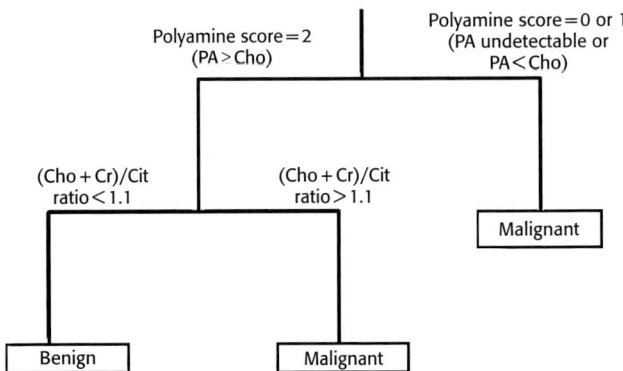

Figure 10.4. The CART-based decision-making tree for voxel-by-voxel analysis of MRSI data. Adapted with permission from Shukla-Dave *et al.* [36].

were aligned to obtain voxels with maximum inclusion of cancer tissue. Both (Cho+Cr)/Cit and Cho/(normal Cho (nCho)) correlated with grade, and the difference between Cho/nCho in low-grade (Gleason sum 5 or 6) and high-grade (Gleason sum 7 or 8) cancer was significant ($p < 0.0001$). While (Cho+Cr)/Cit values had quite a bit of overlap, Cho levels appeared more distinct at different grades [46]. Our group analyzed ^{1}H MRSI data in a set of 94 patients who had whole-mount step-section pathology [47]. Figure 10.5 contains representative data

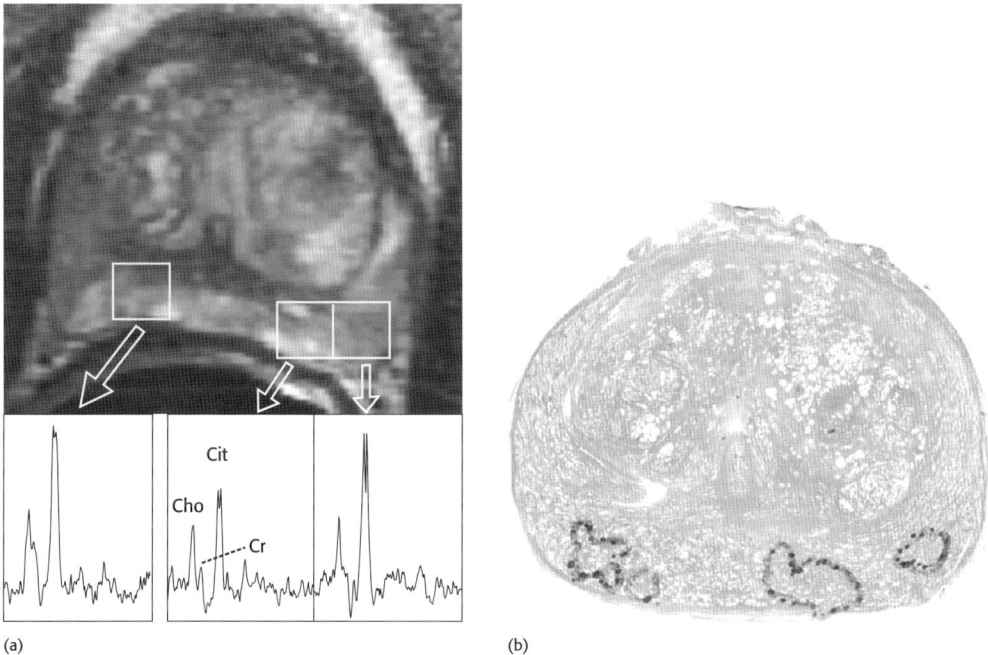

Figure 10.5. Proton MR images, ^{1}H MR spectra and step-section pathology tumor maps for patients with cancer in the peripheral zone. (a) Gleason score 3 + 3 cancer. Axial T$_2$-weighted ^{1}H MR image with cancer voxels highlighted and corresponding ^{1}H MR spectra below. Cho, Cr, Cit as defined in Figure 10.1. (b) Whole-mount step-section tumor map corresponding to the prostate section shown in (a) with Gleason grade 3 + 3 areas outlined. Citrate is present in the tumor voxels and Cho is moderately elevated. (c) Gleason score 4 + 4 cancer. Axial T$_2$-weighted ^{1}H MR image with cancer voxels highlighted and corresponding ^{1}H MR spectra below. (d) Whole-mount step-section tumor map corresponding to the prostate section shown in (c) with Gleason grade $\geq$ 4 + 4 area outlined. Cho is elevated in the tumor voxels and citrate is low or absent. Axial T$_2$-weighted ^{1}H MR image parameters: TR, 4000 ms; effective TE, 102 ms; echo-train length, 12; field of view, 14 cm; acquisition matrix, 256 $\times$ 192; slice thickness, 3 mm; gap, 0 mm; averages, 3. MRSI acquisition parameters: PRESS volume excitation with BASING water and lipid suppression; 16 $\times$ 8 $\times$ 8 chemical shift imaging; MRSI field of view, 100 mm $\times$ 50 mm $\times$ 50 mm; 6.25 mm resolution; TR, 1 s; TE, 130 ms; 1 average (17-min scan time). Adapted with permission from Zakian et al. [47]. See color plate section for full color version of parts (b), (d).

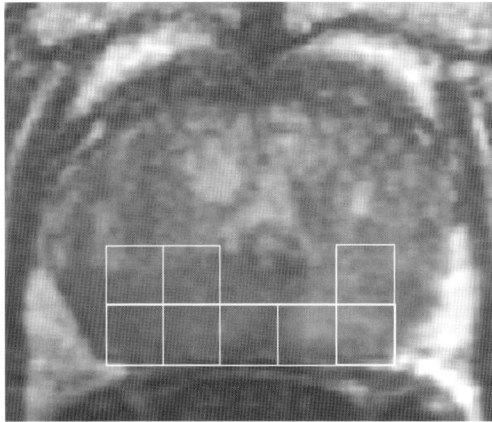

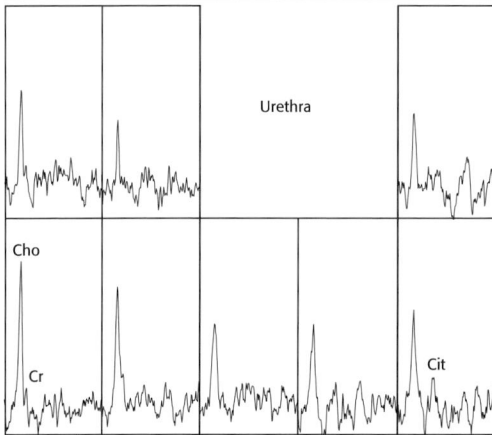

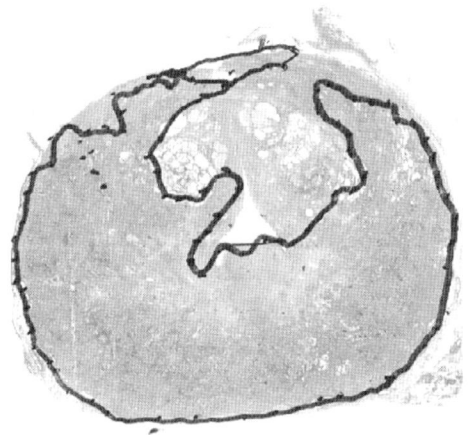

(c)   (d)

Figure 10.5. (cont.)

for tumors with Gleason scores of 3 + 3 and ≥4 + 4, respectively. When the metabolite ratios were analyzed in the peripheral zone, a positive correlation was found between (Cho + Cr)/Cit and Gleason score for individual lesions as well as between (Cho + Cr)/Cit and the overall gland Gleason score. In addition, tumor size, as indicated by the number of suspicious voxels making up the lesion, also correlated with Gleason score. The sensitivity of MRSI for detection of Gleason 3 + 3 lesions was low (44%), whereas the sensitivity for higher grade tumors was much higher (86.7% for Gleason score 4 + 3, and 89.5% for Gleason score ≥4 + 4) [47]. Thus, ^{1}H MRSI is particularly effective in detecting high-grade prostate cancers. A recent study reported moderate correlation between a MRSI score (incorporates (Cho + Cr)/Cit and Cho/Cr) and Gleason score in both peripheral zone and central gland tumors providing further evidence of the relationship between proton metabolites and prostate cancer [39]. In a single study, the number of voxels per slice considered suspicious for cancer by MRSI based on an elevated (Cho + Cr)/Cit ratio was found to predict whether a patient had extracapsular extension [48]. In a retrospective MRSI study the tumor volume as defined by the number of MRSI-positive voxels was positively correlated with lesion Gleason grade [47]. A retrospective study by Shukla-Dave *et al.* to predict the probability of insignificant prostate cancer was performed on 220 patients with clinically low-risk cancer (PSA <20 ng/ml, Gleason score ≤6) who underwent combined MRI/MRSI prior to radical prostatectomy [49]. At pathology, 41% of patients had insignificant cancer; both MRI (AUC 0.803) and MRI/MRSI (AUC 0.854) models incorporating clinical, biopsy, and MR data performed significantly better than the basic (AUC 0.574) and more comprehensive medium (AUC 0.726) clinical models, which incorporated only biopsy and clinical data. The new MRI- and MRI/MRSI-containing models performed better than the clinical models for predicting the probability of insignificant prostate cancer [49]. After appropriate validation, the new MRI and MRI/MRSI models might help in counseling patients who are considering choosing deferred therapy.

Role of magnetic resonance spectroscopic imaging after definitive therapy

Magnetic resonance imaging/Magnetic resonance spectroscopic imaging has been used to monitor the gland after therapy to detect local recurrence. In cases where the patient has undergone external beam radiation therapy (EBRT), shrinkage of the gland and atrophy of the glandular architecture reduces the T_2 contrast in the prostate, limiting the usefulness of MRI [50]. Reduction in proton metabolite levels results in reduced or absent metabolite peaks in proton spectra (metabolic atrophy) in the irradiated gland. Coakley *et al.* studied patients with prostate-specific antigen (PSA) relapse after EBRT for localized prostate cancer using MRI/MRSI. While MRI did not detect local recurrence effectively, MRSI recurrence, defined as a group of three or more voxels with elevated Cho (signal-to-noise ratio >5:1), gave a sensitivity and specificity of 89% and 82%, respectively, for detection of recurrence as verified by biopsy [50]. Pickett *et al.* used MRI/MRSI to follow treatment effect in the prostate gland in 55 patients who underwent EBRT [51]. Complete metabolic atrophy (no detectable metabolites in the voxel) occurred at a mean of 40.3 months in the whole patient population, and patients with lower amounts of cancer found by baseline MRI/MRSI had a shorter time to complete metabolic atrophy than patients with large amounts of cancer at baseline. In patients who received only EBRT (no hormone therapy), a comparison of time to total resolution of disease (TRD) on MRSI with PSA nadir found that MRSI mean TRD (34 months) was less than nadir PSA (40.3 months). In patients who underwent biopsy due to either positive MRSI or increased PSA, MRSI correctly detected cancer in the four positive biopsy cases and did not identify cancer in seven negative biopsy cases (i.e., 100% agreement between MRSI and biopsy). Seven patients with negative biopsy and negative MRSI had increased PSA. The area under the ROC curve for MRSI detection of tumor after EBRT was 0.8. This study indicates the potential of MRSI for monitoring local recurrence after EBRT and also for targeting post radiation therapy biopsy.

Pucar *et al.* [52] have attempted to detect post radiation therapy recurrence by MRI/MRSI in patients who subsequently underwent salvage radical prostatectomy with whole-mount, step-section pathology. In these patients, residual citrate was sometimes noted, as well as the presence of choline, so that (Cho + Cr)/Cit was calculated, when possible, and voxels containing only Cho with a signal-to-noise ratio > 3:1 were also tabulated. While voxels corresponding to cancerous regions on pathology maps tended to have higher (Cho + Cr)/Cit values or were more likely to contain a Cho peak, benign regions also demonstrated Cho or (Cho + Cr)/Cit greater than the cut-off value for cancer. Pathologic examination of the whole-mount sections revealed the presence of viable-appearing glands, which could produce citrate, and in some cases it was possible to assign a Gleason score to the tumor while in other cases it was not. These findings suggest varying effectiveness of radiation therapy within the gland or variation in dose. Pickett *et al.* followed 65 patients for 48 months and noted a steady progression to complete metabolic atrophy (>95% of all voxels having no metabolite peaks with a signal-to-noise ratio >5:1) in all patients [53]. Time to metabolic atrophy was similar in patients treated with permanent prostate implantation (PPI) alone, PPI + EBRT and PPI + EBRT + hormone therapy (range 20–28 months). Time to PSA nadir was longer than time to metabolic atrophy in the PPI-alone group, comparable in the PPI + EBRT group, and shorter than time to metabolic atrophy in the group given PPI + EBRT + hormone therapy. While patients exhibited PSA "blips" or bounces following PPI before the eventual PSA nadir, the MRSI data indicated ongoing metabolic atrophy, suggesting a possible role for monitoring treatment response and/or recurrence. A more recent study from the same group indicated that metabolic atrophy and time to resolution of spectroscopic abnormality occur more rapidly in low-risk patients treated with PPI compared to those treated with EBRT [54]. In another study MRSI was used to predict treatment outcome in high-risk patients with prostate cancer [55]. Patients were treated with chemotherapy/hormone therapy, underwent radical prostatectomy (RP) or radiation therapy, and were followed for PSA relapse (follow-up, 19–43 months). An MRSI risk score on a scale of 0–3 was derived from the volume and degree of metabolic abnormality. The results suggested that tumor metabolic assessment may indicate treatment outcome in high-risk patients with prostate cancer. Although MRSI did not provide added prognostic value to MRI in this small number of patients, MRSI may increase the confidence of the clinician in assessing risk on MRI by contributing supporting metabolic data.

Other emerging technologies

Magnetic resonance imaging with MRSI has gained acceptance as part of clinical radiological practice in prostate cancer pre-treatment evaluation in selected centers/institutions around the world. Furthermore, the other tools that are being investigated for their utility in prostate cancer are DWI and DCE MRI. For details on these newer techniques see also Chapter 9 on MRI.

Diffusion-weighted imaging

Diffusion-weighted imaging is a non-invasive technique sensitive to molecular translation of water in biologic tissues due to the random thermal motion of molecules. By means of apparent diffusion coefficients (ADCs), DWI quantifies the combined effect of both diffusion and capillary perfusion. The primary application of DWI has been in brain imaging [56]. Recently a number of investigators have reported the potential usefulness of DWI for detecting prostate cancer because it shows a lower ADC value than the normal peripheral zone tissue [57, 58, 59, 60, 61]. Due to its relatively short acquisition time and the availability of standard post-processing tools provided by manufacturers, DWI is being widely investigated in prostate cancer imaging. However, technical issues such as susceptibility artifacts on echo planar imaging sequences that can degrade the quality of diffusion-weighted images should be kept in mind. Parallel imaging techniques (such as SENSE (sensitivity encoding) [62] and SMASH (simultaneous acquisition of spatial harmonics) [63]) can be used to reduce distortion and improve image quality in DWI.

Dynamic contrast-enhanced magnetic resonance imaging

In dynamic contrast-enhanced MRI (DCE MRI), injection of gadopentetate dimeglumine (Gd-DTPA) intravenously is followed by the agent passing from the intravascular space to the interstitial space at a rate that depends on perfusion and tissue permeability. Currently, DCE MRI of the prostate is still limited to the research setting, as many technical issues remain to be resolved and the methods for acquiring and analyzing data are yet to be fully standardized. Futterer *et al.*, for instance, acquire data covering the prostate using 3D T_1-weighted spoiled gradient echo images during an intravenous bolus injection of a paramagnetic gadolinium chelate – 0.1 mmol of Gd-DTPA per kilogram of body weight administered by power injector at 2.5 ml/s and followed by a 15-ml saline flush [42]. Prostate cancer, like other cancers, shows early enhancement as well as an early washout of signal. Quantitative parameters such as K^{trans} (transfer constant), v_e (interstitial fluid space volume fraction), and k_{ep} (rate constant) provide better characterization of prostate cancer and benign prostatic tissue than MRI alone. Reported studies on the use of contrast-enhanced MRI for prostate cancer have focused on staging [64, 65], localization [42], evaluation of vascular characteristics [66], discrimination of prostate cancer in the peripheral zone from normal peripheral zone tissue and stromal and glandular BPH [67], and measurement of the effects of androgen deprivation on prostatic morphology and vascular permeability [68]. These studies suggest the many ways in which DCE MRI could be used to augment the value of a prostate MRI exam.

Conclusion

Magnetic resonance imaging provides excellent anatomic details which help in the detection, staging and better management of prostate cancer. Magnetic resonance spectroscopic imaging has shown promise and is gaining acceptance in prostate cancer imaging as a complementary tool to standard anatomic MRI. Biomarkers detected *in vivo* such as choline, polyamine, and citrate play a role in characterization of the tissue, and assessment of aggressiveness. However, in a clinical setting, one of the major limitations of proton MRSI at 1.5 T is the low sensitivity of the metabolites at millimolar concentrations, which demands relatively large voxel sizes (6–7 mm in-plane resolution on a 1.5-T scanner) to obtain an adequate signal-to-noise ratio within a patient-tolerable scan time. The great hope for MRSI is that higher magnetic field strength will mitigate or even remove some of the difficulties associated with spectroscopy at 1.5 T. Initial reports are promising with increased signal-to-noise ratio, spectral dispersion, and spatial resolution at 3 T being demonstrated [33, 34, 69]. Whether this leads to improved cancer detection or assessment of aggressiveness remains to be seen. Additionally the tools such as DWI and DCE MRI are at present investigational and need further research to prove their worth in the clinical realm. While further investigation is needed, assessment of the prostate in the future will most likely consist of a multiparametric approach incorporating T_1- and T_2-weighted MRI, MRSI and/or DWI/DCE MRI, thus maximizing the information to be gained for staging, prognosis, and treatment assessment in this very common disease.

REFERENCES

1. E. B. Cornel, G. A. Smits, G. O. Oosterhof, *et al.*, Characterization of human prostate cancer, benign prostatic hyperplasia and normal prostate by in vitro 1H and 31P magnetic resonance spectroscopy. *J Urol*, **150** (1993), 2019–24.

2. A. H. Fowler, A. A. Pappas, J. C. Holder, *et al.*, Differentiation of human prostate cancer from benign hypertrophy by in vitro 1H NMR. *Magn Reson Med*, **25** (1992), 140–7.

3. J. Kurhanewicz, R. Dahiya, J. M. Macdonald, *et al.*, Citrate alterations in primary and metastatic human prostatic adenocarcinomas: 1H magnetic resonance spectroscopy and biochemical study. *Magn Reson Med*, **29** (1993), 149–57.

4. L. L. Cheng, C. Wu, M. R. Smith, *et al.*, Non-destructive quantitation of spermine in human prostate tissue samples using HRMAS 1H NMR spectroscopy at 9.4 T. *FEBS Lett*, **494** (2001), 112–16.

5. M. G. Swanson, D. B. Vigneron, Z. L. Tabatabai, *et al.*, Proton HR-MAS spectroscopy and quantitative pathologic analysis of MRI/3D-MRSI-targeted postsurgical prostate tissues. *Magn Reson Med*, **50** (2003), 944–54.

6. M. van der Graaf, R. G. Schipper, G. O. Oosterhof, *et al.*, Proton MR spectroscopy of prostatic tissue focused on the detection of spermine, a possible biomarker of malignant behavior in prostate cancer. *Magma*, **10** (2000), 153–9.

7. P. Narayan, P. Jajodia, J. Kurhanewicz, *et al.*, Characterization of prostate cancer, benign prostatic hyperplasia and normal prostates using transrectal 31phosphorus magnetic resonance spectroscopy: a preliminary report. *J Urol,* **146** (1991), 66–74.

8. M. G. Swanson, A. S. Zektzer, Z. L. Tabatabai, *et al.*, Quantitative analysis of prostate metabolites using 1H HR-MAS spectroscopy. *Magn Reson Med*, **55** (2006), 1257–64.

9. M. W. Dewhirst, H. D. Sostman, K. A. Leopold, *et al.*, Soft-tissue sarcomas: MR imaging and MR spectroscopy for prognosis and therapy monitoring. Work in progress. *Radiology*, **174** (1990), 847–53.

10. M. J. Fulham, A. Bizzi, M. J. Dietz, *et al.*, Mapping of brain tumor metabolites with proton MR spectroscopic imaging: clinical relevance. *Radiology*, **185** (1992), 675–86.

11. M. A. Heesters, R. L. Kamman, E. L. Mooyaart, *et al.*, Localized proton spectroscopy of inoperable brain gliomas: response to radiation therapy. *J Neurooncol*, **17** (1993), 27–35.

12. J. A. Koutcher, D. Ballon, M. Graham, *et al.*, P-31 NMR spectra of extremity sarcoma: diversity of metabolic profiles and changes in response to chemotherapy. *Magn Reson Med*, **16** (1990), 19–34.

13. D. Q. McBride, B. L. Miller, D. L. Nikas, *et al.*, Analysis of brain tumors using 1H magnetic resonance spectroscopy. *Surg Neurol*, **44** (1995), 137–44.

14. A. Rutter, H. Hugenholtz, J. K. Saunders, *et al.*, One-dimensional phosphorus-31 chemical shift imaging of human brain tumors. *Invest Radiol*, **30** (1995), 359–66.

15. P. E. Sijens, M. V. Knopp, A. Brunetti, *et al.*, ¹H MR spectroscopy in patients with metastatic brain tumors: a multicenter study. *Magn Reson Med*, **33** (1995), 818–26.

16. T. A. Smith, S. Eccles, M. G. Ormerod, *et al.*, The phosphocholine and glycerophosphocholine content of an oestrogen-sensitive rat mammary tumour correlates strongly with growth rate. *Br J Cancer*, **64** (1991), 821–6.

17. E. O. Aboagye, Z. M. Bhujwalla, Malignant transformation alters membrane choline phospholipid metabolism of human mammary epithelial cells. *Cancer Res*, **59** (1999), 80–4.

18. J. Kurhanewicz, D. B. Vigneron, H. Hricak, *et al.*, Three-dimensional H-1 MR spectroscopic imaging of the in situ human prostate with high (0.24–0.7-cm³) spatial resolution. *Radiology*, **198** (1996), 795–805.

19. M. D. Schnall, B. Lenkinski, B. Milestone, *et al.*, Localized 1H spectroscopy of the human prostate in vivo; Presented at SMRM Ninth Annual Scientific Meeting; New York, NY, USA (1990), p. 288.

20. J. Frahm, H. Bruhn, M. L. Gyngell, *et al.*, Localized high-resolution proton NMR spectroscopy using stimulated echoes: initial applications to human brain in vivo. *Magn Reson Med*, **9** (1989), 79–93.

21. P. Bottomley, Selective volume method for performing localized NMR spectroscopy. US Patent (1984), 4 480 228.

22. J. Kurhanewicz, D. B. Vigneron, S. J. Nelson, *et al.*, Citrate as an in vivo marker to discriminate prostate cancer from benign prostatic hyperplasia and normal prostate peripheral zone: detection via localized proton spectroscopy. *Urology*, **45** (1995), 459–66.

23. F. Schick, H. Bongers, S. Kurz, *et al.*, Localized proton MR spectroscopy of citrate in vitro and of the human prostate in vivo at 1.5 T. *Magn Reson Med*, **29** (1993), 38–43.

24. T. R. Brown, B. M. Kincaid, K. Ugurbil, NMR chemical shift imaging in three dimensions. *Proc Natl Acad Sci USA*, **79** (1982), 3523–6.

25. A. Heerschap, G. J. Jager, M. van der Graaf, *et al.*, Proton MR spectroscopy of the normal human prostate with an endorectal coil and a double spin-echo pulse sequence. *Magn Reson Med*, **37** (1997), 204–13.

26. G. M. Bydder, J. M. Pennock, R. E. Steiner, *et al.*, The short TI inversion recovery sequence – an approach to MR imaging of the abdomen. *Magn Reson Imaging*, **3** (1985), 251–4.

27. A. Haase, J. Frahm, W. Hanicke, *et al.*, 1H NMR chemical shift selective (CHESS) imaging. *Phys Med Biol*, **30** (1985), 341–4.

28. J. Star-Lack, S. J. Nelson, J. Kurhanewicz, *et al.*, Improved water and lipid suppression for 3D PRESS CSI using RF band selective inversion with gradient dephasing (BASING). *Magn Reson Med*, **38** (1997), 311–21.

29. R. G. Males, D. B. Vigneron, J. Star-Lack, *et al.*, Clinical application of BASING and spectral/spatial water and lipid suppression pulses for prostate cancer staging and localization by in vivo 3D 1H magnetic resonance spectroscopic imaging. *Magn Reson Med*, **43** (2000), 17–22.

30. A. A. Schricker, J. M. Pauly, J. Kurhanewicz, *et al.*, Dualband spectral-spatial RF pulses for prostate MR spectroscopic imaging. *Magn Reson Med*, **46** (2001), 1079–87.

31. T. K. Tran, D. B. Vigneron, N. Sailasuta, *et al.*, Very selective suppression pulses for clinical MRSI studies of brain and prostate cancer. *Magn Reson Med*, **43** (2000), 23–33.

32. T. W. Scheenen, D. W. Klomp, S. A. Roll, *et al.*, Fast acquisition-weighted three-dimensional proton MR spectroscopic imaging of the human prostate. *Magn Reson Med*, **52** (2004), 80–8.

33. A. P. Chen, C. H. Cunningham, J. Kurhanewicz, *et al.*, High-resolution 3D MR spectroscopic imaging

of the prostate at 3 T with the MLEV-PRESS sequence. *Magn Reson Imaging*, **24** (2006), 825–32.

34. A. P. Chen, C. H. Cunningham, E. Ozturk-Isik, *et al.*, High-speed 3T MR spectroscopic imaging of prostate with flyback echo-planar encoding. *J Magn Reson Imaging*, **25** (2007), 1288–92.

35. J. A. Jung, F. V. Coakley, D. B. Vigneron, *et al.*, Prostate depiction at endorectal MR spectroscopic imaging: investigation of a standardized evaluation system. *Radiology*, **233** (2004), 701–8.

36. A. Shukla-Dave, H. Hricak, C. Moskowitz, *et al.*, Detection of prostate cancer with MR spectroscopic imaging: an expanded paradigm incorporating polyamines. *Radiology*, **245** (2007), 499–506.

37. O. Akin, E. Sala, C. S. Moskowitz, *et al.*, Transition zone prostate cancers: features, detection, localization, and staging at endorectal MR imaging. *Radiology*, **239** (2006), 784–92.

38. K. L. Zakian, S. Eberhardt, H. Hricak, *et al.*, Transition zone prostate cancer: metabolic characteristics at 1H MR spectroscopic imaging – initial results. *Radiology*, **229** (2003), 241–7.

39. J. J. Futterer, T. W. Scheenen, S. W. Heijmink, *et al.*, Standardized threshold approach using three-dimensional proton magnetic resonance spectroscopic imaging in prostate cancer localization of the entire prostate. *Invest Radiol*, **42** (2007), 116–22.

40. L. Breiman, J. Friedman, R. Olshen, *et al.*, *Classification and Regression Trees*. Belmont, CA: Wadsworth, 1984.

41. P. R. Carroll, F. V. Coakley, J. Kurhanewicz, Magnetic resonance imaging and spectroscopy of prostate cancer. *Rev Urol*, **8**: Suppl 1 (2006), S4–S10.

42. J. J. Futterer, S. W. Heijmink, T. W. Scheenen, *et al.*, Prostate cancer localization with dynamic contrast-enhanced MR imaging and proton MR spectroscopic imaging. *Radiology*, **241** (2006), 449–58.

43. H. Hricak, New horizons in genitourinary oncologic imaging. *Abdom Imaging*, **31** (2006), 182–7.

44. H. Hricak, P. L. Choyke, S. C. Eberhardt, *et al.*, Imaging prostate cancer: a multidisciplinary perspective. *Radiology*, **243** (2007), 28–53.

45. S. E. Seltzer, D. J. Getty, C. M. Tempany, *et al.*, Staging prostate cancer with MR imaging: a combined radiologist-computer system. *Radiology*, **202** (1997), 219–26.

46. J. Kurhanewicz, D. B. Vigneron, R. G. Males, *et al.*, The prostate: MR imaging and spectroscopy. Present and future. *Radiol Clin North Am.* **38** (2000), 115–38.

47. K. L. Zakian, K. Sircar, H. Hricak, *et al.*, Correlation of proton MR spectroscopic imaging with Gleason score based on step-section pathologic analysis after radical prostatectomy. *Radiology*, **234** (2005), 804–14.

48. K. K. Yu, J. Scheidler, H. Hricak, *et al.*, Prostate cancer: prediction of extracapsular extension with endorectal MR imaging and three-dimensional proton MR spectroscopic imaging. *Radiology*, **213** (1999), 481–8.

49. A. Shukla-Dave, H. Hricak, M. W. Kattan, *et al.*, The utility of magnetic resonance imaging and spectroscopy for predicting insignificant prostate cancer: an initial analysis. *BJU Int*, **99** (2007), 786–93.

50. F. V. Coakley, H. S. Teh, A. Qayyum, *et al.*, Endorectal MR imaging and MR spectroscopic imaging for locally recurrent prostate cancer after external beam radiation therapy: preliminary experience. *Radiology*, **233** (2004), 441–8.

51. B. Pickett, J. Kurhanewicz, F. Coakley, *et al.*, Use of MRI and spectroscopy in evaluation of external beam radiotherapy for prostate cancer. *Int J Radiat Oncol Biol Phys*, **60** (2004), 1047–55.

52. D. Pucar, A. Shukla-Dave, H. Hricak, *et al.*, Prostate cancer: correlation of MR imaging and MR spectroscopy with pathologic findings after radiation therapy – initial experience. *Radiology*, **236** (2005), 545–53.

53. B. Pickett, R. K. Ten Haken, J. Kurhanewicz, *et al.*, Time to metabolic atrophy after permanent prostate seed implantation based on magnetic resonance spectroscopic imaging. *Int J Radiat Oncol Biol Phys*, **59** (2004), 665–73.

54. B. Pickett, J. Kurhanewicz, J. Pouliot, *et al.*, Three-dimensional conformal external beam radiotherapy

compared with permanent prostate implantation in low-risk prostate cancer based on endorectal magnetic resonance spectroscopy imaging and prostate-specific antigen level. *Int J Radiat Oncol Biol Phys*, **65** (2006), 65–72.

55. D. Pucar, J. A. Koutcher, A. Shah, *et al.*, Preliminary assessment of magnetic resonance spectroscopic imaging in predicting treatment outcome in patients with prostate cancer at high risk for relapse. *Clin Prostate Cancer*, **3** (2004), 174–81.

56. B. Geijer, S. Holtas, Diffusion-weighted imaging of brain metastases: their potential to be misinterpreted as focal ischaemic lesions. *Neuroradiology*, **44** (2002), 568–73.

57. P. Gibbs, M. D. Pickles, L. W. Turnbull, Diffusion imaging of the prostate at 3.0 tesla. *Invest Radiol*, **41** (2006), 185–8.

58. K. Hosseinzadeh, S. D. Schwarz, Endorectal diffusion-weighted imaging in prostate cancer to differentiate malignant and benign peripheral zone tissue. *J Magn Reson Imaging*, **20** (2004), 654–61.

59. B. Issa, In vivo measurement of the apparent diffusion coefficient in normal and malignant prostatic tissues using echo-planar imaging. *J Magn Reson Imaging*, **16** (2002), 196–200.

60. C. Sato, S. Naganawa, T. Nakamura, *et al.*, Differentiation of noncancerous tissue and cancer lesions by apparent diffusion coefficient values in transition and peripheral zones of the prostate. *J Magn Reson Imaging*, **21** (2005), 258–62.

61. R. Shimofusa, H. Fujimoto, H. Akamata, *et al.*, Diffusion-weighted imaging of prostate cancer. *J Comput Assist Tomogr*, **29** (2005), 149–53.

62. K. P. Pruessmann, M. Weiger, M. B. Scheidegger, *et al.*, SENSE: sensitivity encoding for fast MRI. *Magn Reson Med*, **42** (1999), 952–62.

63. D. K. Sodickson, M. A. Griswold, P. M. Jakob, SMASH imaging. *Magn Reson Imaging Clin N Am*, 7:2 (1999), 237–54, vii–viii.

64. J. J. Futterer, S. W. Heijmink, T. W. Scheenen, *et al.*, Prostate cancer: local staging at 3-T endorectal MR imaging – early experience. *Radiology*, **238** (2006), 184–91.

65. A. R. Padhani, C. J. Gapinski, D. A. Macvicar, *et al.*, Dynamic contrast enhanced MRI of prostate cancer: correlation with morphology and tumour stage, histological grade and PSA. *Clin Radiol*, **55** (2000), 99–109.

66. D. L. Buckley, C. Roberts, G. J. Parker, *et al.*, Prostate cancer: evaluation of vascular characteristics with dynamic contrast-enhanced T1-weighted MR imaging – initial experience. *Radiology* **233** (2004), 709–15.

67. S. M. Noworolski, R. G. Henry, D. B. Vigneron, *et al.*, Dynamic contrast-enhanced MRI in normal and abnormal prostate tissues as defined by biopsy, MRI, and 3D MRSI. *Magn Reson Med*, **53** (2005), 249–55.

68. A. R. Padhani, A. D. MacVicar, C. J. Gapinski, *et al.*, Effects of androgen deprivation on prostatic morphology and vascular permeability evaluated with MR imaging. *Radiology*, **218** (2001), 365–74.

69. T. W. Scheenen, S. W. Heijmink, S. A. Roell, *et al.*, Three-dimensional proton MR spectroscopy of human prostate at 3 T without endorectal coil: feasibility. *Radiology*, **245** (2007), 507–16.

11

Nuclear medicine: diagnostic evaluation of metastatic disease

Neeta Pandit-Taskar and Steven M. Larson

Introduction

Nuclear medicine is a highly sensitive technique for detecting metastatic disease at sites throughout the body using radiotracers as biomarkers of cancer biology. Radioactive signals from these radiotracers are detected by sophisticated radioactivity-detector imaging systems including single-photon-emission computerized tomography (SPECT) and positron-emission tomography (PET). In this way nuclear medicine imaging is an example of "functional" or "molecular imaging" in which the imaging itself is based on a biochemical or physiologic property of the imaged tissue. For the patient with prostate cancer, nuclear medicine techniques, when used judiciously, are an important part of optimized cancer care; for example, bone scans are very commonly used to detect and follow up skeletal metastatic disease.

The clinical states model of Scher and Heller provides a useful guide to the possible progression of prostate cancer from a localized disease to widely spread tumor [1, 2, 3] (Figure 11.1).

From the standpoint of natural history and chance of progression in the individual patient, prostate cancer is one of the most variable of all tumors. The cancer itself may behave in a highly indolent matter and be localized in the prostate gland for years, with the patient's death being due to other diseases. Then again, a localized tumor may rapidly progress, become widely metastatic within a short time and lead to death.

Fortunately, clinical trials are now resolving key management questions based on objective features of cancer histology and biochemistry. Epidemiologic studies that compared watchful waiting with radical prostatectomy in clinically localized prostate cancer now provide clear guidelines, whereby locally progressing lesions are

Prostate Cancer, eds. Hedvig Hricak and Peter T. Scardino. Published by Cambridge University Press.

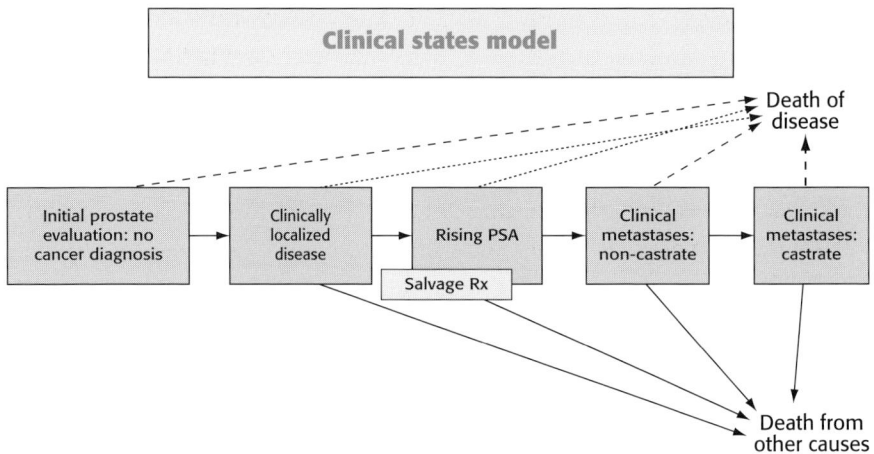

Figure 11.1. The clinical states model of Scher and Heller [2].

better served by surgery in patients who are surgical candidates [4, 5]. Also, after the patient has undergone surgical prostatectomy about 35% may recur, with the initial findings being an elevated prostate-specific antigen (PSA). Patient characteristics that predict for early recurrence include a short PSA doubling time [6, 7]. The ability of nuclear medicine techniques to identify disease sites early depends on the differences in biochemical status between tumor tissue and normal tissue and therefore all factors that influence disease progression and tumor biology affect the results of imaging. It is perhaps no surprise that from the standpoint of proven clinical utility, nuclear medicine techniques are most useful in the most advanced clinical states or aggressive forms of prostate cancer, to detect and monitor the progress of metastatic disease and perhaps also to detect response to therapy.

The nuclear bone scan

The bone scan is one of the best established techniques in nuclear medicine and is widely used for detecting metastatic disease from a large variety of human tumors, particularly the prostate and breast because of the tendency of these to metastasize to bone leading to osteoblastic lesions. The technique is performed by injecting a radiopharmaceutical that localizes in the hydroxyapatite crystals of bone. The radiopharmaceuticals used are radioactive forms of minerals that are normally concentrated by the skeleton as part of the natural biochemical homeostasis of living bone, which involves bone formation, turnover, and repair. A radioisotope most commonly used is technetium ($^{99\,m}$Tc), which is complexed with phosphate compounds and allows rapid binding within the bone matrix. Common radio-pharmaceutical preparations include $^{99\,m}$Tc methylene diphosphate ($^{99\,m}$Tc MDP) or $^{99\,m}$Tc ethylene diphosphate ($^{99\,m}$Tc EDP). Other alternative radioisotope forms that may be used are bone-seeking minerals, such as fluorine-18 (^{18}F). To acquire images, regardless of the preparation, the patient receives an intravenous injection of the radiotracer and after an optimum period of uptake by the skeleton (typically 2–3 h) the patient undergoes whole-body imaging using a gamma camera. The mechanism of uptake within the skeleton relates to the rapid accretion of minerals by the bone. The skeleton is in a continual state of building and destruction, reflected by the rapid exchange of minerals within the hydroxyapatite crystal structure of bone. If there is a cancer in the vicinity of the crystal structure, there is almost always rapid bone turnover at the site caused by the secretion of a variety of osteolytic and osteoblastic factors by the tumor cells. Bone scan images, therefore, show a "hotspot" where there is tumor present superimposed on areas of normal uptake in regions that are not affected by the cancer.

Prostate cancer

Prostatic cancer has a special tropism to bone and this has been explained by anatomic factors such as Bateson's plexus – an internal vertebral network of blood vessels that communicates between the pelvic bones and vertebra.

Prostate cancer is also strongly influenced by specific qualities of cancer cell and tumor physiology. The bone is clearly the most common site of advanced prostate cancer, with about 65% of patients having bone metastasis as their sole manifestation of spread of the disease. As many as 85% of patients will have bone metastasis at some time during the course of their disease. Typically, this is an ominous development in the natural history of the tumor and 45% of patients are likely to die within 2 years of developing metastatic disease to bone.

The initial diagnosis of spread to bony skeleton is often made by the bone scan. A typical $^{99\,m}$Tc MDP image, obtained 2–3 h after intravenous injection of $^{99\,m}$Tc MDP, is shown in Figure 11.2a. Generally, the radioactivity is taken up throughout the skeleton and the entire bony skeleton can be identified. In addition, there are relatively hypermetabolic zones or "hotspots" within the skeleton at sites where the uptake is greater; generally due to increased osteoblastic process. The "hotspots" represent sites of metastatic disease from prostate cancer.

As a cautionary note, it should be noted that the bone scan may be made abnormal by conditions other than metastatic disease; for example, other common

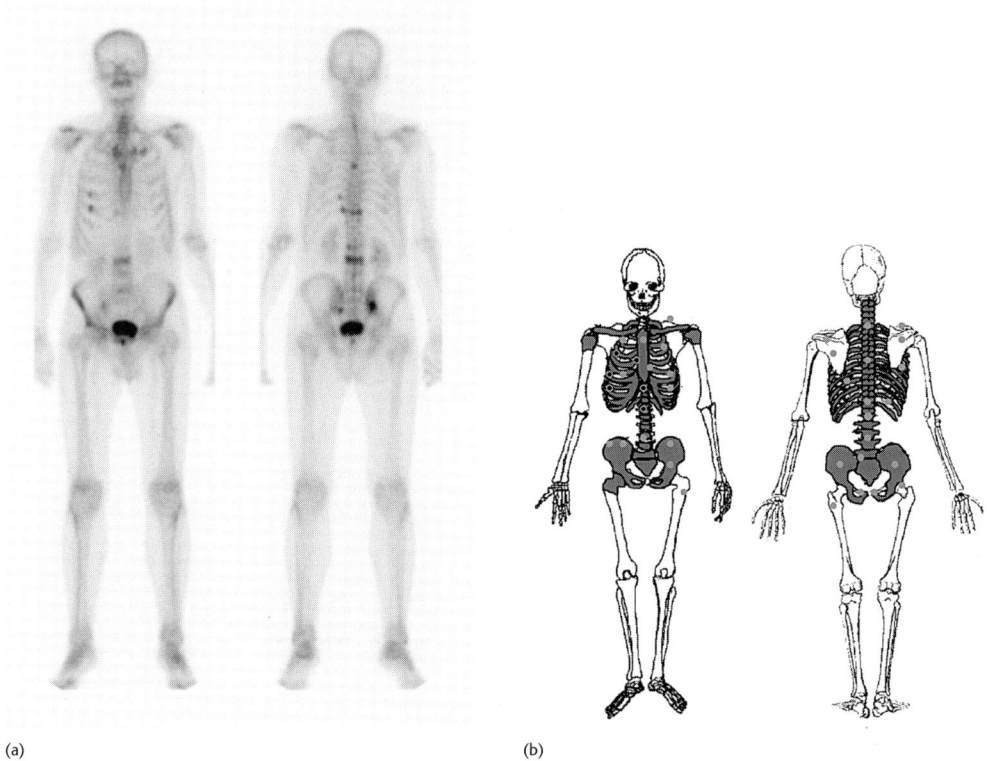

Figure 11.2. (a) Patient with prostate cancer. A bone scan was obtained using ^{99m}Tc methylene diphosphonate, a standard bone-scanning agent. Whole-body anterior (left) and posterior (right) images show uptake in the mid-thoracic and lumbar spine, the right anterior ribs, and the right sacroiliac joint. (b) The initial distribution of prostatic carcinoma metastases to bones corresponds to the distribution of the red bone marrow within the bones. See color plate section for full color version of part (b).

tumors of bone, fibrous dysplasia, Paget's disease, and trauma, particularly fracture and inflammatory and degenerative arthritis, can all lead to increased uptake of the radiotracer at the sites of disease and appear as "hotspots." For this reason, most authorities recommend that the bone scan cannot be routinely used in all clinical states of prostate cancer, but should be used only when there is a strong clinical suspicion for metastatic spread. In a patient with a diagnosis of prostate cancer this suspicion might be derived from an elevated PSA or increased alkaline phosphatase, indicating a likely involvement of bone. A PSA level greater than 10 ng/ml and an alkaline phosphatase level greater than 60 units l are commonly used thresholds above which a bone scan is recommended in the work-up of a patient with prostate cancer. Certain bone scan patterns are more suspicious of metastatic disease than of benign disease and should be borne in mind as the bone scan is being interpreted. As shown in Figure 11.2a, b bony metastasis tends to occur in its earliest form within the axial skeleton, i.e., in vertebrae, pelvis, as well as other sites of axial skeleton, that contain the red bone marrow in adults. For example, a single "hotspot" involving the rib has only about a 10% chance of being metastatic. This is because of the tendency for ribs to be affected more commonly by trauma, leading to increased uptake. In such cases, correlation with other radiographic imaging such as plain X ray and clinical history is recommended to establish traumatic etiology. However, a single area of uptake in the vertebrae, as long as it is in the body of the vertebra and not associated with the presence of degenerative joint disease, has an 85% chance of being metastatic. Also, it is now recognized that metastatic involvement begins within the red bone marrow, and only after a few weeks does the bone begin to respond with reactive changes and hypermetabolism adjacent to the metastasis. Therefore, very early metastases can be missed on the bone scan but may be detected on direct imaging methods, such MRI techniques that can visualize the tumor directly.

The bone scan as a quantitative tool: the bone scan index

We have developed a quantitative tool, called the bone scan index (BSI), which is an estimate of overall skeletal involvement measured as a sum of all sites of abnormal involvement by metastatic disease of the bony skeleton. This tool is very useful for stratifying patients with prostate cancer, and for monitoring treatment response (Figure 11.3) [8, 9].

In developing the BSI we made use of "reference man" information which gives the weight of the total skeleton and of individual bones. Using this method the fraction of skeletal weight within an individual bone could be determined. For example, if you consider all the bones of the skull, over 14% of the weight of the skeleton is actually within those bones. For estimating BSI, a qualitative estimate is made to assess the involvement of each bone in terms of the percentage involvement, and then with the use of a spreadsheet the total fraction of the skeleton involved is calculated.

Monitoring the time-dependent effects of bony involvement by metastatic disease in prostate cancer

The BSI can be very useful in follow-up of metastatic bone disease to monitor progression or treatment response. Figure 11.4 shows the time course of development

May 13,1998   April 29,1999   June 17,1999   August 17,1999
BSI=0%   BSI=0.59%   BSI=7.7%   BSI=5.4%
                                                    (post-treatment)

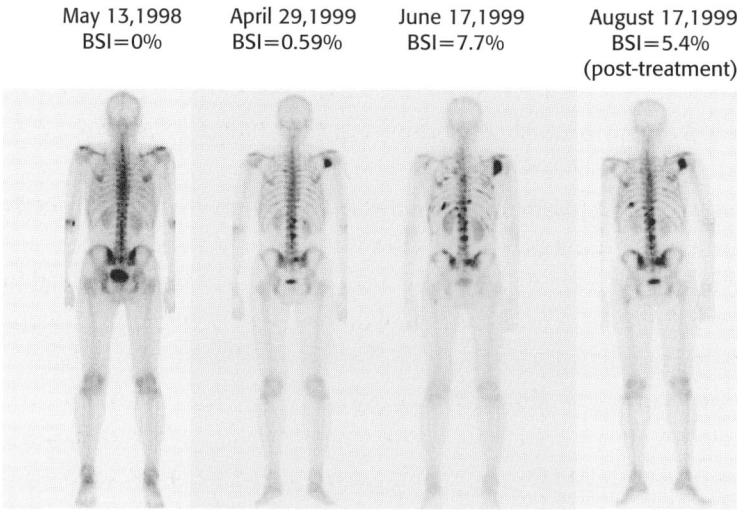

Figure 11.3. Progression of metastatic involvement by prostate cancer may occur quickly and involve multiple bones. This pattern of spread has been called the "exponential growth pattern" (see Figure 11.4).

Progression of bone involvement by prostate cancer

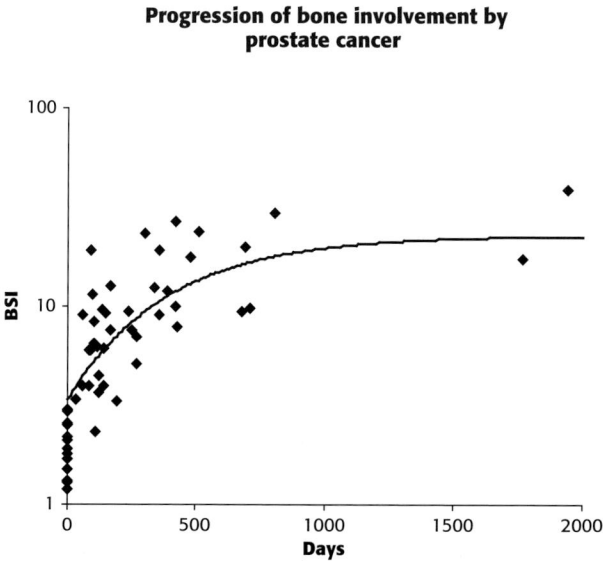

Figure 11.4. The bone scan index (BSI) of castrate-resistant prostate cancer patients plotted as a function of time. The time course follows Gompertzian kinetics, indicating that there was a rapid growth phase early in the course with a gradual diminution therafter.

of bone metastasis by prostate cancer in a group of patients with well-established tumor. Patients with more than 3% of the bony skeleton involved in metastatic prostate cancer were chosen for monitoring the time course of progression. The rate of progression was determined by monitoring the change of percentage of tumor involvement of the skeleton (Figure 11.4) over time. The time course of progression follows Gompertzian kinetics with rapid growth at the early times of observation, reaching a plateau at later times. It is possible to calculate that at the time when the average BSI was 3% the doubling time for tumor within the bone was 45 days. Because the mechanism of uptake of radiotracer in the bone scan is due to a secondary effect on the bone, the actual extent of the bone that has been involved by the tumor over time can be assessed by the accelerated metabolism, which persists for months and years as a signature of the sites within the bony skeleton. Not surprisingly, the extent of metastatic involvement of bone as measured by the BSI is strongly inversely correlated with patient survival. However, as illustrated in Figure 11.3, the BSI is not a particularly good indicator of treatment response. This is because the changes in bone reverse very slowly and the reactive changes persist for longer so that the scan changes are relatively slow to show healing. Instead the BSI's main utility is in documenting the extent to which tumor has involved bone in the past in patients, in monitoring the time course of progression, and in stratifying patients in terms of the percentage of bone involved by tumor over the course of their disease.

Direct measures of tumor metabolism in metastatic disease

$[^{18}F]$-2-Fluoro-2-deoxy-D-glucose (or FDG) is widely used in the staging and detection of malignant tumor in a host of specific tumor diagnoses. This tracer takes advantage of the accelerated glycolysis that is a feature of the malignant state. In the United States, PET-FDG imaging is one of the most rapidly growing diagnostic imaging techniques in patients being studied predominantly for oncologic indications. Most commonly, FDG has been used for the detection and staging of tumors, but indications are now growing to include the monitoring of treatment response, as, for example, in lymphomas and breast cancer. In the United States most insurance companies reimburse for PET imaging of selected tumor types. These include, lung, colorectal, head and neck, thyroid, melanoma, and lymphoma including Hodgkin's disease (HD) and non-Hodgkin's lymphoma (NHL). In 2000, the Food and Drug Administration (FDA) made a general ruling that FDG was useful for imaging glycolysis and those tumor types for which glycolysis was increased in growth and proliferation.

[^{18}F]-2-Fluoro-2-deoxy-D-glucose in castrate-resistant prostate cancer for detecting tumor burden and to monitor treatment response

Uptake of FDG in the castrate-resistant form of disease is greatly increased during the stage of progressing cancer [10], as opposed to hormone-suppressed disease [11].

In a study at our center we explored the use of FDG-PET imaging in advanced-disease patients with rising PSA levels and progressive disease as a way to monitor treatment response. In 9 (75%) of 12 cases in which serial PET scans were available, the standard uptake value (SUV) changed in parallel with the PSA level. Changes in the SUV on serial scanning correlated well with the PSA changes [10].

A lesional analysis comparing abnormalities on FDG-PET with those on CT/ MRI or bone scan for 157 lesions, in 17 patients, showed 71% detection on both FDG and bone scan with 31 (23%) seen only on bone scan (134 lesions), and 8 (6%) seen only on PET. All lesions except one that were seen only on bone scan with negative FDG-PET imaging represented stable disease, while all lesions seen only on PET scan proved to be active disease. We therefore think that FDG-PET actually discriminates active osseous disease from quiescent lesions that may be persistently detected by other imaging due to associated changes [10].

Figure 11.5a illustrates a series of follow-up FDG-PET scans (left) and bone scans (right) in a patient. There is extensive involvement of the axial skeleton including the ribs, with tumor location corresponding to the sites of uptake in the pre-treatment studies, as shown in the upper panel of the images, and corresponding to the hypermetabolic metastatic lesions in bones. A follow-up FDG-PET scan can be useful for patients treated with chemotherapy (Figure 11.5a, b). A response may be indicated by the resolution of a number of disease sites, with non-visualization of lesions or with a drop in SUV in index lesions seen on baseline study. This change on FDG-PET scanning has been found to correlate with the PSA decline, reflecting the extensive nature of the metabolic changes in tumor sites caused by treatment that lead to diminishing intensity of uptake on the post-treatment scans [10]. In contrast, the post-treatment bone scan (Figure 11.5a) may not change over the treatment interval, reflecting the fact that although the bone scan is a good indicator of the extent of tumor involvement over time, it is a relatively poor response parameter, and in fact may be misleading as to the true status and direction of the response. Moreover, bone

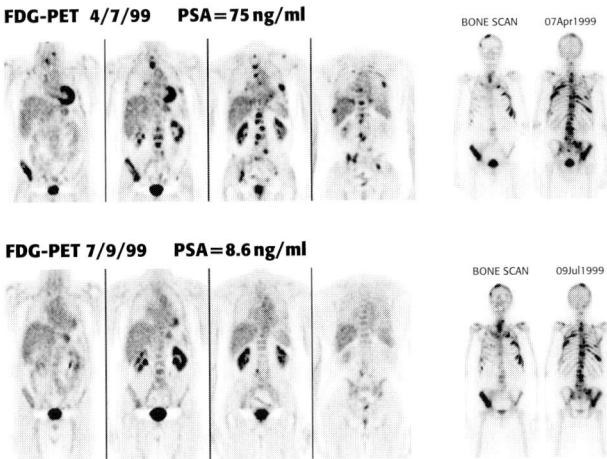

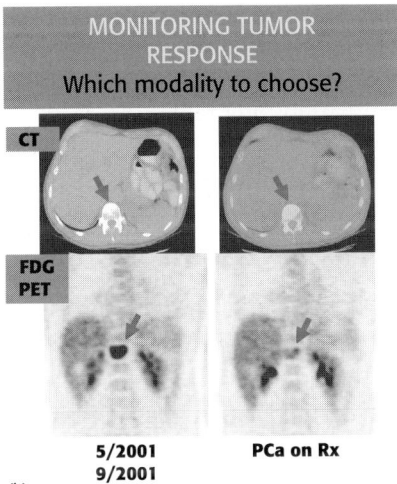

Figure 11.5. (a) Comparison of FDG imaging and bone scan imaging in a patient with castrate-resistant prostate cancer. A follow-up FDG-PET scan following treatment with taxane (lower panel) showed resolution of uptake in right iliac crest, multiple vertebrae and pelvic bones, correlating with the 90% PSA decline, reflecting the extensive nature of the metabolic changes in tumor sites, causing diminishing intensity of uptake on the post-treatment scans. The post-treatment bone scan (right lower panel), however, did not change in appearance following the treatment. (b) Comparison of PET-FDG and CT in castrate-independent prostate cancer. Note the effect of treatment as revealed by the two modalities, which shows what could be misinterpreted as a contradictory effect. The FDG-PET is definitely less in terms of activity, suggesting response, and the CT scan shows a larger region of sclerosis, suggesting progression.

scans in a post-therapy setting can show an increase in tracer uptake instead of a decrease, due to treatment-induced changes in blood flow and increased osteoblast activity associated with healing, which causes an increase in uptake of the tracer at the sites of lesions. This gives a false impression of "worsening" or an increase in tumor burden, even though this is nothing but a reactive change or a "flare response." In such patients, FDG-PET may be helpful for a more accurate assessment of response to therapy [12]. For this reason, we studied the use of FDG-PET imaging in monitoring treatment response [13]. We found that FDG-PET is the single most reliable biomarker parameter in predicting treatment response in castrate-resistant prostate cancer. Although more extensive clinical trials need to be done, including tumors treated with other drugs of a variety of mechanisms, these results are the first definite indication that FDG-PET can be used reliably in patients with prostate cancer for treatment response monitoring.

In approaching the evaluation of response, we used the SUV_{Max} as the treatment parameter. Because there may be heterogeneous changes from one site to another, we used measurements from multiple lesions (up to five) and the average SUV_{Max} over these five lesions as the treatment parameter. European criteria for the measurement of response based on SUV [14] suggest that a greater than 25% drop in SUV, the response parameter, would indicate a partial metabolic response. Progression could be diagnosed when there was an increase of 25% or more in SUV.

Imaging based on FDG has expanded rapidly around the world, in part because of the development of novel instrumentation that combines the PET scanner and a high-resolution CT scan in the same gantry. This allows for simultaneous imaging of FDG distribution with a CT scan, which can be viewed as fused or superimposed images through dedicated image-processing and viewing software. For this reason we now have the opportunity to directly compare anatomic and functional imaging obtained at the same time. As an example (Figure 11.5b), a patient with castrate-resistant metastatic disease in bone was treated, and follow-up CT and FDG-PET studies were done. In the baseline study there is active metabolism of FDG at L1 that decreased over time, so that by the follow-up study there is a more than 25% reduction in SUV_{Max}, indicating a partial metabolic response. However, the follow-up CT scan shows a contrasting change in parallel, namely that there is now a larger area of sclerosis in the vertebra at the site of the blastic lesion. We believe this is evidence that CT scan changes during therapy are unlikely to be reliable indicators of treatment response. Nonetheless, the value of having anatomic localization is obvious in helping plan site-directed biopsies in these patients.

Detection of disease in patients with prostate-specific antigen relapse after radical prostatectomy

A retrospective study was performed at our center in 91 patients with PSA relapse following prostatectomy. This compared FDG-PET with PSA values, other clinical parameters, and conventional imaging. Positron-emission tomography was true-positive in 31% of patients, and identified lesions in the prostate, bones and lymph nodes, and one lesion of liver metastasis. When correlated with PSA, mean PSA was higher in PET-positive than in PET-negative patients, and a PSA of 2.4 ng/ml and a

PSA velocity of 1.3 ng/ml per year provided the best trade-off between the sensitivity (80%; 71%) and specificity (73%; 77%) of PET-positive lesions in a receiver operating characteristic curve analysis. The probability for disease detection increased with PSA levels [15].

Radiolabeled antibody imaging: current status and future prospects

Over the last decade there has been a great deal of interest in the use of antibodies for imaging of prostate cancer, and Cytogen, a US company, has obtained approval from the FDA for ProstaScint® imaging for diagnosis. The antibody has high affinity binding to an internal epitope on prostate-specific membrane antigen (PSMA). Relatively recent reviews have appeared summarizing the role of ProstaScint® imaging in prostate cancer [16]. After more than a decade of experience ProstaScint® imaging is still controversial, and its role has not been clearly defined. In part this may be because images were relatively difficult to interpret due to background vascular activity. A number of techniques have been used, such as dual isotope imaging with labeled red cells for separating out the vascular distribution. Another limitation appears to be due to a relatively unusual appearance of very prominent uptake in the central abdomen, which could not be directly related to lymph node involvement by prostate cancer. A recent study by Haseman et al. provides evidence that central abdominal uptake of ProstaScint® in patients with prostate cancer is correlated with a significantly higher probability of metastatic involvement in comparison with patients who do not have this uptake [17]. However, another recent study by Nagda et al. indicates that patients with central abdominal uptake were neither more nor less likely to fail brachytherapy for PSA recurrence [18]. The exact role for ProstaScint® imaging in assessing the extent of local tumor, or in PSA recurrence and in salvage therapy requires additional study.

Future applications of molecular imaging in prostate cancer: meeting pressing needs

Currently, it appears that diagnostic imaging applications, especially for nuclear medicine, are useful only in advanced disease. The next section will review potential future applications of molecular imaging in prostate cancer that are likely to have important future benefit, either in other clinical stages besides advanced disease or in providing knowledge that may be of benefit in treating prostate cancer.

Understanding the biology of progressive disease: androgen receptor imaging agents

Castrate-resistant prostate cancer is the lethal form of the disease and there is growing evidence that the androgen receptor plays an important role in initiating this progressive phase of the illness [19].

We are currently studying the expression of the androgen receptor and castrate-independent disease, using 16β-[^{18}F]fluoro-5α-dihydrotestosterone (FDHT), an analog of dihydrotestosterone, which is the predominant androgen at the cellular level in humans. This radiotracer was developed by Katzenellenbogen and Welch, and was shown to have favorable biologic properties in baboons [20]. This agent has been shown to be highly concentrated in androgen-receptor-bearing tumors of castrate-resistant patients at Memorial Sloan-Kettering Cancer Center [21] and Washington University in St. Louis [22]. The *in vivo* biodistribution of this radiotracer is illustrated in Figure 11.6 in a patient with metastatic castrate-resistant prostate cancer. Radiotracer binds avidly to sex-binding globulin in the blood. Metabolism is through the liver with excretion of metabolites into the gut. There is very rapid localization into tumors, with standardized uptake values that are comparable to FDG uptake within the tumors of the range of 5–10. Clearance of the active compounds from the blood is rapid, with a metabolic half-time of 8–10 min, and maximal tumor uptake at 15–20 min after injection. Although the FDG uptake and FDHT uptake are normally concordant in advanced tumors, it is clear that glycolysis and androgen receptor expression are modulated by different stimuli, since the uptake of the two tracers differs distinctly in individual patients, in terms of both time of onset in the course of illness and magnitude of expression in an individual metastasis. We are currently monitoring biologic correlates of expression of androgen receptor in a cohort of patients with castrate-resistant prostate cancer.

Discovery of new tracers with potential application to imaging local regional and PSA-relapse clinical states

[^{11}C]Methionine

Amino acid transport is often markedly upregulated in human cancers and [^{11}C] methionine was introduced as a tracer for prostate cancer by Nilsson *et al.* [23]. The initial pilot study showed excellent sensitivity for detection of known bony metastasis from castrate-resistant prostate cancer [24]. Macapinlac *et al.* [25] confirmed this work in a larger series of patients and compared it to FDG, showing that [^{11}C]

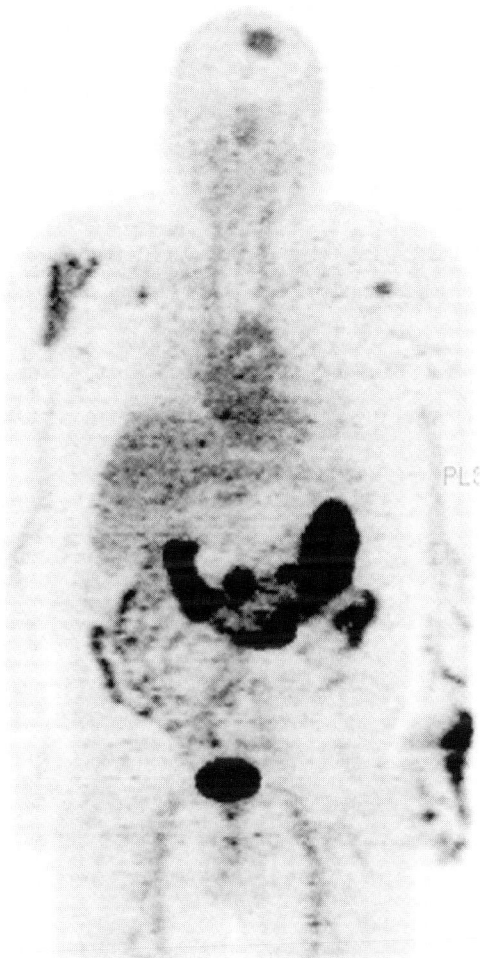

Figure 11.6. Castrate-resistant prostate cancer. Biodistribution of the androgen receptor agent FDHT. Reprojection image, 1 h after intravenous injection.

methionine is more sensitive in detecting metabolically active disease in the bones of patients with prostate cancer.

In 12 patients with prostate cancer who had increasing levels of PSA and evidence of new or progressive disease, the sensitivity of [^{18}F]FDG-PET was 48% (167/348 lesions) as against 72.1% (251/348 lesions) by [^{11}C]methionine PET. [^{11}C]Methionine PET identified significantly more lesions than [^{18}F]FDG-PET ($p < 0.01$). Some lesions (26%) had no detectable metabolism of [^{18}F]FDG or [^{11}C]methionine due to possible necrosis or dormant disease. About 95% of metabolically active sites metabolized [^{11}C]methionine while [^{18}F]FDG uptake was more variable (65%). These findings suggest possible different biologic characteristics of the lesions in prostate cancer. It is

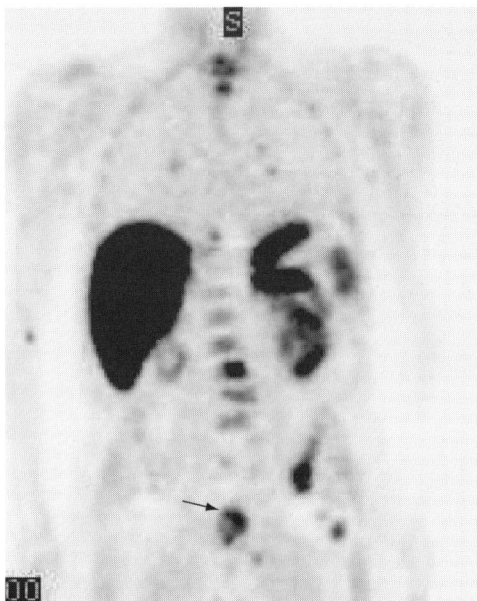

Figure 11.7. [^{11}C]Methionine in castrate-resistant prostate cancer. Coronal image showing uptake in L3, left iliac and prostate bed (arrow).

speculated that a time-dependent metabolic cascade may occur in advanced prostate cancer, with initial uptake of [^{11}C]methionine in dormant sites followed by increased uptake of [^{18}F]FDG during progression of disease [24].

The tracer has excellent characteristics for imaging, being rapidly cleared from the blood and taken up in the tumor with high uptake (Figure 11.7). In addition, [^{11}C]methionine is only minimally excreted in the urine and so it is easier to detect recurrence of the prostate cancer with this tracer [24, 25].

[^{18}F]FACBC ([^{18}F]-1-Amino-3-fluorocyclobutane-1-carboxylic acid)

Among the more promising of the recent radiotracers, the non-natural amino acid [^{18}F]-1-amino-3-fluorocyclobutane-1-carboxylic acid ([^{18}F]FACBC) has recently been applied in a relatively small group of prostate cancer patients. The importance of this tracer is that good uptake is seen in both local regional and distant metastases (Figure 11.8). The fact that it is a fluorinated tracer also makes it more likely that the tracer will be widely applied if it fulfils its initial promise [26].

Other radiotracers for metastases

[^{18}F]Choline [27, 28, 29] and [^{18}F]acetate [27, 30, 31, 32, 33] are two additional radiotracers that show promise in staging locoregional prostate cancer.

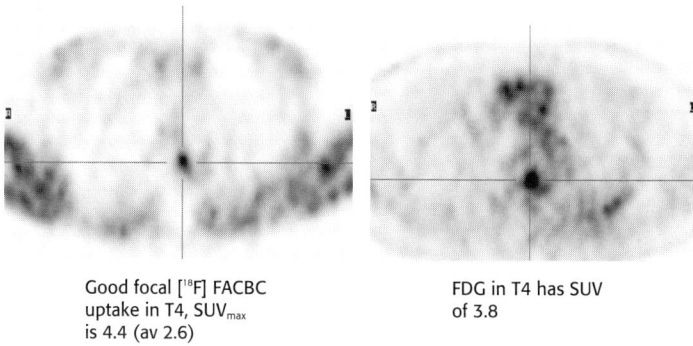

Good focal [^{18}F] FACBC
uptake in T4, SUV$_{max}$
is 4.4 (av 2.6)

FDG in T4 has SUV
of 3.8

Figure 11.8. [^{18}F]FACBC in prostate cancer. Comparison to FDG.

However, no definitive conclusion can be drawn from the current studies and to determine utility additional larger studies must be done in well-defined cohorts of patients.

The promise of radiolabeled antibody imaging as "virtual immunohistochemistry"

Prostate-specific membrane antigen (PSMA) is a well- characterized antigen that is expressed on virtually all prostate cancers. ProstaScint® binds to the internal domain of PSMA and has been employed in the imaging of prostate cancer, as discussed above. Although ProstaScint® has a number of clinical advocates, there is perhaps an equal number who are disappointed in its ability to identify metastatic disease.

It is known that the antibody on which ProstaScint® is based, 7E11, binds to epitopes that are normally internal within the cell. There is a strong possibility that other antibodies may recognize more favorable epitopes, which are external to the cell and thus more easily targeted to viable cancer by radiolabeled antibody *in vivo*. Antibodies that target the external epitopes have been developed and appear to recognize a larger number of sites on prostate cancer cells, and to have a higher degree of localization in animal models [34]. One of these antibodies, J591, has been used extensively in early clinical trials as a carrier and has shown excellent targeting to metastatic tumor *in vivo* [35, 36].

There is little doubt that one of the most promising areas of molecular imaging is the use of specific antibodies that target key biomolecules on human tumors. Figure 11.9 shows an example of excellent targeting of lutetium-177-labeled J591 in a patient with castrate-resistant prostate cancer.

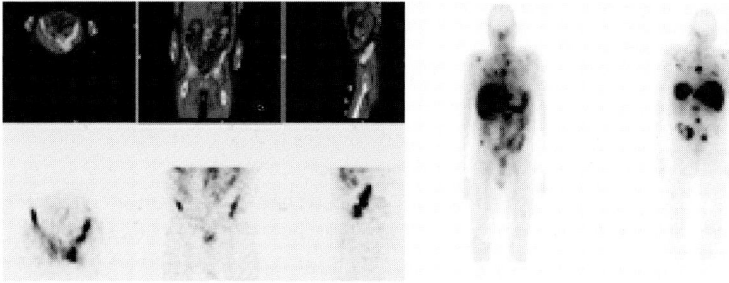

72 male with prostate cancer with bone metastasis. Post-treatment with ^{177}Lu huJ59-labeled antibody. Images show localization of the tracer in metastatic bone lesions.

Figure 11.9. [^{177}Lu]J591 imaging in castrate-resistant prostate cancer.

Time will tell whether reliable images of the quality of that displayed in Figure 11.9 will find their way into clinical medicine to improve staging for both osseous and soft-tissue metastases in prostate cancer.

Conclusion

Nuclear medicine techniques are widely used in the clinical management of prostate cancer to estimate the extent of metastatic involvement in bone. Recently, positron-emission tomography (PET) has become widely available and has been applied to the assessment of castrate-resistant prostate cancer. At Memorial Sloan-Kettering Cancer Center we use FDG-PET as a way to stage the advanced patient and to monitor response to treatment. In the future it is likely that new molecular imaging radiotracers will be developed which will target important biochemical functions in the tumor and become important in clinical management. Candidate tracers include [^{18}F]choline, [^{18}F]acetate, and [^{18}F]FACBC. Although ProstaScint® has been something of a disappointment, the development of improved antibodies and novel radiotracers makes it likely that in the future prostate cancer will be staged with optimized antibody formulations.

REFERENCES

1. H. I. Scher, M. Eisenberger, A. V. D'Amico, et al., Eligibility and outcomes reporting guidelines for clinical trials for patients in the state of a rising prostate-specific antigen: recommendations from the Prostate-Specific Antigen Working Group. *J Clin Oncol*, **22** (2004), 537–56.

2. H. I. Scher, G. Heller, Clinical states in prostate cancer: toward a dynamic model of disease progression. *Urology*, **55** (2000), 323–7.

3. H. I. Scher, M. J. Morris, W. K. Kelly, *et al.*, Prostate cancer clinical trial end points: "RECIST"ing a step backwards. *Clin Cancer Res*, **11** (2005), 5223–32.

4. A. Bill-Axelson, L. Holmberg, M. Ruutu, *et al.*, Radical prostatectomy versus watchful waiting in early prostate cancer. *N Engl J Med*, **352** (2005), 1977–84.

5. L. Holmberg, A. Bill-Axelson, F. Helgesen, *et al.*, A randomized trial comparing radical prostatectomy with watchful waiting in early prostate cancer. *N Engl J Med*, **347** (2002), 781–9.

6. S. J. Freedland, E. B. Humphreys, L. A. Mangold, *et al.*, Risk of prostate cancer-specific mortality following biochemical recurrence after radical prostatectomy. *JAMA*, **294** (2005), 433–9.

7. S. J. Freedland, E. B. Humphreys, L. A. Mangold, *et al.*, Death in patients with recurrent prostate cancer after radical prostatectomy: prostate-specific antigen doubling time subgroups and their associated contributions to all-cause mortality. *J Clin Oncol*, **25** (2007), 1765–71.

8. P. Sabbatini, S. M. Larson, A. Kremer, *et al.*, Prognostic significance of extent of disease in bone in patients with androgen-independent prostate cancer. *J Clin Oncol*, **17** (1999), 948–57.

9. M. Imbriaco, S. M. Larson, H. W. Yeung, *et al.*, A new parameter for measuring metastatic bone involvement by prostate cancer: the Bone Scan Index. *Clin Cancer Res*, **4** (1998), 1765–72.

10. M. J. Morris, T. Akhurst, I. Osman, *et al.*, Fluorinated deoxyglucose positron emission tomography imaging in progressive metastatic prostate cancer. *Urology*, **59** (2002), 913–18.

11. S. D. Yeh, M. Imbriaco, S. M. Larson, *et al.*, Detection of bony metastases of androgen-independent prostate cancer by PET-FDG. *Nucl Med Biol*, **23** (1996), 693–7.

12. J. A. Schneider, C. R. Divgi, A. M. Scott, *et al.*, Flare on bone scintigraphy following Taxol chemotherapy for metastatic breast cancer. *J Nucl Med*, **35** (1994), 1748–52.

13. M. J. Morris, T. Akhurst, S. M. Larson, *et al.*, Fluorodeoxyglucose positron emission tomography as an outcome measure for castrate metastatic prostate cancer treated with antimicrotubule chemotherapy. *Clin Cancer Res*, **11** (2005), 3210–16.

14. H. Young, R. Baum, U. Cremerius, *et al.*, Measurement of clinical and subclinical tumour response using [^{18}F]-fluorodeoxyglucose and positron emission tomography: review and 1999 EORTC recommendations. European Organization for Research and Treatment of Cancer (EORTC) PET Study Group. *Eur J Cancer*, **35** (1999), 1773–82.

15. H. Schöder, K. Herrmann, M. Gönen, *et al.*, 2-[^{18}F]fluoro-2-deoxyglucose positron emission tomography for the detection of disease in patients with prostate-specific antigen relapse after radical prostatectomy. *Clin Cancer Res*, **11**:13 (2005), 4761–9.

16. A. A. Mohammed, I. S. Shergill, M. T. Vandal, *et al.*, ProstaScint and its role in the diagnosis of prostate cancer. *Expert Rev Mol Diagn*, **7** (2007), 345–9.

17. M. K. Haseman, S. A. Rosenthal, S. L. Kipper, *et al.*, Central abdominal uptake of indium-111 capromab pendetide (ProstaScint) predicts for poor prognosis in patients with prostate cancer. *Urology*, **70** (2007), 303–8.

18. S. N. Nagda, N. Mohideen, S. S. Lo, *et al.*, Long-term follow-up of ^{111}In-capromab pendetide (ProstaScint) scan as pretreatment assessment in patients who undergo salvage radiotherapy for rising prostate-specific antigen after radical prostatectomy for prostate cancer. *Int J Radiat Oncol Biol Phys*, **67**:3 (2007), 834–40.

19. C. D. Chen, D. S. Welsbie, C. Tran, *et al.*, Molecular determinants of resistance to antiandrogen therapy. *Nat Med*, **10** (2004), 33–9.

20. T. A. Bonasera, J. P. O'Neil, M. Xu, *et al.*, Preclinical evaluation of fluorine-18-labeled androgen receptor ligands in baboons. *J Nucl Med*, **37** (1996), 1009–15.

21 S. M. Larson, M. Morris, I. Gunther, *et al.*, Tumor localization of 16beta-^{18}F-fluoro-5alpha-dihydrotestosterone versus 18F-FDG in patients with progressive, metastatic prostate cancer. *J Nucl Med*, **45** (2004), 366–73.

22. F. Dehdashti, J. Picus, J. M. Michalski, *et al.*, Positron tomographic assessment of androgen receptors in prostatic carcinoma. *Eur J Nucl Med Mol Imaging*, **32** (2005), 344–50.

23. S. Nilsson, K. Kalner, C. Ginman, *et al.*, C-11 methionine positron emission tomography in the management of prostatic carcinoma. *Antibody Immunoconj Radiopharm*, **8** (1995), 23–38.

24 R. Nunez, H. A. Macapinlac, H. W. Yeung, *et al.*, Combined ^{18}F-FDG and ^{11}C-methionine PET scans in patients with newly progressive metastatic prostate cancer. *J Nucl Med*, **43** (2002), 46–55.

25. H. A. Macapinlac, J. L. Humm, T. Akhurst, *et al.*, Differential metabolism and pharmacokinetics of L-[1-(11)C]-methionine and 2-[(18)F] fluoro-2-deoxy-D-glucose (FDG) in androgen independent prostate cancer. *Clin Positron* Imaging, **2** (1999), 173–81.

26. D. M. Schuster, J. R. Votaw, P. T. Nieh, *et al.*, Initial experience with the radiotracer anti-1-amino-3-^{18}F-fluorocyclobutane-1-carboxylic acid with PET/CT in prostate carcinoma. *J Nucl Med*, **48** (2007), 56–63.

27. T. Powles, I. Murray, C. Brock, *et al.*, Molecular positron emission tomography and PET/CT imaging in urological malignancies. *Eur Urol*, **51** (2007), 1511–20; discussion 1520–1.

28. M. Heinisch, A. Dirisamer, W. Loidl, *et al.*, Positron emission tomography/computed tomography with F-18-fluorocholine for restaging of prostate cancer patients: meaningful at PSA <5 ng/ml? *Mol Imaging Biol*, **8** (2006), 43–8.

29. W. Langsteger, M. Heinisch, I. Fogelman, The role of fluorodeoxyglucose, ^{18}F-dihydroxyphenylalanine, ^{18}F-choline, and ^{18}F-fluoride in bone imaging with emphasis on prostate and breast. *Semin Nucl Med*, **36** (2006), 73–92.

30. H. Vees, F. Buchegger, S. Albrecht, *et al.*, ^{18}F-choline and/or ^{11}C-acetate positron emission tomography: detection of residual or progressive subclinical disease at very low prostate-specific antigen values (<1 ng/ml) after radical prostatectomy. *BJU Int*, **99** (2007), 1415–20.

31. N. Oyama, T. R. Miller, F. Dehdashti, *et al.*, ^{11}C-acetate PET imaging of prostate cancer: detection of recurrent disease at PSA relapse. *J Nucl Med*, **44** (2003), 549–55.

32. N. Oyama, J. Kim, L. A. Jones, *et al.*, MicroPET assessment of androgenic control of glucose and acetate uptake in the rat prostate and a prostate cancer tumor model. *Nucl Med Biol*, **29** (2002), 783–90.

33. N. Oyama, H. Akino, H. Kanamaru, *et al.*, ^{11}C-acetate PET imaging of prostate cancer. *J Nucl Med*, **43** (2002), 181–6.

34. P. M. Smith-Jones, S. Vallabahajosula, S. J. Goldsmith, *et al.*, In vitro characterization of radiolabeled monoclonal antibodies specific for the extracellular domain of prostate-specific membrane antigen. *Cancer Res*, **60** (2000), 5237–43.

35. M. J. Morris, C. R. Divgi, N. Pandit-Taskar, *et al.*, Pilot trial of unlabeled and indium-111-labeled anti-prostate-specific membrane antigen antibody J591 for castrate metastatic prostate cancer. *Clin Cancer Res*, **11** (2005), 7454–61.

36. N. H. Bander, Technology insight: monoclonal antibody imaging of prostate cancer. *Nat Clin Pract Urol*, **3** (2006), 216–25.

12

Imaging recurrent prostate cancer

Tamar Sella and Darko Pucar

Introduction

In the setting of recurrent prostate cancer (PCa), awareness and understanding of clinical findings are essential for accurate imaging interpretation. Accordingly, this text will first address the principles of recurrent PCa management. Subsequently, the principles of recurrent PCa evaluation with computed tomography (CT), magnetic resonance imaging (MRI), transrectal ultrasound (TRUS), and TRUS-guided biopsy will be described. Nuclear medicine methods are reviewed in Chapter 11.

Management principles of recurrent prostate cancer

General principles

Prostate cancer is usually suspected based on the detection of an abnormal serum prostate-specific antigen (PSA) value (≥4 ng/ml is the most commonly used criterion) and diagnosed by TRUS-guided systematic prostate biopsy [1]. With systematic biopsy, one or more cores are obtained from each prostate sextant regardless of TRUS findings [2]. Although optional additional cores can be obtained from regions that are abnormal on TRUS or other imaging modalities, image-guided biopsy is currently accepted only as an adjunct to systematic biopsy [2]. Biopsy results are used to assign the Gleason grade [3]. Digital rectal examination (DRE) findings are used to determine clinical tumor stage; however, due to earlier detection by PSA testing, PCa is now non-palpable in about two-thirds of patients and the clinical stage often underestimates the pathologic tumor stage [4, 5] (Table 12.1).

Newly diagnosed PCa is designated as "primary" PCa and its treatment modalities are designated as "primary" treatments. In the PSA era, about 85% of

Prostate Cancer, eds. Hedvig Hricak and Peter T. Scardino. Published by Cambridge University Press.
© Cambridge University Press 2009.

Table 12.1. Treatment modalities for local primary and recurrent prostate cancer after radiation therapy (RT)

Anticipated pathologic stage (pT)[a]	Clinical correlates for local primary PCa[b]	Primary therapy[c]	Clinical and imaging correlates for local recurrent PCa after RT	Salvage therapy[d]
pT2	Low-risk: clinical stage T1–T2a and Gleason score 6 and PSA <10 ng/ml	Conventional: EBRT, brachytherapy, RP Experimental: HIFU, cryosurgery	Advanced risk stratification not possible; pre-RT clinical stage T1–T2, NX or N0, post-RT imaging negative for osseous metastases and lymph node involvement, post-RT positive TRUS-guided prostate biopsy, and post-RT PSA <10 ng/ml suggest local recurrence and no metastatic disease	SRP, salvage brachytherapy, salvage HIFU, salvage cryosurgery
pT2 or pT3a	Intermediate-risk: clinical stage T2b–T2c or Gleason score 7 or PSA 10–20 ng/ml	EBRT, RP		
pT3a–pT4, N0 or N1	High-risk: clinical stage T3a or Gleason score 8–10 or PSA >20 ng/ml	EBRT, RP in selected patients		
pT3b–pT4, N0 or N1	Very high risk: clinical stage T3b–T4	EBRT		

Source: Modified from PROS-2, PROS-3, and PROS-6, *NCCN Practice Guidelines in Oncology – Prostate Cancer* v2.2007 available at online at: http://www.nccn.org/professionals/physician_gls/default.asp [4].

[a] pT2. Tumor confined to prostate that involves < ½ of prostate lobe (pT2a), > ½ prostate lobe (pT2b), both prostate lobes (T2c); pT3a (unilateral) and pT3b (bilateral) extracapsular extension (ECE) – tumor penetration through the prostate fibrous capsule into periprostatic fat; pT3c, seminal vesicle invasion; pT4, bladder neck, sphincter, rectum, levator muscle, or pelvic sidewall invasion; N1, involvement of regional obturator, internal and external iliac lymph nodes.

[b] Clinical stage T1. Non-palpable tumor detected on transurethral resection of prostate (T1a,b) or systematic biopsy (T1c); clinical stages T2–T4 defined as corresponding pathologic stages described above; Gleason score – sum or primary and secondary Gleason grade.

[c] The details are available in NCCN *Practice Guidelines in Oncology – Prostate Cancer* v2.2007, algorithms PROS-2 and PROS-3; in certain situations radical prostatectomy is combined with pelvic lymph node dissection, and external beam radiation therapy is combined with brachytherapy, pelvic lymph node dissection, or androgen deprivation.

[d] The details are available in NCCN *Practice Guidelines in Oncology – Prostate Cancer*, algorithm PROS-6, which is Figure 12.1 in this text. All salvage treatments listed are experimental but SRP is most studied; since risk is difficult to assess prior to SRP, some surgeons routinely perform pelvic lymph node dissection.

Abbreviations: PCa, prostate cancer; EBRT, external beam radiation therapy; RP, radical prostatectomy; SRP, salvage radical prostatectomy; HIFU, high-intensity focused ultrasound.

patients have local primary PCa that can be treated with definitive (curative) local therapy [2, 4, 6, 7]. The most common forms of conventional local therapy for localized PCa are radical prostatectomy (RP) and one of two forms of radiation therapy (RT): external beam RT (EBRT) and brachytherapy. Additional experimental treatment modalities for localized PCa, such as cryotherapy and high-intensity focused ultrasound (HIFU), are emerging [4] (Table 12.1). In general, all local treatment modalities can be used for clinically low-risk patients who are likely to have primary local PCa confined to the prostate, while EBRT and RP are used to treat intermediate-risk and high-risk patients who might have local PCa spreading to periprostatic structures [4] (Table 12.1). Patients with pre-treatment evidence of systemic disease are usually not treated with these forms of local therapy, with the exception of the use of EBRT for palliation when obstructive symptoms occur.

Following primary local treatment, serial PSA follow-up is performed at 3- to 12-month intervals. Recurrent PCa is suspected when the PSA value rises, particularly if a rising trend appears in several sequential values. This clinical situation is referred to as PSA relapse, biochemical relapse or biochemical failure [4]. After primary RP or RT, approximately 30%–50% of patients will have PSA relapse at 5 years [8, 9]. The definition of PSA relapse depends on the treatment modality utilized to treat the primary PCa. Since prostate tissue is the only source of PSA, the post-RP PSA level should be essentially undetectable and PSA relapse is defined either as failure to achieve undetectable PSA following surgery or detectable and rising PSA on two or more subsequent measurements if PSA was initially undetectable [4]. The threshold for detectable PSA is not standardized with values ranging between 0.05 and 0.4 ng/ml in the literature. Following primary RT, PSA usually sharply declines but does not become undetectable since prostatic tissue is left in situ; PSA relapse is defined according to The American Society for Therapeutic Radiology and Oncology (ASTRO) Consensus Panel as a rise ≥2 ng/ml above the PSA nadir (lowest PSA value after RT), regardless of whether the patient is on androgen-deprivation therapy (ADT) [10]. There is no standard definition for PSA relapse after primary experimental treatments; however, since these treatments leave the prostate in situ, the ASTRO criteria for post-RT PSA failure are frequently used, with or without modifications.

Locally recurrent PCa can be treated with local salvage treatment modalities, i.e., with salvage radiation therapy (SRT) after primary RP [11], or with salvage radical prostatectomy (SRP), cryosurgery, HIFU, or brachytherapy after RT [8, 12, 13] (Table 12.1). Although all salvage therapies are experimental, SRT and SRP have been used the most extensively. These salvage techniques are not indicated if there is evidence of metastatic disease. Androgen-deprivation therapy and other systemic therapies are utilized for metastatic PCa or if the patient is unable or unwilling to undergo local treatment, but systemic therapies are not curative for either primary or recurrent PCa [4, 14, 15]. Furthermore, local salvage treatments for recurrent PCa are associated with a higher frequency of adverse effects compared with local primary treatments. Thus, developing reliable diagnostic tests to prove local and exclude metastatic recurrent PCa is critical for treatment selection [8, 11].

No single clinical or imaging test is sufficiently accurate to reliably predict the local extent of primary or recurrent PCa. Complex algorithms that combine pre-treatment and post-treatment clinical (i.e., PSA, clinical stage, Gleason score) and imaging parameters have been developed to assist in predicting the most likely tumor extent and accordingly the most effective treatment option [4]. The radiologists interpreting prostate studies must be familiar with these algorithms, particularly with those used at their institutions. They should collect all relevant clinical parameters and if necessary discuss the goals of imaging studies with the referring clinicians before giving their interpretation. The National Comprehensive Cancer Network (NCCN) *Practice Guidelines in Oncology – Prostate Cancer* are widely recognized algorithms, presented here [4] (Table 12.1, Figures 12.1, 12.2).

Patient selection for imaging of recurrent PCa after radiation therapy

Patients with PSA relapse or positive DRE after RT are first stratified according to whether they are candidates for local salvage therapy (NCCN PCa guidelines v2.2007, PROS-6 algorithm) (Figure 12.1) [4]. Those who are not candidates for local salvage therapy might be assessed for metastatic diseases with technetium 99 m-diphosphonate bone scintigraphy (bone scan) and CT of the abdomen and pelvis in order to facilitate a decision between observation and ADT.

Patients who are candidates for local salvage therapy include those with a pre-treatment clinical stage T1–T2, NX or N0; life expectancy >10 years, and current PSA <10 ng/ml. These patients will undergo assessment for local recurrence versus metastatic disease, since patients with biopsy-proven locally recurrent PCa and no evidence of metastatic disease can be treated with local salvage therapy [4, 8]. Imaging methods that can assist in detection of local recurrence or salvage treatment planning include TRUS, conventional prostate T_1- and T_2-weighted MRI, experimental MRI techniques (such as MR spectroscopy, diffusion-weighted imaging and dynamic contrast-enhanced MRI), ^{18}F-2-fluoro-D-deoxyglucose (^{18}F-FDG)-PET/CT, monoclonal antibody imaging with the prostate-specific

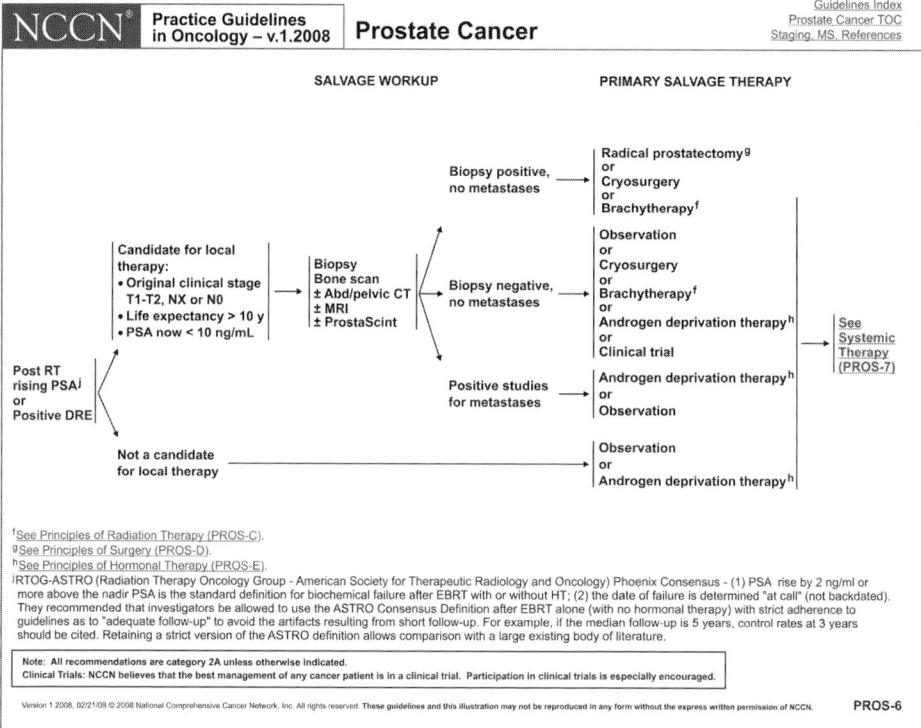

Figure 12.1. PROS-6 NCCN Practice Guidelines in Oncology for Prostate Cancer v2.2007: Reprinted from online publication available at: http://www.nccn.org/professionals/physician_gls/default.asp.

membrane antigen (PSMA) antibody ^{111}In-capromab pendetide (ProstaScint®, Cytogen Corporation, Princeton, NJ, USA), and novel experimental nuclear medicine techniques.

Patient selection for imaging of recurrent prostate cancer after radical prostatectomy

Patients with PSA relapse or persistent PSA after RP are initially evaluated with a battery of diagnostic tests which may include prostate bed biopsy, abdominal and pelvic CT or MRI, and nuclear medicine methods, with the goal again being to differentiate between local recurrence and distant metastases (NCCN PCa guidelines v2.2007, PROS-5 algorithm) (Figure 12.2) [4]. If distant metastases are detected, ADT is initiated; however, distant metastases are very unlikely (<5%) to be detected if PSA is less than 10 ng/ml [2, 16, 17]. A definite local recurrence is also often not diagnosed when PSA failure is determined (<25%) [11]. Thus, the

NCCN® Practice Guidelines in Oncology – v.2.2007   **Prostate Cancer**

Guidelines Index
Prostate Cancer TOC
Staging, MS, References

POST-RADICAL PROSTATECTOMY RECURRENCE

SALVAGE WORKUP

PRIMARY SALVAGE THERAPY

High probability of benefit from RT:
Gleason score ≤ 7, PreRT PSA ≤ 2, positive margins
or
Gleason score ≤ 7, PreRT PSA ≤ 2, negative margins, PSADT > 10 months
or
Gleason score 8-10, PreRT PSA ≤ 2, positive margins, PSADT > 10 months
→ RTf

Failure of PSA to fall to undetectable

± Bone Scan
± Biopsy
± CT/MRI
± ProstaScint

Lower probability of benefit from RT:
Seminal vesicle invasion
Lymph node metastases
Not in one of above categories
→ RTf
or
Androgen deprivation therapyh

PSA detectable and rising on 2 or more subsequent determinations

See Systemic Therapy (PROS-7)

Distant metastases →
Androgen deprivation therapyh
or
Observation

f See Principles of Radiation Therapy (PROS-D).
h See Principles of Hormonal Therapy (PROS-F).

Note: All recommendations are category 2A unless otherwise indicated.
Clinical Trials: NCCN believes that the best management of any cancer patient is in a clinical trial. Participation in clinical trials is especially encouraged.

PROS-5

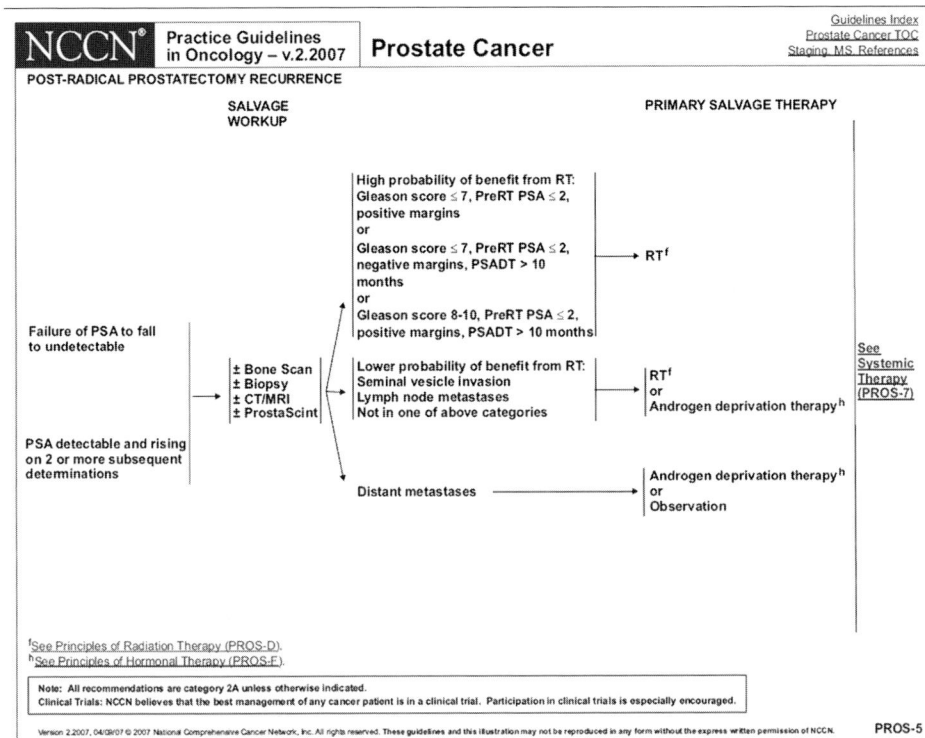

Figure 12.2. PROS-5 NCCN Practice Guidelines in Oncology for Prostate Cancer v2.2007: Reprinted from online publication available at: http://www.nccn.org/professionals/physician_gls/default.asp.

majority of patients comprise a heterogeneous population with suspected local recurrence with no clear evidence of either local recurrence or distant metastases; an elevated PSA will be the only evidence of tumor progression in up to two-thirds of patients with biochemical relapse after RP [18]. Amongst this group, patients who have a high probability of benefiting from SRT are those with no pre-surgical or surgical evidence of seminal vesicle or lymph node involvement and three of the four following favorable predictors: Gleason score ≤7, pre-RT PSA ≤2.0 ng/ml, positive surgical margins, and post-surgical PSA doubling time >10 months. Patients not meeting these criteria have a lower probability of benefiting from SRT and can be treated with either SRT or systemic therapy [4, 11].

A local recurrence is more likely to be confirmed with biopsy when abnormal soft tissue in the post-RP bed is detected with either DRE or imaging [11]. Imaging modalities that can aid in the detection, progression monitoring, and SRT planning of post-RP recurrence include TRUS, MRI, and nuclear medicine methods.

Evaluation for metastatic recurrent prostate cancer

Even when a local recurrence is identified, there may also be concurrent metastatic disease. Therefore, metastases must always be ruled out before local curative therapy is considered.

The most common presentations of metastatic disease in PCa are nodal and osseous metastases. The regional lymphatic drainage of the prostate accompanies the veins, and passes primarily to obturator, internal iliac, external iliac, common iliac, and presacral lymph nodes [19]. Computed tomography is commonly considered the imaging modality of choice for detecting lymphadenopathy in PCa patients; however, conventional MRI is comparable to CT in detecting lymphadenopathy. Enlarged lymph nodes are readily detected on non-contrast-enhanced T_1-weighted images. Lymphadenopathy is classically defined as the presence of one or more nodes with a short axis diameter greater than 1 cm. This size criterion has limited value for detection of positive nodal disease, as nodal enlargement due to metastases occurs relatively late in the progression of PCa, usually when the PSA level is high (>20 ng/ml), or rising rapidly (>2 ng/ml per month) [2]. Since nodal metastases are often microscopic, neither CT nor conventional MRI can be used to reliably rule them out. Reported CT sensitivity for the detection of lymph node metastases varies, ranging from 25% to 78%, with a specificity ranging from 77% to 98% [20, 21, 22]. One study found a sensitivity of 78% and a specificity of 97% when the size criterion was reduced to 0.6 cm [23], but this smaller size limit has not been widely adopted. The use of MRI with ultrasmall superparamagnetic iron oxide nanoparticles (USPIO) is showing promise in improving the detection of lymphadenopathy. These nanoparticles are injected intravenously 24 h before MRI scanning. They slowly extravasate from the blood vessels to the interstitial space and are transported via the lymphatics to lymph nodes, where they are taken up by normal macrophages and cause a signal drop on a T_2^*-weighted sequence. In metastatic lymph nodes, the normal macrophages are replaced by metastatic cells that do not take up the USPIO, and therefore the T_2^*-weighted signal drop does not occur [24]. Utilizing this experimental technique, PCa lymph node metastases as small as 3 mm can be detected, and reported sensitivity and specificity exceed 90% [24]. Additionally, benign reactive enlarged lymph nodes can be differentiated from metastatic ones.

Prostate cancer metastases most commonly present in the bones, usually in the axial skeleton. Approximately 65%–75% of patients with metastatic PCa will have osseous metastases. The risk of having osseous metastases correlates with PSA elevation, both at diagnosis and after treatment. The Tc bone scan is considered the standard method for detecting osseous metastases. In pre-treatment PCa, the bone scan is rarely positive until PSA levels are high, around 30 ng/ml [16]. In patients treated with RT or RP, the incidence of positive bone scans was only 0.2%–1.4% at PSA levels below 5 ng/ml [25]. Some studies suggest that MRI may be superior to Tc bone scan in demonstrating metastases in the axial skeleton, and should be used as a supplementary form of imaging in questionable cases [26, 27]. One recent study found that MRI of the axial skeleton had higher sensitivity and specificity (100% and 88%) than Tc bone scan (46% and 32%) for detecting osseous metastases in patients with high-risk PCa and that routine screening with MRI might eventually prove to be more cost-effective [28]. Osseous metastases from PCa may be osteoblastic, osteolytic, or both, but the majority are purely osteoblastic. Therefore, they appear as low-signal-intensity lesions on both T_1- and T_2-weighted MRI (Figure 12.3). Both Tc bone scanning and MRI are superior to CT in diagnosing bone metastases.

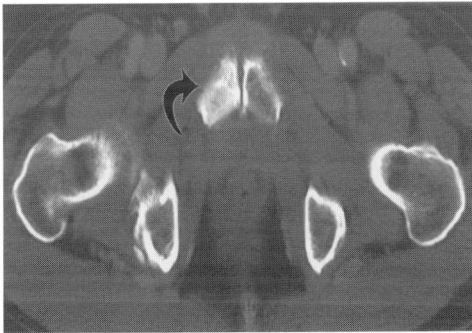

(a)

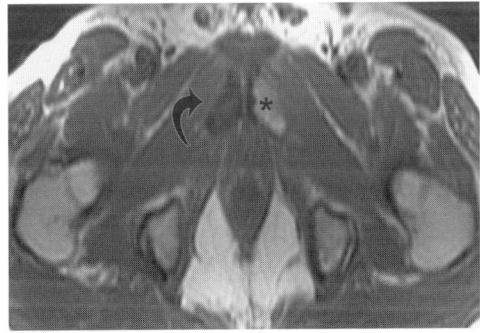

(b)

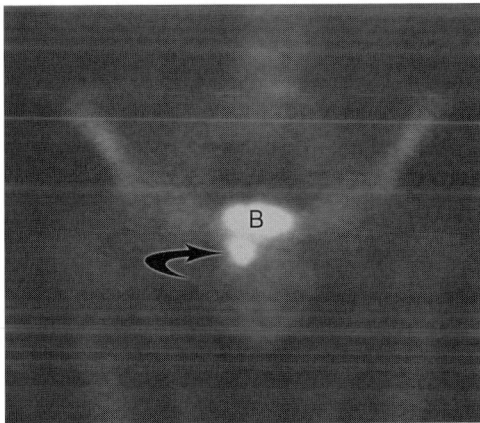

(c)

Figure 12.3. Bone metastasis of prostate cancer (PCa) on computed tomography (CT), magnetic resonance imaging (MRI), and technetium (T_c) bone scan. Axial CT (a) shows a sclerotic lesion (arrow) in the right side of the pubic symphysis, consistent with an osteoblastic metastasis of PCa. The same lesion (arrow) is shown on an axial T_1-weighted image (b). Normal bone marrow has a high signal intensity (SI) on T_1-weighted images due to fat content, as demonstrated in the left side of the pubic symphysis (*). In a sclerotic metastasis, the normal fatty content is replaced with calcified tissue, resulting in decreased SI (arrow). An anterior coronal projection of the corresponding T_c bone scan (c) shows increased tracer uptake in the right pubic symphysis (arrow), confirming a metastasis. Metastases in this location may sometimes be obscured on bone scan by the excreted tracer found in the bladder (B) on coronal projections.

Detection of nodal and osseous metastases is also possible with a growing array of nuclear medicine studies (see Chapter 11).

Imaging of local recurrence after radiation therapy

Digital rectal examination, transrectal ultrasound (TRUS), and TRUS-guided biopsy

Early detection and treatment of local recurrence is of paramount importance for a favorable outcome. Despite up to 70% of men with PSA relapse after RT having no evidence of metastasis [29] and promising disease control rates with SRP (about 50% freedom from PSA relapse at 5 years and 75% disease-specific survival at 10 years) [8], SRP is infrequently utilized because of difficulties in the detection of local recurrence with DRE, TRUS and TRUS-guided biopsy [30, 31, 32] and because it is associated with more adverse effects than primary RP [8]. Although PCa can be detected as a hypoechoic nodule on gray-scale TRUS, the accuracy of TRUS (49% sensitivity, 57% specificity) is not superior to that of DRE (73% sensitivity, 66% specificity) in predicting a positive post-RT biopsy [32]. At present, TRUS is primarily used to guide systematic sextant biopsy, with the option to obtain additional samples from regions that look suspicious on TRUS [2]. A false-negative rate of 20% is reported for first biopsy attempts in patients systematically followed-up with post-RT prostate biopsies [31]. Additionally, insufficient knowledge of the time required for tumor to become non-viable after radiation can complicate the interpretation of positive biopsies [30, 31]. It is, however, recommended that salvage therapy be considered for patients with rising PSA if viable tumor (without significant treatment effect) is detected on biopsy 2 years after RT [8]. Even when DRE, TRUS, and sextant biopsy do detect local recurrence in patients with PSA relapse, they typically underestimate the disease burden [33], creating uncertainty in salvage therapy planning and potentially limiting its success. In the detection of post-RT local recurrence, the utility of multi-parametric additions to conventional gray-scale TRUS, such as color and power Doppler or intravascular microbubble agents, has not been assessed.

Prostate magnetic resonance imaging

A conventional prostate MRI is essentially a pelvic MRI optimized for detection of PCa. On a 1.5-T scanner, images are usually acquired with a combination of an external phased-array coil and an endorectal coil [2]. High-resolution (3-mm slice thickness) axial, coronal, and sagittal T_2-weighted images of the prostate and seminal vesicles are utilized to detect PCa. In an untreated prostate gland, PCa appears as a nodule of low signal intensity (SI) contrasting with the surrounding high-SI healthy prostate glandular tissue. This is presumed to be due to hypercellularity in the PCa contrasting with the fluid-filled lumina of acini in healthy prostate tissue [34]. T_1-weighted images obtained from the aortic bifurcation to the symphysis pubis (5-mm slice thickness) do not provide sufficient soft-tissue contrast to detect PCa but are used to detect post-biopsy hemorrhage that can mimic PCa on T_2-weighted images, and to detect pelvic lymph node involvement and bone metastases [2, 17]. At present, prostate MRI is considered the most accurate imaging method for cancer detection and local staging in the untreated prostate [2, 35].

Post-RT changes in the pelvis visible on MRI were initially described in the late 1980s [36, 37]. Post-RT changes and toxic effects were more likely to present on MRI when the dose was above 45 Gy, and were described in the bladder, anorectum, perivesical fat, perirectal fascia, presacral space, uterus, prostate, pelvic side wall muscles, and bone marrow of the sacral spine [36, 37] (Table 12.2, Figure 12.4). Changes in the prostate gland following RT are presumably caused by RT-induced glandular atrophy and fibrosis and result in a decrease in prostate size, diffusely decreased T_2-weighted SI in the prostate gland and seminal vesicles, and decreased differentiation between the peripheral and transition zones [37, 38] (Figures 12.4, 12.5, 12.6, 12.7). Since these early studies were completed, radiation dosages have changed. Modern RT uses much higher doses (typically 80–85 Gy for EBRT, 145 Gy for ^{125}iodine and 125 Gy for ^{103}palladium brachytherapy) with dose modulation to limit the toxicity to the bladder, urethra, and rectum [4]. More recent studies describe brachytherapy-induced intraprostatic changes on MRI in all patients, and radiation changes to the levator ani muscle and urogenital diaphragm in the majority of patients, but no correlation between post-brachytherapy urinary symptoms and changes on MRI in the periurethral tissue or urogenital diaphragm [38]. Further investigation is necessary to determine if RT-induced changes in radiosensitive structures around the prostate can predict toxicity in modern RT of the prostate.

For a long time, prostate MRI was presumed to be of limited value for PCa detection after RT due to an assumption that a diffuse reduction in T_2-weighted SI in benign irradiated prostate tissue would mask a focal reduction in T_2-weighted SI in PCa. However, recent studies have shown that the decrease in T_2-weighted SI of PCa is great enough to allow detection of PCa nodules by experienced radiologists, who accurately predicted the location of PCa on sextant biopsy [39, 40] or on

Table 12.2. Post-radiation therapy changes and toxicities in the pelvis

Anatomic part	Post-radiation therapy changes and toxicities
Bladder	Wall thickness >5 mm, high T_2-weighted SI of the outer wall, fistulas and sinus tracts
Anorectum	Wall thickness >6 mm, high T_2-weighted SI of the outer muscle layer, outer muscle layer indistinguishable from submucosa, fistulas and sinus tracts
Perirectal fascia	Increased width >3 mm at S4–S5 level
Presacral space	Increased width >15 mm at S4–S5 level
Uterus	Decrease in uterine size, decreased T_2-weighted SI of the myometrium, decreased thickness and T_2-weighted SI of the endometrium, loss of uterine zonal anatomy
Prostate	Decrease in prostate size, diffusely decreased T_2-weighted SI in prostate and seminal vesicles, decreased differentiation between peripheral and transitional zone
Perivesical fat	Decreased non-homogenous T_1-weighted SI
Pelvic sidewall muscles	Increased T_2-weighted SI
Bone marrow of sacral spine	Increased T_1-weighted SI

Source: Modified from article by Sugimura *et al.* [37].
Abbreviation: SI, signal intensity.

post-SRP pathology step-sections [34, 41] (Table 12.3, Figures 12.4, 12.5, 12.6, 12.7). In a study on sextant tumor localization by imaging that used whole-mount post-SRP step-section pathology as the reference standard, T_2-weighted MRI and MRSI, which detects cancer based on elevation of the PCa marker choline and reduction of the healthy tissue marker citrate, had higher sensitivities than TRUS-guided sextant biopsy and DRE (68% and 78% vs. 48% and 16%, respectively). Due to RT-induced cancer-like metabolic changes in the benign gland, MRSI was less specific (78%) than the other three tests, which each had a specificity above 90% [34] (Table 12.3). Another study showed the utility of T_2-weighted MRI for re-staging recurrent PCa before SRP [41] (Table 12.3). Some studies also demonstrated that adding MRSI or dynamic contrast-enhanced MRI (DCE MRI), which detects early nodular enhancement and early washout of gadolinium contrast in PCa, could further improve the detection of recurrence after RT [39, 40, 41, 42] (Table 12.3, Figure 12.6). However, MRSI and DCE MRI for post-RT recurrent PCa are still experimental techniques requiring the use of specialized acquisition

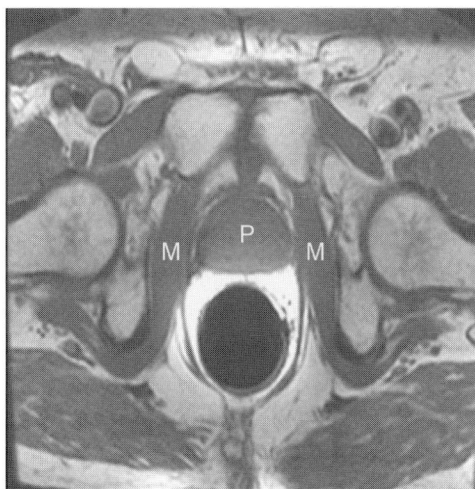

(a)

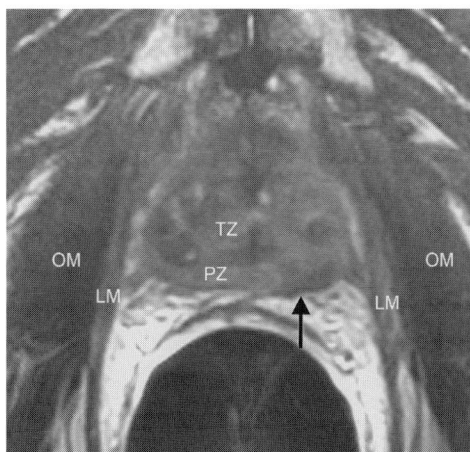

(b)

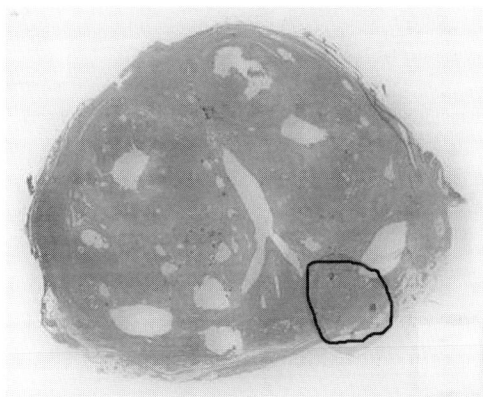

(c)

Figure 12.4. Radiation-therapy-induced changes and tumor detection after external beam radiation therapy (EBRT). A 73-year-old patient with local recurrence after EBRT. (a) Transverse T_1-weighted MR image at the level of prostate midgland (P). All visualized osseous structures display high marrow signal intensity (SI) consistent with the effect of radiation. The prostate has uniform SI similar to adjacent muscles (M). This is a typical appearance of both untreated and treated prostate on T_1-weighted images that do not have the soft-tissue contrast necessary to identify prostate zonal anatomy or detect PCa. No regions of high SI are identified within the prostate to suggest hemorrhage. (b) Transverse T_2-weighted MR image at the level of prostate midgland. RT-induced increase in T_2-weighted SI is severe in the levator muscles (LM) and mild in the obturator muscles (OM). Diffusely decreased T_2-weighted signal and decreased differentiation between peripheral (PZ) and transition zone (TZ) represent RT changes in the prostate. However, PCa can be still identified as a focal nodular region of even more reduced SI in the left PZ (arrow). (c) Pathologic axial slice corresponding to T_2-weighted MRI image. The tumor is located in the region identified as suspicious on MRI. See color plate section for full color version of part (c).

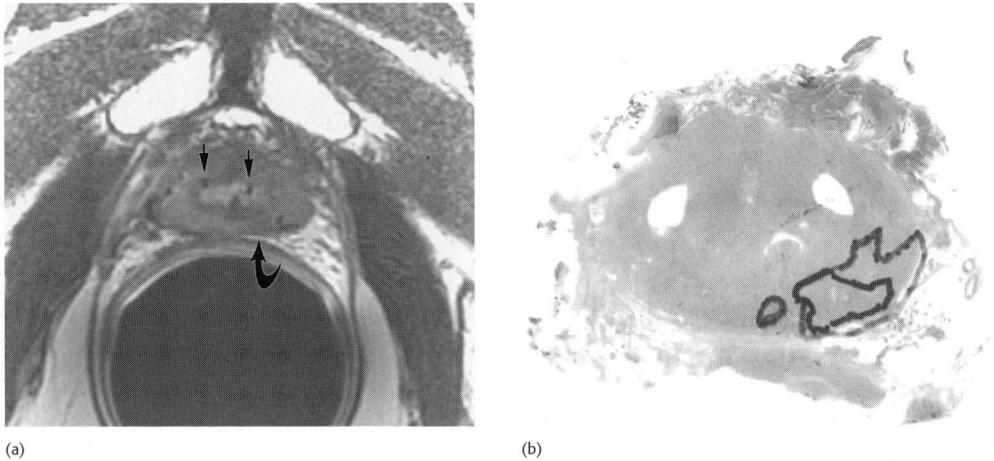

(a)   (b)

Figure 12.5. Detection of subtle tumor after brachytherapy – a value of multiplanar imaging.
A 67-year-old patient with local recurrence after brachytherapy. (a) Transverse T_2-weighted image at the
level of prostate midgland shows scattered small SI voids corresponding to brachytherapy seeds
(short arrows) and prominent RT-induced changes in the prostate that has diffusely decreased SI. A very
subtle region indicative of possible tumor is seen on the left side (curved arrow). (b) Pathologic axial
slice demonstrates a tumor corresponding to the suspicious imaging findings. See color plate section for
full color version of part (b).

and processing software and are performed only in selected research-orientated
institutions [2].

In 2002, a study that compared pre-RT and post-RT DRE and TRUS, without
reported pathologic confirmation, suggested that post-RT recurrence usually originates from the primary tumor [43]. A recent study that compared T_2-weighted
pre-RT and post-RT MRI images with post-SRP pathology confirmed this observation
[44] (Figure 12.7). These two studies support the emerging therapeutic approach of
boosting the radiation dose within the primary tumor using imaging guidance [45].
Furthermore, awareness that most recurrences occur at the site of the primary tumor,
and that extracapsular extension and seminal vesicle invasion are most likely to
originate from that site might aid in post-RT tumor detection and re-staging. The
second study found that T_2-weighted MRI had limited precision in tumor volume
estimation, with the ratios between tumor volumes on step-section pathology and
post-RT MRI ranging between 0.52 and 2.80 [44]. This suggests that generous
treatment margins should be planned if focal salvage therapy for tumor recurrence
is attempted in the future. Currently, the alternatives to SRP, such as cryotherapy or
HIFU, generally treat the entire prostate gland [12, 13].

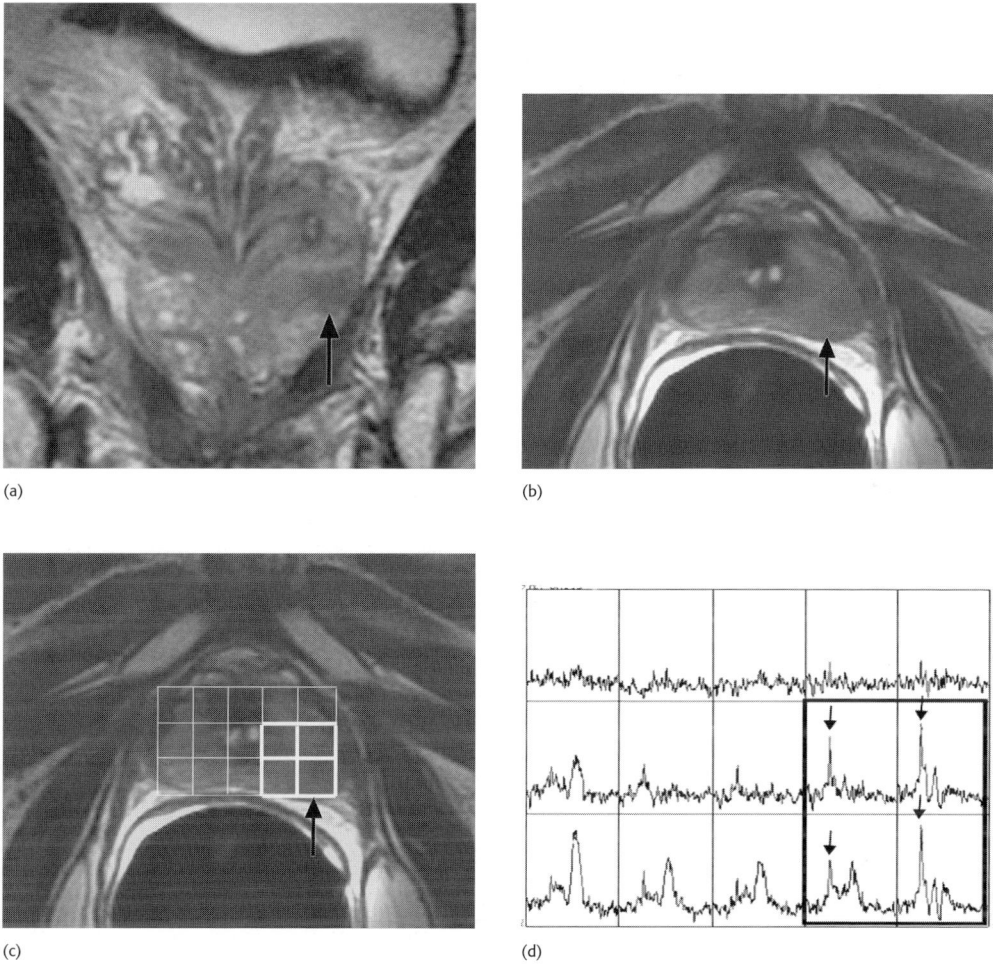

(a)

(b)

(c)

(d)

Figure 12.6. Multiplanar and multiparametric tumor detection after EBRT. A 70-year-old man with rising PSA following ERBT. Decreased SI suspicious for tumor is noted in the left midgland on coronal (a) and axial (b) T_2-weighted images (arrows). Grid overlay on axial image (c) corresponds to proton MR spectral array (d). On MRSI the tumor is detected based on elevated choline peaks (black arrows) in the left PZ voxels; the low-level scattered residual choline in the voxels on the right side is non-specific (d). MRSI was obtained using commercially available acquisition and processing software from GE Medical Systems that utilizes the point resolved spectroscopy (PRESS) voxel excitation technique, with an in-plane spatial resolution of 6.9 mm, spectral-spatial pulses for water and lipid suppression within the PRESS-selected volume, and very selective outer voxel suppression pulses to reduce contamination from surrounding tissues. MRSI is an experimental technique without universally excepted criteria for tumor detection after RT.

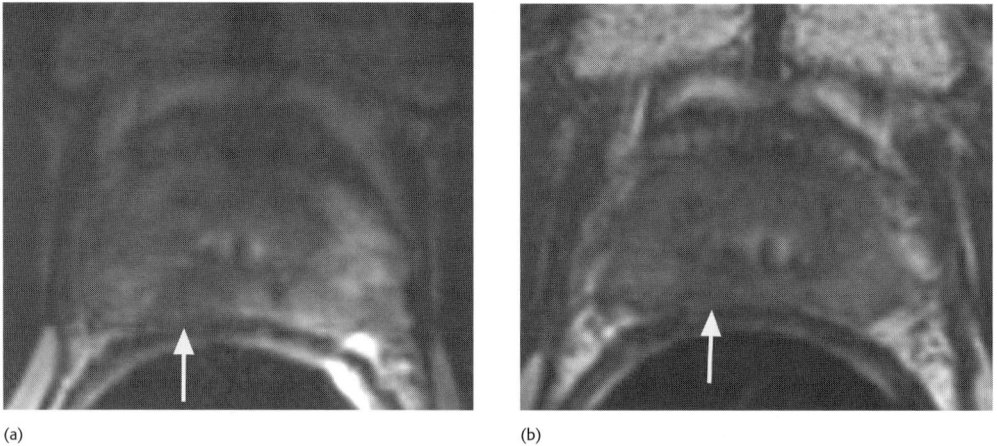

(a)   (b)

Figure 12.7. Modified from article by Pucar D *et al.*, *Int J Radiat Oncol Biol Phys*, 69 (2007), 62–69 [44]. Prostate cancer local recurrence after EBRT at the site of primary tumor. Corresponding axial pre-RT (a) and post-RT (b) T_2-weighted MRI images in a patient with post-EBRT local recurrence. The tumor is strikingly similar in location and appearance on pre-RT MRI, and post-RT MRI. Location of the tumor was confirmed on step-section pathology obtained at salvage radical prostatectomy.

It seems plausible that monitoring the primary tumor site with MRI after RT could lead to earlier detection of recurrence than is possible with PSA measurements. However, this hypothesis has not been tested, and, at present, MRI is neither recommended nor reimbursed for post-RT follow-up in the absence of rising PSA values [2, 4]. This may be partly due to post-RT changes interfering with the interpretation of imaging examinations, if performed in proximity to treatment. A study that followed low-risk post-RT patients (Gleason score ≤ 6, PSA ≤ 10 ng/ml) with serial MRSI examinations found that the median times to resolution of radiation-induced spectroscopic abnormalities were 32.2 months after EBRT and 24.8 months following brachytherapy; however, no cases of recurrent PCa were reported in this study [46].

In summary, the addition of MRI to DRE and TRUS-guided biopsy permits evaluation for pelvic osseous metastases and lymphadenopathy and could potentially aid in the detection and re-staging of post-RT local recurrence.

Imaging of local recurrence after radical prostatectomy

TRUS- and DRE-guided biopsies

Transrectal ultrasound is the most available and most commonly performed imaging technique used in post-RP patients with suspected recurrence. The description

Table 12.3. Prostate MRI in detection of post-RT local recurrence

	Number of patients	Number of readers	Parameter	Units of analysis	Test	Sensitivity (%)[c]	Specificity (%)[c]	Accuracy (AUC)[c]
Studies with post-SRP step-section pathology as the standard of reference								
Pucar et al. [34]	9	1 radiologist	Tumor location for all tests	6 PZ sextants for all tests	T_2-weighted MRI[a]	68	96	–
	9	1 spectroscopist			MRSI[a]	77	78	–
	8	NA			Systematic biopsy	45	95	–
	9	NA			DRE	16	96	–
Sala et al. [41]	45 for all parameters	2 radiologists read all parameters	Tumor location	4 quadrants	T_2-weighted MRI[a] for all parameters	76 or 58[d]	73 or 81[d]	0.75[d]
						55 or 36[d]	65 or 81[d]	0.61[d]
			ECE	4 quadrants		86 or 64[d]	84 or 91[d]	0.87[d]
						64 or 39[d]	76 or 86[d]	0.76[d]
			SVI	2 sides		58 or 53[d]	96 or 96[d]	0.76[d]
						42 or 32[d]	96 or 96[d]	0.70[d]
Studies with TRUS-guided systematic biopsy as the standard of reference								
Coakley et al. [42]	21 for both tests	2 radiologists	Tumor location for both tests	2 PZ sides for both tests	T_2-weighted MRI[a]	–	–	0.49
						–	–	0.51
		1 spectroscopist			MRSI[a]	89	82	0.81
Rouviere et al. [40]	22 for both tests	3 radiologists read both tests	Tumor location for both tests	10 sectors (6 PZ sextants, 2 TZ sides, 2 SV sides) for both tests	T_2-weighted MRI[b]	26	86	0.60
						42	64	0.54
						44	80	0.64

Table 12.3. (cont.)

Number of patients	Number of readers	Parameter	Units of analysis	Test	Sensitivity (%)[c]	Specificity (%)[c]	Accuracy (AUC)[c]
				DCE MRI[b]	70	85	0.79
					74	73	0.73
					74	74	0.74
Haider et al. [39]	1 radiologist read both tests	Tumor location for both tests	6 sextants for both tests	T$_2$-weighted MRI[b]	38	80	0.74
33 for both tests				DCE MRI[b]	72	85	0.83

[a] With endorectal coil.

[b] Without endorectal coil.

[c] In studies where the same test is read by multiple readers, the sensitivity, specificity, and accuracy for each reader are given in a separate row.

[d] Two cutoffs are used, the first and second values represent sensitivity or specificity for more sensitive/less specific and less sensitive/more specific cutoffs, respectively.

Abbreviations: DRE, digital rectal examination; ECE, extracapsular extension; PZ, peripheral zone; SV, seminal vesicle; TZ, transition zone; SVI, seminal vesicle invasion; SRP, Salvage radical prostatectomy; AUC, area under the curve; MRI, magnetic resonance imaging; MRSI, magnetic resonance spectroscopic imaging; TRUS, transrectal ultrasound; DCE dynamic contrast-enhanced.

of normal versus pathologic features of the vesicourethral anastomosis (VUA) following prostatectomy [47, 48] has enabled this modality to play a significant role for the post-RP patient, detecting sites suspicious for local recurrence and directing biopsies. The sensitivity of TRUS-guided biopsies (66%–75%) is greater than that of DRE-guided biopsies (29%–50%) in the post-RP patient [49, 50, 51] and increases with higher PSA levels at the time of recurrence [52]. Thus, only 25% of patients with PSA <1 ng/ml had TRUS-guided biopsy-proven recurrence, compared to 53% of patients with PSA levels >2 ng/ml [51]. Similarly, the positive predictive value of TRUS-guided biopsy has also been shown to improve with increasing PSA levels [49, 51, 52]. However, the negative predictive value is independent of size, reported as only 67% for TRUS-guided biopsies even in patients with PSA >2 ng/ml [51], likely due to the influence of sampling error at biopsy. The specificity of TRUS-guided biopsies (67%–86%) is lower than that of DRE-guided biopsies (76%–100%); this may be due to postoperative changes seen on TRUS being mistaken for recurrence [51, 53, 54].

More recent advances in TRUS of post-RP patients include the use of color and power Doppler to detect vascularity. Both of these techniques have been shown to improve sensitivity, specificity, positive predictive value, and negative predictive value (86%–93%, 100%, 100%, 75%–82%, respectively) [53, 54]. The use of experimental intravascular microbubble contrast agents in TRUS of post-RP patients may have the potential to further improve the utility of this modality for detecting local recurrences and differentiating them from postoperative changes. A single novel study reports contrast-enhanced color Doppler TRUS detection of 10/10 biopsy-proven local recurrences, a detection rate comparable to that of contrast-enhanced MRI [55].

Pelvic magnetic resonance imaging
Since PSA is secreted only by prostatic tissue, detectable PSA following RP may be attributed to residual benign prostatic tissue, local recurrence of PCa or metastatic disease [56, 57]. With its superior soft-tissue resolution, MRI is the most accurate imaging modality for depicting the first two possibilities. Additionally, routine MRI protocols for the post-RP patient include sequences that can evaluate for pelvic lymphadenopathy and pelvic osseous metastases, the most common sites of early metastasis. Thus, pelvic MRI may be regarded as a single examination for evaluating the post-RP patient with biochemical relapse. For reasons discussed above, the use of endorectal MRI is currently limited to select centers.

The conventional MRI protocol for post-RP patients is similar to that described above for post-RT patients and is described elsewhere [58]. The combination of an external and an endorectal coil improves the detection of local recurrence of PCa [59]. Magnetic resonance imaging has the ability to cover the entire post-prostatectomy fossa and detect recurrences that are located beyond the region routinely imaged on TRUS. Transrectal ultrasound readily depicts the peri-anastomotic and retrovesicle regions; however, it has been reported that 30% of MRI-depicted recurrences lie beyond these locations, within retained tips of seminal vesicles or at the anterior or lateral surgical margins [58]. Because of the anatomic detail and wide coverage of the pelvis that MRI provides, it is increasingly used in directing salvage RT when a recurrence is depicted [60].

The reported sensitivity and the specificity of MRI for depicting local recurrences are 95%–100% and 100%, respectively [58, 61]. To interpret post-RP MRI studies accurately, it is necessary to become familiar with the normal appearance of the post-prostatectomy fossa, as well as potential pitfalls. Recurrent PCa presents as a lobulated mass with intermediate SI on T_1-weighted images, similar to that of adjacent pelvic muscles, and intermediate SI on T_2-weighted images, slightly higher than that of muscle (Figure 12.8). When intravenous contrast is administered, PCa recurrence enhances [61], though the use of DCE MRI studies for detecting local recurrence following RP is still under investigation. The intermediate SI on T_2-weighted images is key to differentiating a local recurrence of PCa from post-surgical fibrosis, which demonstrates low T_2-weighted signal intensity [58, 61].

Changes in the post-RP fossa on MRI that may mimic local recurrence include post-surgical fibrosis, residual prostatic tissue, retained seminal vesicles, and peri-urethral injections of collagen used for post-surgical urinary incontinence [62] (Table 12.4, Figure 12.9). Prostatic tissue may be left behind unintentionally after surgery, most commonly in the apical region. Alternatively, prostatic tissue may be left behind intentionally, being spared along with an adjacent pelvic structure with the goal of maintaining continence or potency (i.e., in bladder-neck-sparing RP). Benign prostatic tissue has been documented in up to 15% of TRUS-guided biopsies of post-RP patients [56]. Residual prostatic tissue may complicate the monitoring of PSA following RP, as well as be confusing on DRE and imaging. Rarely, retained prostatic tissue could be a sight of retained or recurrent cancer (Figure 12.10). Completely or partially retained seminal vesicles are another recognized post-RP finding which may be confusing on follow-up. Though they do not secrete PSA, and are not responsible for biochemical failure, retained seminal vesicles may be mistaken for recurrence on DRE, TRUS, or CT. Magnetic resonance imaging often has the ability to distinguish retained seminal vesicles from local recurrence, especially if they are intact and fluid filled (Figure 12.11) [63].

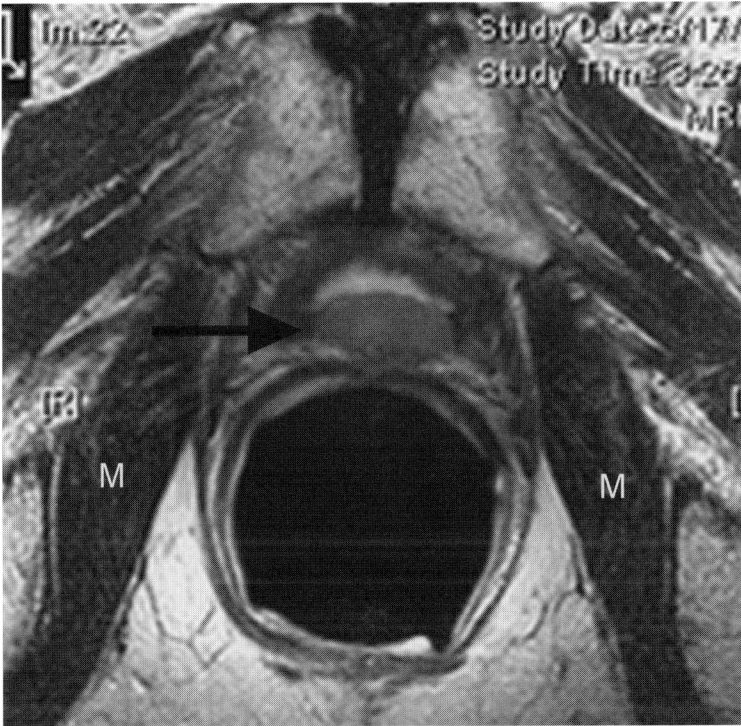

Figure 12.8. Local recurrence after radical prostatectomy detected by MRI. Axial T$_2$-weighted MR image shows a local recurrence in the prostatectomy bed in the retrovesicle region (arrow). The signal intensity (SI) of the recurrent tumor is higher than that of adjacent pelvic muscles (M) on T$_2$-weighted images. The increased SI and mass-like configuration distinguish this recurrence from post-surgical fibrosis in the surgical bed.

Advanced MRI techniques, including MR spectroscopy and DCE MRI, have not yet been systematically evaluated for detection of post-RP recurrence.

Nuclear medicine imaging for local recurrence

The main role of nuclear medicine in patients with suspected PCa recurrence is in the evaluation for metastatic disease (discussed in detail in Chapter 11). However, a variety of nuclear medicine techniques are currently being evaluated for detection of local recurrence in post-RP patients. These studies use combined PET/CT and various radiotracers. ^{18}F-FDG, the most common radiotracer used in cancer imaging, has shown low sensitivity and specificity in the past [64]; however, using newer generations of PET scanners with higher spatial resolution, ^{18}F-FDG can detect local disease in selected patients [65]. New, experimental radiotracers, including [^{11}C] or [^{18}F]choline, [^{11}C] or [^{18}F]acetate or [^{18}F] FACBC, appear

Table 12.4. Magnetic resonance characteristics of pelvic findings which may mimic a local recurrence of prostate cancer in a post-RP patient

	T2W SI [a]	T1W SI [a]	Enhancement with IV contrast	Characteristic features
Local recurrence	Intermediate	Intermediate	Yes	Lobulated mass
	Hyperintense to muscle	Isointense to muscle		Adjacent to surgical clips
Post-surgical fibrosis	Low	Intermediate	No	Abundant at the anastomosis
	Isointense to muscle	Isointense to muscle		
Retained prostatic tissue	High for PZ tissue	Intermediate	Yes	May show PZ and TZ differentiation
	Hyperintense to muscle	Isointense to muscle		
Injected periurethral collagen	Intermediate	Intermediate	No	Bilateral symmetrical
	Hyperintense to muscle	Isointense to muscle		Regular borders
Retained seminal vesicles	High (if not fibrotic)	Intermediate	Yes	Convoluted shape
	Hyperintense to muscle	Isointense to muscle		Fluid filled (SI like bladder) – if not fibrotic

[a] Signal intensity relative to the adjacent pelvic muscles.
Abbreviations: SI, signal intensity; PZ, peripheral zone; TZ, transition zone; T1W, T_1-weighted; T2W, T_2-weighted.

more promising for the detection of both local and metastatic recurrent PCa [66, 67, 68, 69]. Monoclonal antibody imaging with the prostate-specific membrane antigen (PSMA) antibody ^{111}In-capromab pendetide (ProstaScint®) is controversial. It demonstrates low sensitivity for detecting local recurrences and bone metastases [70]; therefore, we believe that it has no added benefit over other imaging modalities in evaluating post-RP recurrence. A new antibody, J591, which is directed against the extracellular domain of PSMA, is currently undergoing experimental investigation and appears more promising [70].

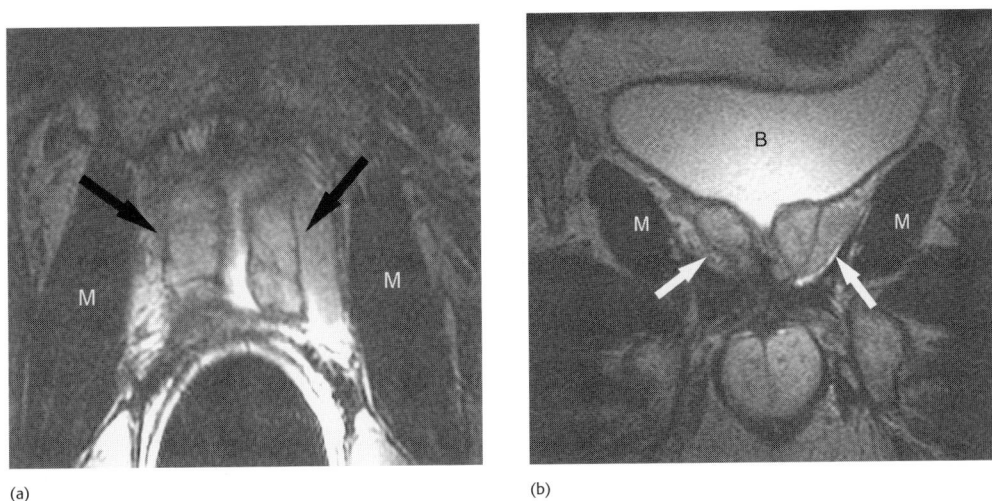

(a)   (b)

Figure 12.9. Injected collagen for post-surgical incontinence depicted on MRI. Axial (a) and coronal (b) T_2-weighted images of a post-prostatectomy patient who had periurethral collagen injection for incontinence. Compared to adjacent pelvic muscles (M) the injected collagen (arrows) has increased signal intensity, which may be similar to the signal intensity of a local recurrence; however, the regular shape, location, and symmetry of the collagen on both sides of the urethra help distinguish it from recurrent tumor. B, urinary bladder.

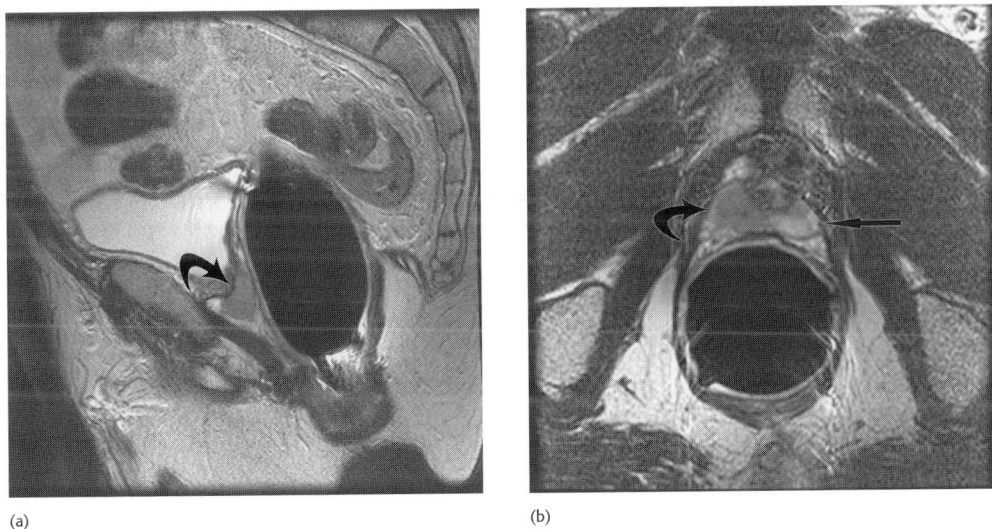

(a)   (b)

Figure 12.10. Retained prostatic tissue with recurrent tumor depicted on MRI. Retained apical prostatic tissue is noted on sagittal (a) and axial (b) T_2-weighted MR images in this patient 1 year following radical retropubic prostatectomy with rising PSA levels. The MR appearance resembles that of the apex of the prostate gland in a patient who has not undergone surgery. On the axial image (b) normal peripheral zone tissue with high signal intensity is seen on the left (straight arrow), while low-signal-intensity residual or recurrent tumor is seen on the right (curved arrow). The left side of the residual prostatic apex, with tumor (curved arrow), is depicted on the sagittal image.

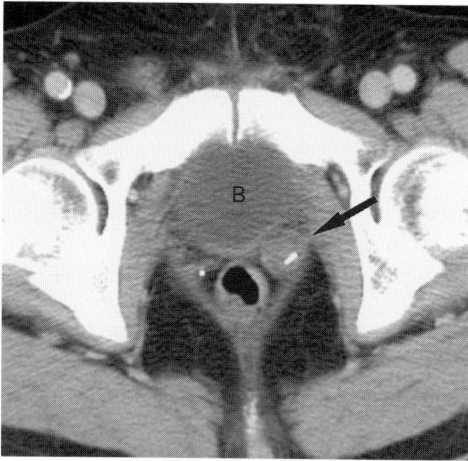

(a)

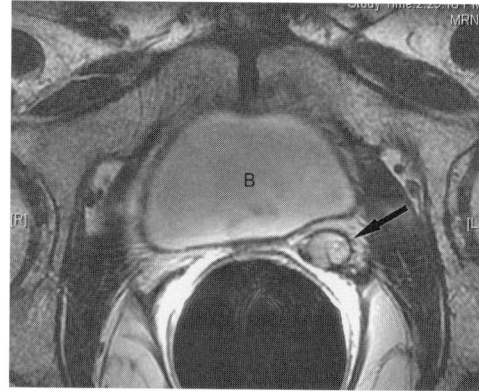

(b)

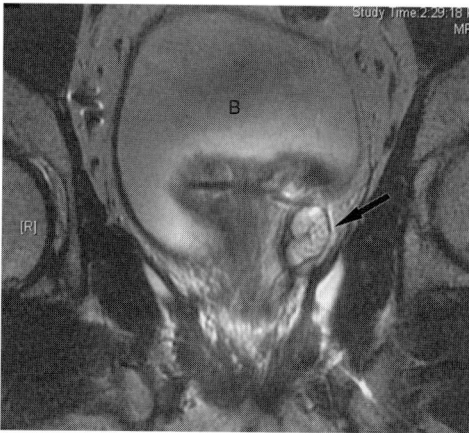

(c)

Figure 12.11. Retained seminal vesicle mistaken for local recurrence on CT. Axial CT image shows a round soft-tissue mass (arrow) in the left retrovesicle location, adjacent to surgical clips, in a post-RRP patient. The PSA level was not elevated; however, on digital rectal exam (DRE) a palpable nodule was noted in the same position. Based on the DRE and CT findings, local recurrence was suspected, and an MRI was performed to confirm this. Axial (b) and coronal (c) T_2-weighted MR images show the abnormality to be a retained left seminal vesicle (arrow). The seminal vesicle has a convoluted appearance and is filled with fluid content with high signal intensity, similar to that of the contents of the urinary bladder (B). This appearance is the same as the characteristic MR appearance of normal seminal vesicles in patients who have not undergone any treatment.

Conclusion

With systemic therapies for recurrent PCa being non-curative, the identification of patients with isolated local recurrence amenable to salvage treatment is critical. The addition of conventional T_1- and T_2-weighted and experimental MRI sequences to DRE and TRUS-guided biopsy may improve the detection of recurrent PCa and the planning of salvage treatment. Therefore, we recommend the use of prostate MRI if a radiologist experienced in its interpretation is available.

ACKNOWLEDGMENT

The authors thank Ada Muellner, BA, for editing the manuscript.

REFERENCES

1. I. M. Thompson, D. P. Ankerst, Prostate-specific antigen in the early detection of prostate cancer. *CMAJ*, **176**:13 (2007), 1853–8.
2. H. Hricak, P. L. Choyke, S. C. Eberhardt, *et al.*, Imaging prostate cancer: a multidisciplinary perspective. *Radiology*, **243**:1 (2007), 28–53.
3. J. I. Epstein, W. C. Allsbrook, Jr., M. B. Amin, *et al.*, Update on the Gleason grading system for prostate cancer: results of an international consensus conference of urologic pathologists. *Adv Anat Pathol*, **1** (2006), 57–9.
4. J. Mohler, R. J. Babaian, R. R. Bahnson, NCCN Clinical Practice Guidelines in Oncology – Prostate Cancer, v 1.2008. 2008.
5. A. W. Partin, L. A. Mangold, D. M. Lamm, *et al.*, Contemporary update of prostate cancer staging nomograms (Partin Tables) for the new millennium. *Urology*, **58**:6 (2001), 843–8.
6. American Cancer Society. *Cancer facts and figures 2006*. Atlanta, GA; 2006, Publication No. 500806.
7. C. J. Mettlin, G. P. Murphy, C. J. McDonald, *et al.*, The National Cancer Database Report on increased use of brachytherapy for the treatment of patients with prostate carcinoma in the U.S. *Cancer*, **86**:9 (1999), 1877–82.
8. A. J. Stephenson, J. A. Eastham, Role of salvage radical prostatectomy for recurrent prostate cancer after radiation therapy. *J Clin Oncol* **23**:32 (2005), 8198–203.
9. A. J. Stephenson, P. T. Scardino, J. A. Eastham, *et al.*, Preoperative nomogram predicting the 10-year probability of prostate cancer recurrence after radical prostatectomy. *J Natl Cancer Inst*, **98**:10 (2006), 715–17.
10. M. Roach, 3rd, G. Hanks, H. Thames, Jr., *et al.*, Defining biochemical failure following radiotherapy with or without hormonal therapy in men with clinically localized prostate cancer: recommendations of the RTOG-ASTRO Phoenix Consensus Conference. *Int J Radiat Oncol Biol Phys*, **65**:4 (2006), 965–74.
11. A. J. Stephenson, S. F. Shariat, M. J. Zelefsky, *et al.*, Salvage radiotherapy for recurrent prostate cancer after radical prostatectomy. *JAMA*, **291**:11 (2004), 1325–32.
12. C. Chaussy, S. Thuroff, X. Rebillard, *et al.*, Technology insight: high-intensity focused ultrasound for urologic cancers. *Natl Clin Pract Urol*, **2**:4 (2005), 191–8.
13. N. J. Touma, J. I. Izawa, J. L. Chin, Current status of local salvage therapies following radiation failure for prostate cancer. *J Urol*, **173**:2 (2005), 373–9.
14. G. D. Grossfeld, Y. P. Li, Carroll PR. Patterns of failure after primary local therapy for prostate cancer and rationale for secondary therapy. *Urology*, **60**:3 Suppl. 1 (2002), 57–62; discussion 62–3.
15. D. G. McLeod, Hormonal therapy: historical perspective to future directions. *Urology*, **61**:2 Suppl 1 (2003), 3–7.
16. M. L. Cher, F. J. Bianco, Jr., J. S. Lam, *et al.*, Limited role of radionuclide bone scintigraphy in patients with prostate specific antigen elevations after radical prostatectomy. *J Urol*, **160**:4 (1998), 1387–91.
17. H. Hricak, H. Schoder, D. Pucar, *et al.*, Advances in imaging in the postoperative patient with a rising prostate-specific antigen level. *Semin Oncol*, **30**:5 (2003), 616–34.
18. J. I. Epstein, G. Pizov, P. C. Walsh, Correlation of pathologic findings with progression after radical retropubic prostatectomy. *Cancer*, **71**:11 (1993), 3582–93.
19. R. H. Flocks, D. Culp, R. Porto, Lymphatic spread from prostatic cancer. *J Urol*, **81**:1 (1959), 194–6.

20. J. Rorvik, O. J. Halvorsen, G. Albrektsen, *et al.*, Lymphangiography combined with biopsy and computer tomography to detect lymph node metastases in localized prostate cancer. *Scand J Urol Nephrol*, **32**:2 (1998), 116–19.

21. J. W. Walsh, M. A. Amendola, K. F. Konerding, *et al.*, Computed tomographic detection of pelvic and inguinal lymph-node metastases from primary and recurrent pelvic malignant disease. *Radiology*, **137**:1 Pt 1 (1980), 157–66.

22. J. S. Wolf, Jr., M. Cher, M. Dall'era, *et al.*, The use and accuracy of cross-sectional imaging and fine needle aspiration cytology for detection of pelvic lymph node metastases before radical prostatectomy. *J Urol*, **153**:3 Pt 2 (1995), 993–9.

23. R. H. Oyen, H. P. Van Poppel, F. E. Ameye, *et al.*, Lymph node staging of localized prostatic carcinoma with CT and CT-guided fine-needle aspiration biopsy: prospective study of 285 patients. *Radiology*, **190**:2 (1994), 315–22.

24. J. O. Barentsz, J. J. Futterer, S. Takahashi, Use of ultrasmall superparamagnetic iron oxide in lymph node MR imaging in prostate cancer patients. *Eur J Radiol*, **63**:3 (2007), 369–72.

25. K. S. Warren, G. W. Chodak, W. A. See, *et al.*, Are bone scans necessary in men with low prostate specific antigen levels following localized therapy? *J Urol*, **176**:1 (2006), 70–3; discussion 73–4.

26. G. M. Freedman, W. G. Negendank, G. R. Hudes, *et al.*, Preliminary results of a bone marrow magnetic resonance imaging protocol for patients with high-risk prostate cancer. *Urology*, **54**:1 (1999), 118–23.

27. D. I. Rosenthal, Radiologic diagnosis of bone metastases. *Cancer*, **80**:8 Suppl (1997), 1595–607.

28. F. E. Lecouvet, D. Geukens, A. Stainier, *et al.*, Magnetic resonance imaging of the axial skeleton for detecting bone metastases in patients with high-risk prostate cancer: diagnostic and cost-effectiveness and comparison with current detection strategies. *J Clin Oncol*, **25**:22 (2007), 3281–7.

29. G. K. Zagars, A. Pollack, A. C. von Eschenbach, Prostate cancer and radiation therapy – the message conveyed by serum prostate-specific antigen. *Int J Radiat Oncol Biol Phys*, **33**:1 (1995), 23–35.

30. L. Cheng, J. C. Cheville, D. G. Bostwick, Diagnosis of prostate cancer in needle biopsies after radiation therapy. *Am J Surg Pathol*, **23**:10 (1999), 1173–83.

31. J. Crook, S. Malone, G. Perry, *et al.*, Postradiotherapy prostate biopsies: what do they really mean? Results for 498 patients. *Int J Radiat Oncol Biol Phys*, **48**:2 (2000), 355–67.

32. J. Crook, S. Robertson, G. Collin, *et al.*, Clinical relevance of trans-rectal ultrasound, biopsy, and serum prostate-specific antigen following external beam radiotherapy for carcinoma of the prostate. *Int J Radiat Oncol Biol Phys*, **27**:1 (1993), 31–7.

33. E. Rogers, M. Ohori, V. S. Kassabian, *et al.*, Salvage radical prostatectomy: outcome measured by serum prostate specific antigen levels. *J Urol*, **153**:1 (1995), 104–10.

34. D. Pucar, A. Shukla-Dave, H. Hricak, *et al.*, Prostate cancer: correlation of MR imaging and MR spectroscopy with pathologic findings after radiation therapy-initial experience. *Radiology*, **236**:2 (2005), 545–53.

35. M. Mullerad, H. Hricak, K. Kuroiwa, *et al.*, Comparison of endorectal magnetic resonance imaging, guided prostate biopsy and digital rectal examination in the preoperative anatomical localization of prostate cancer. *J Urol*, **174**:6 (2005), 2158–63.

36. L. Arrive, Y. C. Chang, H. Hricak, *et al.*, Radiation-induced uterine changes: MR imaging. *Radiology*, **170**:1 Pt 1 (1989), 55–8.

37. K. Sugimura, B. M. Carrington, J. M. Quivey, *et al.*, Postirradiation changes in the pelvis: assessment with MR imaging. *Radiology*, **175**:3 (1990), 805–13.

38. F. V. Coakley, H. Hricak, A. E. Wefer, *et al.*, Brachytherapy for prostate cancer: endorectal MR imaging of local treatment-related changes. *Radiology*, **219**:3 (2001), 817–21.

39. M. A. Haider, P. Chung, J. Sweet, *et al.*, Dynamic contrast-enhanced magnetic resonance imaging for localization of recurrent prostate cancer after external beam radiotherapy. *Int J Radiat Oncol Biol Phys*, **70**:2 (2008), 425–30.

40. O. Rouviere, O. Valette, S. Grivolat, *et al.*, Recurrent prostate cancer after external beam radiotherapy: value of contrast-enhanced dynamic MRI in localizing intraprostatic tumor – correlation with biopsy findings. *Urology*, **63**:5 (2004), 922–7.

41. E. Sala, S. C. Eberhardt, O. Akin, *et al.*, Endorectal MR imaging before salvage prostatectomy: tumor localization and staging. *Radiology*, **238**:1 (2006), 176–83.

42. F. V. Coakley, H. S. Teh, A. Qayyum, *et al.*, Endorectal MR imaging and MR spectroscopic imaging for locally recurrent prostate cancer after external beam radiation therapy: preliminary experience. *Radiology*, **233**:2 (2004), 441–8.

43. N. Cellini, A. G. Morganti, G. C. Mattiucci, *et al.*, Analysis of intraprostatic failures in patients treated with hormonal therapy and radiotherapy: implications for conformal therapy planning. *Int J Radiat Oncol Biol Phys*, **53**:3 (2002), 595–9.

44. D. Pucar, H. Hricak, A. Shukla-Dave, *et al.*, Clinically significant prostate cancer local recurrence after radiation therapy occurs at the site of primary tumor: magnetic resonance imaging and step-section pathology evidence. *Int J Radiat Oncol Biol Phys*, **69**:1 (2007), 62–9.

45. P. Kupelian, J. L. Meyer, Prostate cancer: image guidance and adaptive therapy. *Front Radiat Ther Oncol*, **40** (2007), 289–314.

46. B. Pickett, J. Kurhanewicz, J. Pouliot, *et al.*, Three-dimensional conformal external beam radiotherapy compared with permanent prostate implantation in low-risk prostate cancer based on endorectal magnetic resonance spectroscopy imaging and prostate-specific antigen level. *Int J Radiat Oncol Biol Phys*, **65**:1 (2006), 65–72.

47. N. F. Wasserman, D. A. Kapoor, W. C. Hildebrandt, *et al.*, Transrectal US in evaluation of patients after radical prostatectomy. Part I. Normal postoperative anatomy. *Radiology*, **185**:2 (1992), 361–6.

48. N. F. Wasserman, D. A. Kapoor, W. C. Hildebrandt, *et al.*, Transrectal US in evaluation of patients after radical prostatectomy. Part II. Transrectal US and biopsy findings in the presence of residual and early recurrent prostatic cancer. *Radiology*, **185**:2 (1992), 367–72.

49. A. K. Leventis, S. F. Shariat, K. M. Slawin, Local recurrence after radical prostatectomy: correlation of US features with prostatic fossa biopsy findings. *Radiology*, **219**:2 (2001), 432–9.

50. V. Scattoni, M. Roscigno, M. Raber, *et al.*, Multiple vesico-urethral biopsies following radical prostatectomy: the predictive roles of TRUS, DRE, PSA and the pathological stage. *Eur Urol*, **44**:4 (2003), 407–14.

51. C. Deliveliotis, T. Manousakas, M. Chrisofos, *et al.*, Diagnostic efficacy of transrectal ultrasound-guided biopsy of the prostatic fossa in patients with rising PSA following radical prostatectomy. *World J Urol*, **25**:3 (2007), 309–13.

52. B. Shekarriz, J. Upadhyay, D. P. Wood, Jr., *et al.*, Vesicourethral anastomosis biopsy after radical prostatectomy: predictive value of prostate-specific antigen and pathologic stage. *Urology*, **54**:6 (1999), 1044–8.

53. G. S. Sudakoff, R. Smith, N. J. Vogelzang, *et al.*, Color Doppler imaging and transrectal sonography of the prostatic fossa after radical prostatectomy: early experience. *AJR Am J Roentgenol*, **167**:4 (1996), 883–8.

54. S. Tamsel, R. Killi, E. Apaydin, *et al.*, The potential value of power Doppler ultrasound imaging compared with grey-scale ultrasound findings in the diagnosis of local recurrence after radical prostatectomy. *Clin Radiol*, **61**:4 (2006), 325–30; discussion 323–4.

55. F. M. Drudi, F. Giovagnorio, A. Carbone, *et al.*, Transrectal colour Doppler contrast sonography in the diagnosis of local recurrence after radical prostatectomy – comparison with MRI. *Ultraschall Med*, **27**:2 (2006), 146–51.

56. J. E. Fowler, Jr., J. Brooks, P. Pandey, *et al.*, Variable histology of anastomotic biopsies with detectable prostate specific antigen after radical prostatectomy. *J Urol*, **153**:3 Pt 2 (1995), 1011–14.

57. D. P. Wood, Jr., S. J. Peretsman, T. M. Seay, Incidence of benign and malignant prostate tissue in biopsies of the bladder neck after a radical prostatectomy. *J Urol*, **154**:4 (1995), 1443–6.

58. T. Sella, L. H. Schwartz, P. W. Swindle, *et al.*, Suspected local recurrence after radical prostatectomy: endorectal coil MR imaging. *Radiology*, **231**:2 (2004), 379–85.

59. R. A. Huch Boni, C. Meyenberger, J. Pok Lundquist, *et al.*, Value of endorectal coil versus body coil MRI for diagnosis of recurrent pelvic malignancies. *Abdom Imaging*, **21**:4 (1996), 345–52.

60. R. Miralbell, H. Vees, J. Lozano, *et al.*, Endorectal MRI assessment of local relapse after surgery for prostate cancer: a model to define treatment field guidelines for adjuvant radiotherapy in patients at high risk for local failure. *Int J Radiat Oncol Biol Phys*, **67**:2 (2007), 356–61.

61. J. M. Silverman, T. L. Krebs, MR imaging evaluation with a transrectal surface coil of local recurrence of prostatic cancer in men who have undergone radical prostatectomy. *AJR Am J Roentgenol*, **168**:2 (1997), 379–85.

62. D. D. Maki, M. P. Banner, P. Ramchandani, *et al.*, Injected periurethral collagen for postprostatectomy urinary incontinence: MR and CT appearance. *Abdom Imaging*, **25**:6 (2000), 658–62.

63. T. Sella, L. H. Schwartz, H. Hricak, Retained seminal vesicles after radical prostatectomy: frequency, MRI characteristics, and clinical relevance. *AJR Am J Roentgenol*, **186**:2 (2006), 539–46.

64. C Hofer, C. Laubenbacher, T. Block, *et al.*, Fluorine-18-fluorodeoxyglucose positron emission tomography is useless for the detection of local recurrence after radical prostatectomy. *Eur Urol*, **36**:1 (1999), 31–5.

65. H. Schoder, K. Herrmann, M. Gonen, *et al.*, 2-[^{18}F]Fluoro-2-deoxyglucose positron emission tomography for the detection of disease in patients with prostate-specific antigen relapse after radical prostatectomy. *Clin Cancer Res*, **11**:13 (2005), 4761–9.

66. S. Albrecht, F. Buchegger, D. Soloviev, *et al.*, (11)C-acetate PET in the early evaluation of prostate cancer recurrence. *Eur J Nucl Med Mol Imaging*, **34**:2 (2007), 185–96.

67. M. Cimitan, R. Bortolus, S. Morassut, *et al.*, [(^{18})F]fluorocholine PET/CT imaging for the detection of recurrent prostate cancer at PSA relapse: experience in 100 consecutive patients. *Eur J Nucl Med Mol Imaging*, **33**:12 (2006), 1387–98.

68. V. Scattoni, M. Picchio, N. Suardi, *et al.*, Detection of lymph-node metastases with integrated [(11)C] choline PET/CT in patients with PSA failure after radical retropubic prostatectomy: results confirmed by open pelvic-retroperitoneal lymphadenectomy. *Eur Urol*, **52**:2 (2007), 423–9.

69. D. M. Schuster, J. R. Votaw, P. T. Nieh, *et al.*, Initial experience with the radiotracer anti-1-amino-3-^{18}F-fluorocyclobutane-1-carboxylic acid with PET/CT in prostate carcinoma. *J Nucl Med*, **48**:1 (2007), 56–63.

70. N. H. Bander, Technology insight: monoclonal antibody imaging of prostate cancer. *Nat Clin Pract Urol*, **3**:4 (2006), 216–25.

Index